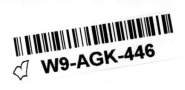

SCHOOL PROGRAMS IN SPEECH-LANGUAGE PATHOLOGY

FOURTH EDITION

SCHOOL PROGRAMS IN SPEECH-LANGUAGE PATHOLOGY

Organization and Service Delivery

JEAN L. BLOSSER

Creative Strategies for Schools

ELIZABETH A. NEIDECKER

Associate Professor Emerita
Bowling Green State University

ALLYN AND BACON

Boston ■ London ■ Toronto ■ Sydney ■ Tokyo ■ Singapore

Executive Editor and Publisher: *Stephen D. Dragin*
Series Editorial Assistant: *Barbara Strickland*
Marketing Manager: *Kathleen Morgan*
Editorial-Production Service: *Chestnut Hill Enterprises, Inc.*
Composition and Prepress Buyer: *Linda Cox*
Manufacturing Manager: *Chris Marson*
Cover Administrator: *Kristina Mose-Libon*
Electronic Composition: *Omegatype Typography, Inc.*

Library of Congress Cataloging-in-Publication Data
Blosser, Jean.
    School programs in speech-language pathology : organization and
service delivery / Jean Blosser, Elizabeth A. Neidecker. — 4th ed.
        p. cm
Rev. ed. of: School programs in speech-language / Elizabeth A.
Neidecker, Jean L. Blosser. 3rd ed. © 1993.
Includes bibliographical references and index.
    ISBN 0-205-31798-7
    1. Speech therapy for children—United States—Curricula. 2. Speech
therapy—Vocational guidance—United States.   I. Neidecker, Elizabeth A.
II. Neidecker, Elizabeth A. School programs in speech-language.   III. Title
    LB3454 .N44 2002
    371.91'42–dc21
                                                                2001022665

Printed in the United States of America
10   9   8   7   6   5   4   3   2   1   06   05   04   03   02   01

This book is dedicated to our families:
Mary, Bill, Renick, Trevor, John
and in memory of
Fred, Alpha, John, and Nancy

CONTENTS

CHAPTER 4

The Speech-Language Pathologist as a Manager   55

CHAPTER 5

Tools of the Trade: Space, Facilities, Equipment, and Materials   79

CHAPTER 6

Documentation and Accountability   96

CHAPTER 7

Case Finding and Case Selection 113

CHAPTER 8

Models of Service Delivery and Scheduling   162

CHAPTER 9

Developing a Relevant Intervention Program   182

CHAPTER 10

Working with Others: Collaboration and Consultation   **231**

CHAPTER 11
Student Teaching   273

CHAPTER 12
Life After College   290

PREFACE

A look at the early history of the profession of speech-language pathology and audiology makes it clear that many changes have occurred since the early 1900s when the public schools of Detroit and Chicago instituted programs to help children with speech and hearing problems. Some of the most profound changes have occurred in the past several decades. And even more changes are taking place today and will continue to occur. Fortunately the profession has not only weathered the changes but has successfully adapted to them.

In this, the Fourth Edition of this book, we hope to help the speech-language pathologist working in the schools adapt to, and profit from, the many changes that are occurring. We hope the information will help students preparing to work in the schools as well as experienced practitioners and clinicians moving to the schools from other settings. The major premise of this book, however, remains the same: the school speech-language pathologist is committed to the idea that good communication skills are necessary to the acquisition of educational skills and knowledge of subject. The school SLP's role is to prevent, alleviate, and remove communication barriers that hinder the student from profiting from the instruction offered in the classroom.

The education of children is a top-rated priority in the United States today. The school SLP can have an important role in this endeavor by enhancing the child's access to a good education and improving his or her quality of life.

Chapter One traces the growth and development of the speech-language pathology profession in the schools, including the philosophy that invited speech-language and hearing programs into the school system, the growth of those programs and the improvement of quality. An evolution of the speech-language pathology profession is presented. The chapter also includes an overview of legislation and the emerging role of the school-based SLP.

Chapter Two includes the role of the Code of Ethics of the American Speech-Language and Hearing Association, as well as professionalism, certification, and licensing, and professional organizations.

Chapter Three discusses legislation impacting service delivery in the schools. New laws, trends in education, and national goals and priorities are covered as well as prevalence and incidence data. The organization of school systems is also presented. Funding for services is discussed, including sources of funding and third-party reimbursement. The role of parents as team members is highlighted.

Chapter Four discusses the SLP's role as a manager and the importance of planning and setting goals. A strategic planning model for developing program changes is presented. The chapter also explores time management and planning program, personal, and treatment goals.

Chapter Five provides a comprehensive description of the facilities for intervention and tools available for use by the SLP. The use of technology for service delivery and record keeping is explored. Suggestions are made for using the Internet to access information or communicate with colleagues and parents. Also included is the importance of providing resources to others, including parents, teachers, and specialists.

Chapter Six explores the importance of documentation and accountability and the driving forces behind the need to include these important elements in speech-language pathology service delivery. Treatment outcomes and the American Speech-Language-Hearing Association National Outcomes Measurement project are described. The essentials of report writing are presented.

Chapter Seven discusses case finding and case selection. It explores alternative methods of assessment including interviewing, observation, functional assessment, curriculum-based assessment, as well as environmental assessment techniques. Information is included to help understand criteria for case selection and caseload management in view of the changing school environment and emerging national educational goals and trends. A section on special populations includes literacy, autism, behavioral disabilities, English as a second language, and transition to work. Highlighted is the SLP's role and strategies for providing service to these groups.

Chapter Eight includes the concept and intent of alternative service delivery options, as well as examples of models. Information on caseload size and composition is provided, as well as eligibility criteria. A decision-making framework based on criteria and guidelines for matching children to service delivery models is discussed. Scheduling and service delivery models within the classroom are presented.

Chapter Nine explains the SLP's role in developing individualized educational plans (IEPs) and individualized family service plans (IFSPs). Also included are methods of providing individualized transition plans (ITP). Particular emphasis is placed on linking treatment to student's academic needs and working with teachers to facilitate development of communication skills required for classroom success.

Chapter Ten focuses on the SLP's role as a collaborative consultant with other professionals and the student's family. The importance of collaborating with others to develop creative solutions to students' communication problems is discussed. The roles and responsibilities of various professionals are included along with methods of developing effective communication and interaction with educators, administrators, family members, and community members.

Chapter Eleven deals with student teaching. It describes the many aspects of the student teaching experience along with practical advice. Goals and tasks to be completed during the experience are incorporated. A discussion of ASHA certification requirements is included.

Chapter Twelve discusses the importance of lifelong learning and actively engaging in the profession on the national, state, and local levels. Career tracks within the profession, especially in the educational setting, are incorporated in the chapter. Ideas for research within the school setting are also included. Preparation for the job search, interviewing techniques, letters of application and the resume are covered in Chapter Twelve.

At the end of each chapter are discussion questions and projects. They are included to help the college student make practical applications of theoretical knowledge and factual information and to stimulate dialogue and discussion with each other and the instructor of the course.

The authors thank Gara Alderman, Jignesh Shah, Casey Keller, Meghan Sullivan, and April Beck for their assistance with this edition.

SCHOOL PROGRAMS IN SPEECH-LANGUAGE PATHOLOGY

CHAPTER ONE

THE GROWTH AND DEVELOPMENT OF THE PROFESSION IN THE SCHOOLS

This chapter provides a historical background of the profession of speech-language pathology and the development of programs within the schools of the United States. The philosophy of education that invited speech, language, and hearing programs into the schools is described. Also discussed is the expansion of school programs, both professionally and geographically. The chapter points out the role of the school pathologist (SLP) in the early days and changes in that role, as well as the factors that influenced those changes. It also considers the prevailing philosophy and legislation mandating equal educational opportunities for all children with disabilities and its implications for both the programs of the future and the roles and responsibilities of the school speech-language pathologist.

EARLY HISTORY

Although people have experienced speech, language, and hearing problems since the early history of humankind, rehabilitative services for children with communication disabilities were not realized until the early part of the twentieth century. The growth of the profession and the establishment of the American Academy of Speech Correction in 1925 reflect the realization of the needs and special problems of individuals with these disabilities.

According to Moore and Kester (1953), the educational philosophy that invited speech correction into the schools was expressed in the preface to a teacher's manual published in 1897, which contained John Dewey's "My Pedagogic Creed." The preface, written by Samuel T. Dutton, superintendent of schools, Brookline, Massachusetts, stated:

> The isolation of the teacher is a thing of the past. The processes of education have come to be recognized as fundamental and vital in any attempt to improve human conditions and elevate society.
>
> The missionary and the social reformer have long been looking to education for counsel and aid in their most difficult undertakings. They have viewed with interest and pleasure the broadening of pedagogy so as to make it include not only experimental physiology and child study, but the problems of motor training, physical culture, hygiene, and the treatment of defectives and delinquents of every class.

The schoolmaster, always conservative, has not found it easy to enter this large field; for he has often failed to realize how rich and fruitful the result of such researches are; but remarkable progress has been made, and a changed attitude on the part of the educators is the result.

Moore and Kester (1953) suggested that child labor laws influenced the growth of speech programs in the schools. Barring children from work forced both the atypical and the typical child to remain in school, and teachers soon asked for help with the exceptional children. A few got help, including assistance with children having speech defects.

According to Moore and Kester (p. 49), it was in 1910 that the Chicago public schools started a program of speech correction. Ella Flagg Young, the superintendent of schools, in her annual report in 1910 said:

> Immediately after my entrance upon the duties of superintendent, letters began to arrive filled with complaints and petitions by parents of stammering children—complaints that the schools did nothing to help children handicapped by stammering to overcome their speech difficulty, but left them to lag behind and finally drop out of the schools; and petitions that something be done for those children. It was somewhat peculiar and also suggestive that these letters were followed by others from people who had given much attention to the study of stammering and wished to undertake the correction of that defect in stammerers attending the public schools. Soon after the schools were opened in the fall, I sent out a note, requesting each principal to report the number of stammerers in the school. It was surprising to find upon receiving the replies that there were recognized as stammerers 1,287 children. A recommendation was made to the committee on school management to the effect that the head of the department of oral expression in the Chicago Teachers' College be authorized to select ten of the members of the graduating class who showed special ability in the training given at the college in that particular subject and should be further empowered to give additional training of these students preparatory to their undertaking, under the direction of the department, the correction of the speech defects of these 1,287 children. The Board appropriated $3,000.00 toward the payment of these students who should begin their work after graduation at the rate of $65 a month during a period extending from February 1 to June 30.
>
> Instead of gathering the children into one building or into classes to be treated for their troubles, a plan was adopted of assigning to the young teacher a circuit and having her travel from school to school during the day. The object of this plan was to protect the young teacher from the depression of spirit and low physical condition that often ensue from continued confinement in one room for several successive hours at work upon abnormal conditions. It was soon found that the term "stammering" had been assumed to be very general in its application and many children who had been reported as stammerers had not the particular defect reported but some other form of speech defect. (pages 48–53)

The superintendent of schools in New York City in 1909 requested an investigation of the need for speech training in the schools. Two years later the following recommendations were presented to the board of education: First, the number of speech handicapped children was to be ascertained and case histories obtained. Second, speech centers were to be established providing daily lessons of from 30 to 60 minutes. Third, English teachers were to be given further training and utilized as instructors. Fourth, a department for training teachers was to be established. It was not until four years later, however, that a director of speech improvement was appointed to carry out the recommendations (Moore and Kester, 1953).

THE MICHIGAN STORY

In their fascinating history of the early years of the Michigan Speech-Language-Hearing Association, Costello and Curtis (1989) described the beginnings of the Detroit public school speech correction program.

> In 1909, Mrs. Frank Reed, of the Reed School of Stammering in Detroit, contacted the superintendent of the Detroit Public Schools and offered to train two teachers, free of charge, in the Reed Method of the Correction of Stammering, provided the program would be incorporated in the Detroit Schools. A survey was made of the need and 247 cases were found. In May 1910, Mrs. Reed's offer was accepted and during the summer two teachers trained. They were Miss Clara B. Stoddard and Miss Lillian Morley. In September 1910, two centers were opened in Detroit, one on the east side and one on the west side of the city. Wednesday was kept free from classes to call on parents, visit children in the regular classroom and for other activities associated with their work. In 1914, classes for children with other speech defects were begun.
>
> In 1916, Miss Stoddard recommended the establishment of a special clinic at which a thorough physical examination and Binet test be given to children who seemed to have special problems. Regular monthly staff meetings were held and the latest literature on speech was reviewed. The cooperation of teachers and parents was enlisted in the correction of speech. The speech department personnel very early recognized the need for medical care for some of the children. A program for the mentally subnormal in special rooms was inaugurated in 1914 (Costello and Curtis, 1989).

EARLY GROWTH

During this same decade there was an increasing number of public school systems employing speech clinicians. Among them were Detroit, Grand Rapids, Cleveland, Boston, Cincinnati, and San Francisco (Paden, 1970). In 1918, Dr. Walter B. Swift of Cleveland wrote an article entitled "How to Begin Speech Correction in the Public Schools" (reprinted in *Language, Speech and Hearing Services in Schools,* April 1972).

To the state of Wisconsin goes the credit for establishing at the University of Wisconsin the first training program for prospective specialists in the field and for granting the first doctor of philosophy degree in the area of speech disorders to Sara M. Stinchfield in 1921. Wisconsin was also the first state to enact enabling legislation for public school speech services and to appoint in 1923 a state supervisor of speech correction, Pauline Camp. Meanwhile, other universities throughout the United States were developing curricula in the area of speech disorders. Until 1940, however, only eight additional states added similar laws to their statute books (Irwin, 1959). By 1963, a study by Haines (1965) indicated that 45 of the states had passed legislation placing speech and hearing programs in the public schools. These laws provided for financial help to school districts maintaining approved programs, supervision by the state, responsibility for administering the law, and the establishment of standards. The laws described minimum standards, which the programs were expected to exceed (Haines, 1965).

The first state supervisors, in cooperation with the school clinicians in their respective states, did a remarkably far-sighted job in establishing statewide programs in regard to the organizational aspects. With no precedents to follow, they established standards that have retained merit through many years. The Vermont program (Dunn, 1949), providing speech and hearing services to children in rural areas, and the Ohio plan (Irwin, 1949) furnish two such examples. They addressed themselves to such topics as finding children who need the services, diagnostic services, caseloads, the scheduling of group and individual therapy sessions, rooms for the therapist, equipment and supplies, planning time, summer residence programs, in-service training of parents and teachers, and periodic rechecks of children.

A PERIOD OF EXPANSION

The decades of the 1940s and the 1950s were times of growth for all aspects of the profession. In 1943 the American Medical Association requested that a list of ethical speech correction schools and clinics be provided for distribution to physicians. During World War II the entire membership was listed in the National Roster of Scientific Personnel. The organization that started life in 1926 as The American Academy of Speech Correction with 25 dedicated and determined individuals changed its name in 1948 to The American Speech and Hearing Association and in 1979 to The American Speech-Language-Hearing Association. Its membership increased from the original 25 persons in 1926 to 330 in 1940, to 1,623 in 1950, and again to 6,249 in 1960. In 1964, the "associate" category was eliminated and there were 11,703 members. By 1975, the membership had climbed to 21,435 with a steady increase until the present time when the membership is approaching 100,000.

The official publication, the *Journal of Speech Disorders,* was first published in 1936 at Ohio State University with G. Oscar Russell as editor. In 1957 the American Speech and Hearing Association established a permanent national office and appointed a professional executive secretary, Kenneth Johnson. In 1959 an employment bulletin, *Trends,* and a monthly professional magazine, *Asha,* were published. Currently there are several journals published by ASHA and other organizations that are devoted to discussion of the nature and treatment of communication disorders.

HEARING HANDICAPPED

Initially, programs for children with hearing impairments in this country were designed for children who were deaf and the needs of those with mild to moderate hearing impairments were, for the most part, neglected. Educational programs for the deaf were first established in the United States in 1817 with the founding of the American School for the Deaf at

Hartford, Connecticut (Bender, 1960). Children who were deaf received their education in residential schools or institutions until the establishment of classrooms in regular schools. The child in the regular classroom with a mild to moderate to possibly a severe hearing loss was dealt with by the classroom teacher. In his book, *Speech Correction Methods,* Ainsworth (1948) pointed out that "substitutions and omissions were frequently found in children with hearing loss and may be attacked with articulatory principles employing also visual and kinaesthetic avenues of approach." During this era, professionals in the schools were "speech correctionists" and dealt with most communication problems as articulatory problems.

Later the "speech correctionist" became a "speech and hearing therapist" and the public school therapists included hard-of-hearing children in their caseloads on the same basis as the child with speech handicaps. There were also classroom teachers of the hard-of-hearing in the public schools.

Concern for the hearing handicapped child in the classroom was indicated by one of the sessions in the 33rd annual convention of the American Speech and Hearing Association held in 1957 in Cincinnati, Ohio. The title of the session was "The Hard of Hearing Child in the Public Schools" and covered such topics as "The Public School Program for the Hard of Hearing in a Large School System," "Types of Public School Programs Presently in Existence in Small School Systems," "The Preparation for Teachers of the Hard of Hearing in the Public Schools," and "The Use of Amplification in Public School Programs for the Hard of Hearing."

SPEECH IMPROVEMENT PROGRAMS

School programs designed to help all children develop the ability to communicate effectively in acceptable speech, voice, and language patterns were first called speech improvement programs. Such programs were usually carried out by the classroom teacher, with the speech-language specialist serving as a consultant and doing demonstration teaching in the classroom. Many such programs were initiated in the 1920s, 1930s, and 1940s and were concentrated on the kindergarten and first-grade levels. One of the purposes was to reduce the number of minor speech problems.

The programs were not considered part of the school clinician's regular duties in many states. However, in some cities, speech improvement programs were carried out successfully despite lack of state support.

It was also during these decades that the public school programs increased and expanded, both professionally and geographically. School clinicians found themselves wearing many hats. In addition to selling the idea of such a program to the school system and the community, the clinician had to

- Keep records and prepare reports
- Identify the children with speech and hearing handicaps
- Schedule them for therapy, after talking with their teachers, at the most convenient time for all concerned
- Provide the diagnosis and the therapy

- Work with the school nurse on locating the children with hearing losses
- Counsel the parents
- Answer many questions from teachers who were often totally unfamiliar with such a program
- Keep the school administration informed
- Confer with persons in other professional disciplines
- Remain healthy, well groomed, trustworthy, modest, friendly, cheerful, courteous, patient, enthusiastic, tolerant, cooperative, businesslike, dependable, prompt, creative, interesting, and unflappable

Furthermore, the clinician had to keep one eye on the clock and the calendar and the other eye on state standards.

LANGUAGE AND SPEECH

Speech-language pathologists have been dealing with children with language problems for many years. Before research and experience sharpened diagnostic tools and awareness, these children were referred to as having "severe articulation disorders," "delayed speech," or "immature language." During the 1940s, 1950, and early 1960s, there was considerable interest among professionals in articulation and speech sounds. The focus changed in the late 1960s and early 1970s to an interest in syntactic structures and sentence forms. The past several decades have increased both knowledge and awareness of language problems. Indeed, the title of the professional organization was changed, in recognition of this, from the "American Speech and Hearing Association" to the "American Speech-Language-Hearing Association."

Along with this growing awareness of language problems was the realization that the school clinician had a commitment to the student whose language is disordered or delayed; the language problem may be the underlying cause of a student's difficulty in mastering reading or arithmetic skills. In addition, language problems may be present in the child who is hearing impaired, mentally retarded, learning disabled, physically handicapped, emotionally disturbed, or environmentally disadvantaged.

IMPROVEMENT IN QUALITY

The growth in numbers of clinicians serving the schools was steady during the 1950s and the 1960s. That era concentrated on the improvement of quality as well as quantity by emphasizing increased training for clinicians through advanced certification standards set by the professional organization.

A major project geared toward improving speech and hearing services to children in the schools was undertaken by the U.S. Office of Education, Purdue University, and the Research Committee of the American Speech and Hearing Association (Steer et al., 1961). The major objectives were to provide authoritative information about current practices in the public schools and to identify unresolved problems. On the basis of these findings, priorities were established for identification of urgently needed research. Hundreds of clinicians, supervisors, classroom teachers, and training institution personnel collaborated to develop a list of topics for further study; research was then distilled by the work groups. The following topics were given the highest priority: the collection of longitudinal data on speech; comparative studies of program organization (with special attention to the frequency, duration, and intensity of therapy); and comparative studies of the use of different remedial procedures with children of various ages presenting different speech, voice, and language problems.

Six additional topics were also identified and assigned a high priority: the development of standardized tests of speech, voice, and language; the development of criteria for selection of primary-grade children for inclusion in remedial programs; comparative studies of speech improvement and clinical programs; comparative studies of group, individual, and combined group and individual therapy programs; studies of the adjustment of children and their language usage in relation to changes in speech accomplished during participation in therapy programs; and comparative studies of different curricula and clinical training programs for prospective public school speech and hearing personnel.

The study also addressed itself to such topics as the professional roles and relationships of the school clinician, the supervision of programs, diagnosis and measurement, and the recruitment of professional personnel to meet the growing needs of children with communication handicaps in the schools.

THE "QUIET REVOLUTION"

School programs changed rapidly in the late 1960s and early 1970s. O'Toole and Zaslow (1969) referred to that time period as the "quiet revolution." SLPs became less quiet as they began talking about breaking the cycle of mediocrity, lowering caseloads, giving highest priority to the most severe cases, scheduling on intensive cycles rather than intermittently, extending programs throughout the summer, utilizing diagnostic teams, and many other issues. The emphasis had shifted, slowly but surely, from quantity to quality.

There were a number of occurrences in the late 1960s and 1970s that attest to the recognition of the public school speech-language specialist as a large and important part of the profession. The American Speech and Hearing Association named a full-time staff member to serve as Associate Secretary for School/Clinic Affairs. In 1971, a new journal was initiated, *Language, Speech and Hearing Services in Schools (LSHSS)*. In addition, ASHA appointed a standing committee on Language, Speech and Hearing Services in Schools. This all attests to the recognition of the public school speech-language specialist as a large and important part of the profession.

It was not only the professional organization's thinking that brought about the many changes. Outside influences—mainly the changes in the philosophy and conditions surrounding the American education system—began to effect changes in the profession. Increases in the population, growing demographic diversity, tightened school budgets, focus on the lack of reading skills in the elementary schools, more attention to special populations such as children who are mentally retarded and socially or economically disadvantaged—all had an impact.

FEDERAL LEGISLATION

In 1954, the U.S. Supreme Court's decision in the case of *Brown v. Board of Education* set into motion a new era and struck down the doctrine of segregated education. This decision sparked such issues as women's rights; the right to education and treatment for the handicapped; and the intrinsic rights of individuals, including blacks and minority groups.

Parent organizations have long been a catalyst in bringing about change, and in the case of children with disabilities they were certainly no exception. According to Reynolds and Rosen (1976)

> Parents of handicapped children began to organize about thirty years ago to obtain educational facilities for their offspring and to act as watchdogs of the institutions serving them. At first, the organizations concentrated on political action; since 1970, however, they have turned to the courts. This fact may be more important than any other in accounting for the changes in special education that are occurring now and are likely to occur in the near future.

THE PARC CASE

An extension of the *Brown v. Board of Education* decision, according to Reynolds and Rosen, was the consent decree established in the case of the Pennsylvania Association for Retarded Children. This decree stated that no matter how serious the handicap, every child has the right to education. The PARC case established the right of parents to become involved in making decisions concerning their child and stipulated that education must be based on programs appropriate to the needs and capacities of each individual child.

MAINSTREAMING

One of the unexpected aftermaths of the PARC case was to place the stamp of judicial approval on mainstreaming. According to Reynolds and Rosen (p. 558)

> Mainstreaming is a set or general predisposition to arrange for the education of children with handicaps or learning problems within the environment provided for all other children—the regular school and normal home and community environment—whenever feasible.

The intent of mainstreaming was to provide handicapped children with an appropriate educational program in as "normal" or "regular" an environment as possible. Thus, depending on the nature and/or severity of the handicapping condition, the child may be in a self-contained classroom or a regular classroom for all or part of the educational program. In other words, the child should be taught in the "least restrictive environment allowed by the condition."

Mainstreaming had special implications for the regular classroom teacher as well as other personnel involved in the education of children with handicaps. Reynolds and Rosen (pp. 557–58) said

Obviously, mainstreaming makes new demands on both regular classroom and special education teachers. In the past, a regular education teacher was expected to know enough about handicapping conditions to be able to identify children with such problems for referral out of the classroom into special education settings. At the same time, special education teachers were trained to work directly with the children with certain specific handicaps (as in the days of residential schools) in separate special settings.

Under mainstreaming, different roles are demanded for both kinds of teachers. The trend for training special education teachers for indirect resource teacher roles rather than narrow specialists is well established in many preparation centers. Concurrently, programs are underway to provide regular education teachers with training in the identification of learning problems. At the local school level, regular and special education teachers in mainstreamed programs are no longer isolated in separate classrooms. They work together in teams to share knowledge, skills, observations, and experiences to enhance the programs for children with special problems, whether the children are permanently or temporarily handicapped. Thus, it has become essential for special teachers to learn the skills of consultation and for both teachers to learn techniques of observation as well as communication.

UNITED STATES DEPARTMENT OF EDUCATION

In 1967, Congress created the Bureau of Education for the Handicapped and began a program of grants to speed the development of educational programs. In 1974, Edwin W. Martin, then director of the Bureau of Education for the Handicapped, in an address to the members of the American Speech and Hearing Association, stated that he did not feel we were successfully integrating our roles as speech and hearing specialists in the educational system. He urged that speech-language pathologists and audiologists in schools must be actively involved in interdisciplinary efforts with parents, learning disability specialists, administrators, guidance counselors, classroom teachers, and all educational colleagues.

Over the years, the Bureau has evolved into its present form as The United States Department of Education. The mission of the department is to ensure equal access to education and to promote education success. The Department is located in Washington DC and consists of many divisions and supports numerous programs and initiatives. The most relevant to the field of speech-language pathology services in the schools is the Office of Special Education and Rehabilitative Services (OSERS). The departments within OSERS support programs that assist in providing education to youngsters with special needs, provides for the rehabilitation of youth and adults with disabilities, and supports research to improve the lives of individuals with disabilities. To carry out its functions, OSERS consists of three major program-related components. The Office of Special Education Programs (OSEP) is responsible for administering projects and programs that relate to the free appropriate public education of all children, youth, and adults with disabilities, from birth through age 21. The Rehabilitation Services Administration (RSA) oversees programs that help individuals with physical or mental disabilities to obtain employment through the provision of support services such as counseling, medical, and psychological services, job training, and other individualized services. The National Institute on Disability Rehabilitation Research (NIDRR) supports a comprehensive program of research related to the rehabilitation of individuals with disabilities. One can learn much about the education-related legislation, the goals of education, and support systems in place for professionals by visiting the U.S. Department of Education's website <http://www.ed.gov>. Generally the United States government defines priorities for education for current time periods. These priorities have impact on the opportunities, findings, and practices for special education including speech-language pathology.

EDUCATION REFORM AND FEDERAL LEGISLATION

Parents, educators, and lawmakers continue to campaign for education reform. Their initiatives, if adopted, inevitably have profound impact on the face of public education. Each initiative ultimately will also impact the practice of speech-language pathology in schools. The past three decades have seen emphasis on several other important initiatives including: inclusion of students with disabilities in all facets of the education system; greater focus on preparing students for the world of work; increased involvement of parents in decision making about educational programming; expanding alternative school funding through the voucher system; and the development of programs to deal with students with emotional disorders and school violence.

Several key federal statutes relating to the education of students with disabilities have been implemented over the past three decades. Among the laws that have had the greatest effect on the course of special education and speech-language pathology service delivery are: The Education for All Handicapped Children Act of 1975 (the original Public Law 94-142); an updated version of PL:94-142 called the Education of the Handicapped Act Amendments of 1986 (Public Law 99-457); the most recent revision called the Individuals with Disabilities Education Act (IDEA) Amendments of 1997 (Public Law 101-476, later revised as 105-17); and the Rehabilitation Act of 1973 (specifically, section 504). These laws are briefly described below. Recommendations for developing quality service delivery programs that are responsive to the goals of these laws will be discussed throughout the book.

Legislation: PL 94-142

The most sweeping and significant change concerning the education of children with disabilities took place on November 29, 1975, when President Gerald Ford signed into law The Education For All Handicapped Children Act (Public Law 94-142). The major intent of the law was to assure full and appropriate education for all children who are disabled between the ages of three and twenty-one. It provided for Individualized Education Programs (IEPs), due process, the use of evaluation procedures for determining eligibility, and education in the least restrictive environment.

The impact of Public Law 94-142 has been both beneficial and substantial. It has changed not only the education of children with handicaps but has had widespread influence on the entire education system. State laws and regulations have been changed, parents have become more involved in the education of their children with handicaps, advocacy groups have influenced education at the local and the state levels, and training institutions and their programs have been affected. Parents and guardians of all children who are disabled are guaranteed legal due process with regard to identification, evaluation, and placement.

Public Law 94-142 has had a pervasive and profound effect on public school speech-language and hearing programs. Before the passage of the law, individual states had enacted legislation *permitting* speech and hearing services in the schools, but PL 94-142 *mandated* services for children with speech-language or hearing impairments. In addition, the law established a legal basis for services and provided financial assistance. The scope of speech-language pathology and audiology services are defined in the provisions of the law and mandate the identification and evaluation of communicatively handicapped children as well as the development of an Individualized Education Program (IEP) and its implementation. The regulations also cover the provision of appropriate administrative and supervisory activities necessary for program planning, management, and evaluation.

Legislation: PL 99-457

In 1986, President Ronald Reagan signed into law Public Law 99-457, amendments to the Education of the Handicapped Act (PL 94-142). These amendments expanded and strengthened the mandate for providing services to children with handicaps by assisting states to plan, develop, and implement statewide interagency programs for all young children with disabilities from birth through age two. The law included those infants and toddlers who are experiencing developmental delays in the areas of physical development, including vision and hearing, language and speech, psychosocial development, or self-help skills. The law also included infants and toddlers who have a diagnosed physical or mental condition that has a high probability of resulting in developmental delay, or children from birth through age two who may experience developmental delays if early intervention is not provided.

Section 619 of PL 99-457 creates enhanced incentives for states to provide a free and appropriate public education for eligible three- to five-year olds with disabilities. Parent training, family services, and variations in child programming are encouraged by law.

Legislation: PL 101-476 and PL 105-17

In 1990, Public Law 94-142 was further amended. The changed legislation was called IDEA (The Individuals with Disabilities Education Act) or Public Law 101-476. The law resulted in some major changes. Two new categories of disability (autism and traumatic brain injury) were added. In addition, "person-first" language was introduced changing all references to handicapped children to "children with disabilities." Another change mandated that schools provide transition services to support movement from school to post-school activities.

IDEA was again revised and signed into law by President William Clinton in 1997 (Public Law 105-17). In May, 1999, the final regulations were in effect. IDEA regulations for Part B of the amendment apply to services in school settings. Individual states have the responsibility to establish their own educational requirements. This legislation will have impact on school programs for the foreseeable future; it will most likely continue to be revised as philosophies and knowledge about education for students with disabilities continue to evolve.

TERMINOLOGY: WHAT'S IN A NAME?

The historical development of school programs in speech, language, and hearing is interestingly revealed in what titles have been used over the years. The earliest professionals called themselves "speech correctionists." Some who had previously worked in school systems in this capacity were known as "speech teachers," although they were more concerned with habilitation than with elocution. During the 1950s and the 1960s we became "speech and hearing therapists" and "speech and hearing clinicians." All these changes caused no end of trouble, especially in trying to explain the professional's role to others.

During the 1970s we became known as "speech pathologists," and in 1977 The American Speech-Language-Hearing Association in a preference survey found that "speech-language pathologist" was the choice of professionals in the field.

How did we get from "speech correctionist" and "speech teacher" to "speech-language pathologist"? The answer is not simple, but perhaps a review of clinical practices may shed some light.

In the 1930s a few universities began programs to train people for clinical roles in public schools and universities. We were "speech correctionists" and "speech teachers." Stuttering problems were the major focus during the earliest days, along with articulation problems. Clinicians were aware of language systems, but problems in that area were treated as speech problems. When faced with students who did not talk, clinicians attempted to stimulate speech by targeting vocal play and babbling. Speech clinicians weren't without their Bryngelson Glaspey Speech Improvement Cards (1941) or Schoolfield's book, *Better Speech and Better Reading* (1937).

Children who did not talk or who had little speech were viewed as having "organic" problems, those related to the brain or neurological system. Children whose problems in communication yielded to therapy were said to have had "functional" problems. Children who had even minimal vocalization, such as cerebral palsied children or hearing-impaired children, were treated as speech problems. It was at this time the titles of "speech therapist" and "speech and hearing therapists" were used.

Very young children with "delayed speech" and mentally retarded children were excluded from therapy as it was thought they had not reached the proper stage of development to benefit from treatment.

This clinical model was followed for about 30 years, until the late 1950s and early 1960s, when Noam Chomsky's "generative grammar" theories set the stage for the beginning of the profession's understanding of language and language behavior. Although Chomsky offered little help in solving clinical problems, it was at this time that B. F. Skinner's behavioral theories appeared. Speech clinicians still used the functional approach to therapy; however, they did include language-handicapped children on their caseloads for the first time.

One result of these two widely divergent schools of thought was to move the speech clinician's focus away from concentration on phonemes and articulation.

During the 1960s and the 1970s, the stimulus-response and reinforcement strategies as well as "precision therapy" methods were used to elicit language and speech. These behavior modification methods were widely accepted and speech clinicians freely dispersed rewards and "reinforcers."

Chomsky's grammar and Skinner's behaviorism systems prepared the way for the profession's move into semantics and pragmatics and the area of child language. During the 1970s the profession expanded the knowledge base and built on the foundations developed in the 1960s. This had the effect of developing new concepts about language behavior and its component parts.

During the early 1980s children previously excluded from therapy were now included. Children with articulation problems, although still a large part of the speech-language pathologist's caseload in the public schools, now included individuals with severe language deficiencies, language-learning disabilities, mental retardation, motor handicaps, and hearing handicaps. Adding impetus to this development was the passage and implementation of Public Law 94-142.

Although some may view the trouble with terminology as an identity crisis affecting an entire profession, it might also be construed as symptomatic of a gradual shift in focus from a preoccupation mainly with articulation problems to an interest in language-learning behavior. It also indicates a widening of the scope of services to include prevention as well as remediation, to hone and fine-tune our individual professional skills, and to see that these skills are delivered in the most efficient and effective way to the appropriate consumer.

THE EMERGING ROLE OF THE SCHOOL SLP

Traditionally, in the United States of America, speech, language, and hearing services have been offered as a part of the school program, and a high percentage of the profession has been employed in the schools. Unlike the systems in other countries where speech, language, and hearing professionals have followed the "medical model" and have provided services through health and medical facilities such as hospitals, in this country we have followed the "educational model" and provide services in the public schools. Our system is undoubtedly a reflection of our democratic philosophy of education that children have a right to education and that our function in the schools is to prevent, remove, and alleviate communication barriers that interfere with the child's ability to profit from the education offered.

Furthermore, the schools constitute an ideal setting in which to provide speech-language intervention services: there is an identified population who are the "consumers" of the services, there are legal mandates for implementing and carrying out the services, and there is local, state, and federal financial support. Competency in oral and written communication is one of the primary objectives of the school system and today many states, with the encouragement of the federal government, have mandated assessment in these areas. Speech, language, and hearing services are the primary support systems in the achievement of these competencies.

Figure 1.1 illustrates the evolution of speech-language pathology service delivery over the past three decades and into the future. For each decade, Row 1 indicates the areas of communication that were the clinicians' focus for treatment. Row 2 shows the roles clinicians have assumed in service delivery. Row 3 lists the emerging issues under professional consideration. This chart shows that changes in service delivery models and the clinicians' role have paralleled the increased understanding of communication disorders.

FIGURE 1.1   The Evolution of SLP Service Delivery Models

	1970s	1980s	1990s	2000s
Focus	Mechanistic view of language	Pragmatics	Functional, interactive communication Preparation for learning, living, and working	Outcomes Quality Efficacy
SLP Role	Specialist model	Expert model	Collaborative-consultative model	Facilitator of the service delivery
Emerging Issues	Language use is important	Language and learning are linked	Inclusion Transition Efficacy Accountability Outcomes	Standards Alternative schools

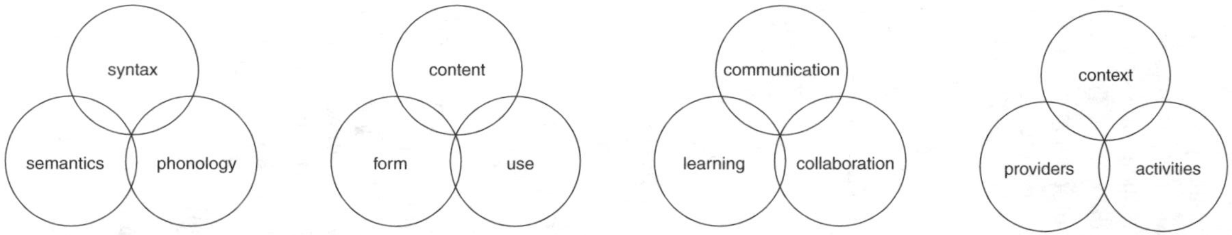

1970s diagram: intersecting circles labeled syntax, phonology, semantics

1980s diagram: intersecting circles labeled content, use, form

1990s diagram: intersecting circles labeled communication, collaboration, learning

2000s diagram: intersecting circles labeled context, activities, providers

As issues have emerged and clinical environments changed, clinicians have attempted to modify their practices in order to adapt to new changes.

The profession is at a new turning point in the evolutionary process. In fact, it appears that the field of speech-language pathology is currently undergoing a metamorphosis in service delivery. Significant changes are taking place in educational settings that are forcing clinicians to reflect on their options for service delivery. In educational forums, public education laws and policies are being rewritten to clarify the meaning and intent of providing services within the classroom setting and in the least restrictive environment. Current perspectives propose an expansion of service delivery options based on a commitment to serve all children in the environment that best fits their individual needs.

At present, speech-language pathologists in school settings are moving toward using inclusive models of service delivery that merge speech and language services with educational programming. Inclusive practices can be described as intervention services that are based on the unique and specific needs of the individual and are provided in a setting that is least restrictive. States are reevaluating services and acceptable service delivery options for all children with special needs. Personnel working in educational settings must demonstrate that their services will support the student so that he or she can participate to the maximum extent possible in social and learning contexts. Based on these directions, the best practice for speech-language pathology service delivery within the school setting would indicate that the general education classroom should be considered the first step in the continuum of service delivery to students with communication disabilities.

Clinical success is defined in terms of helping students reach measurable, functional outcomes so they can participate in community, family, work, and learning activities. Service delivery has been expanded to include families where possible.

Let us look at multiple roles and responsibilities of the school speech-language pathologist. The school-based SLP plans, directs, and provides diagnostic and intervention services to children and youth with communication disabilities. The pathologist works with articulation, language, voice, dysfluency (stuttering), and hearing impairments, as well as speech, language, and hearing problems associated with such conditions as cleft palate, cerebral palsy, intellectual impairment, visual impairment, emotional and behavioral disturbances, autistic behavior, aphasia, and traumatic brain injury.

The speech language pathologist in the schools serves high-risk infants and toddlers from birth to age five in school-operated child development centers, Head Start programs, special schools, centers, classrooms or home settings. Also served are children with severe disabilities in special schools, centers, classes or home settings, and students with multiple impairments, as well as elementary, middle, and secondary school pupils.

An important aspect of the school pathologist's duties is cooperation with other school and health specialists, including audiologists, nurses, social workers, physicians, dentists, special education teachers, psychologists, and guidance counselors. Cooperative planning with these individuals on a regular basis results in effective diagnostic, habilitative, and educational programs for children with communication problems.

The school speech-language pathologist works with classroom teachers and resource teachers to implement and generalize intervention procedures for the child with communication disabilities. Working with parents to help them alleviate and understand problems is also a part of the clinician's function. School administrators are often the key to good educational programming for children, and the school speech-language pathologist works with both principals and superintendents toward that end.

The school pathologist may also be a community resource person, providing public information about communication problems and the availability of services for parents and families and for the personnel in both public and voluntary community agencies.

Many school pathologists are engaged in research related to program organization and management, clinical procedures, and professional responsibility. The field of speech-language pathology is constantly broadening, and the school pathologist must keep abreast of new information by reading professional journals and publications; attending seminars and conventions; enrolling in continuing education programs; and sharing information and ideas with colleagues through state, local, and national professional organizations.

Frequently school pathologists are asked to help university students by serving as supervisors of student teaching and by providing observational opportunities for students-in-training. The supervision of paraprofessionals and volunteers in school programs is also the responsibility of the school pathologist.

Because the school speech-language pathologist is considered an important part of the total educational program, the size, need, and structure of the local school district will have much to do with the organizational model used as well as with the nature of the services provided. Many school pathologists work as itinerant staff. Some will be assigned to a single building, whereas others may work in special classes, resource rooms, in classrooms with teachers, or self-contained classrooms. Often the school pathologist will be either a full- or part-time member of the pupil evaluation team or a resource consultant to teachers, administrators, or other staff members. Many school pathologists are employed as supervisors or administrators of speech and language programs.

The collaborative-consultative role is becoming more and more important, and more is required of the school pathologist in the way of diagnosis of speech, language, and hearing problems. Classroom teachers, special teachers, and personnel in other specialized fields will depend on the school pathologist to provide information on diagnoses, assessment, and treatment of youngsters with communication disorders. In addition, the school-based SLP will be expected to be able to discuss the school curriculum and the impact the communication disability will have on the student's performance and ability to meet educational standards.

FUTURE CHALLENGES

What is the future role of the speech-language pathologist (SLP) in the schools? Speech-language pathologists working in the schools in the future will need to have strategies for coping with change. They will need to be well-educated, skillful, and tolerant individuals who, in addition to their expertise in communication disorders, will have to understand and be aware of the cultural and social backgrounds of their students. They will need to have information about research in evaluating students. They will need to be able to work with computers for record keeping and various aspects of intervention. Working closely with classroom teachers and health professionals in the schools is crucial to a quality program.

Undoubtedly, the federal laws related to special education often serve as a catalyst to programs in the schools and the role of the school speech-language pathologist. Most clinicians agree that the laws have improved the quality of speech, language, and hearing services. It is evident that they have enhanced the access to services and that they have served to augment parental involvement in the educational process.

During interviews with SLPs conducted over the past several years, many of the problems have been identified. First and foremost, SLPs indicate that the changing size and composition of the caseload places new demands on their time, skills, energies, and knowledge base. The type of documentation required to verify compliance with the laws resulted in increased paperwork, and again demands on the clinician's time. Perhaps one of the most difficult matters to resolve is the lack of adequate funding necessary to offer quality programs. The cost of service delivery is high. In most areas of the country, there is an imbalance between monies generated by SLP services and those actually spent to support these programs. As America becomes more consumer-oriented, professionals are required to be more and more accountable for their decisions and actions.

Demands such as these can lead to burnout and stress for clinicians. Staying abreast of new trends in treatment, attending professional conferences, working with professionals from other disciplines, and trying new and different strategies in therapy are all positive steps clinicians can take to maintain their interest and energy. To help alleviate the financial constraints, SLPs can work closely with their administration and advocate for change through their professional organizations and political arenas.

Although there are many problems faced by school SLPs and the profession as a whole, there are also exciting and challenging developments. It is difficult to predict how speech-language pathology will be different in the future, but we can make some educated guesses. The makeup of the caseload in the schools has already shifted from a preponderance of articulation problems to mainly language and learning disabilities. More and more children from diverse backgrounds will be enrolled in the school systems. It will be necessary to develop programs, which meet the growing and diverse needs of our multicultural society. There will be an extension of services to preschool children, and, at the other end of the line, to high school students to prepare them for the world of work and participation in the community and society. Youngsters with severe or multiple disabilities will be placed in regular classrooms and many of these children will have speech and/or language problems.

The role of the SLP as a collaborator and consultant will be greatly expanded, as will the role as a team member in the school in diagnosis, assessment, and placement. The school SLP will be more and more involved in overall education, in the communicative skills of reading, writing, and spelling as well as in speaking and listening. As has been true in the fields of medicine and dentistry, there will be an emergence of specialists in speech-language pathology. Funding streams for services will be altered greatly. Speech-language pathologists will be expected to use technology for record keeping as well as for diagnosis and intervention. They will be expected to work closely with classroom teachers and health professionals.

Strategies for coping with these changes will have to be met by the school SLP as well as by the profession as a whole, and certainly by the professional organization, the American Speech-Language-Hearing Association, and the state speech, language, and hearing groups. Speech-language pathologists will be expected to be highly educated, flexible, and multiskilled. In addition to consulting, evaluating, or providing intervention, SLPs will have to demonstrate knowledge and competency about the social, political, and cultural issues that impact the performance of their roles. Keeping school administrators apprised of their work, their responsibilities, and their program needs is required to conduct a quality school program. The funding for school programs for children with disabilities is an important issue and school SLPs will need to keep abreast of how money is allocated for their programs in their state and local systems.

DISCUSSION QUESTIONS AND PROJECTS

1. How does an understanding of the early role of the school speech-language clinician help in understanding the current role?

2. How has the role of the clinician in the schools changed over the years? Do you think this has any relationship to the titles by which we have been and are presently called?

3. Ask ten of your friends, who are not in the speech-language or hearing field, to comment on the titles by which we have called ourselves and what these titles convey to them. Ask the same questions of elementary education majors at your university.

4. Do you think the changes in the profession were brought about by outside pressures or by internal factors?

5. How do you think the role of the SLP in the schools differs from the role of the SLP in private practice? In a community clinic? In a hospital setting?

CHAPTER TWO

THE PROFESSIONAL SCHOOL SPEECH-LANGUAGE PATHOLOGIST

The Code of Ethics of the American Speech-Language-Hearing Association has established the ground rules for the entire profession. The principles include conduct toward the client, the public, and fellow professionals. Certification is the stamp of approval issued by a responsible agency to the individual meeting specific requirements. It confers the right to practice and the right to be recognized as a professional. It also carries with it the responsibility of exemplary professional behavior.

Organizations are important links facilitating the exchange of new ideas, information, research, recent developments, materials, and professional affairs. School speech-language pathologists will need to be aware of the various organizations and their functions in order to choose the ones with which they will affiliate. Professionalism and professional behavior are discussed in this chapter.

THE CODE OF ETHICS

One of the first tasks of the American Academy of Speech Correction, as the professional organization was first called, was the establishment of a Code of Ethics. Mindful of the fact that there were unscrupulous individuals who would take advantage of persons with handicapping conditions by making rash promises of cures and by charging exorbitant fees, the earliest members of the profession felt it necessary to maintain professional integrity and encourage high standards by formulating a Code of Ethics. As may be expected, it was a difficult task, and throughout the history of the organization the code has been periodically updated to meet current problems; however, it has remained substantially the same. The Code outlines the ASHA member's professional responsibilities to the patient, to coworkers, and to society. Thus, it might be said that accountability has always been one of the profession's highest priorities.

Although the Code was adopted for an association, it serves the entire profession. In the language of the Code the term *individuals* refers to all members of the American Speech-Language-Hearing Association and those nonmembers who hold the Certificate of Clinical Competence.

A code of ethics defines a profession's parameters; it should also protect the rights of the consumer. The ASHA Code addresses confidentiality, the use of persons in research, the supervision of paraprofessionals and of students in training, as well as other matters.

The Code has no legal basis except in states where it has been adopted as part of the licensing requirements.

The American Speech-Language-Hearing Association has established an Ethical Practice Board whose major responsibility is the enforcement of the Code of Ethics. A member of ASHA who is a holder of the Certificate of Clinical Competence and who is found guilty of noncompliance may be dropped from membership and have the Certificate revoked. A nonmember who is found guilty of noncompliance would face revocation of the Certificate. The loss of membership status and/or the revocation of the Certificate of Clinical Competence would follow procedures of due process set up by the Ethical Practice Board. There is also an appeals procedure. A copy of the Board's practices and procedures as well as the appeals procedures are printed in the directory of the American Speech-Language-Hearing Association, 10801 Rockville Pike, Rockville, Maryland 20852. In addition, the Association's Code of Ethics is available on the ASHA website <http://www.asha.org> and reprinted each year in many of ASHA's publications. Examples of cases that have been brought forward for review by the Ethics Board are published and illustrate how the Code of Ethics is interpreted.

The ASHA Code of Ethics was last revised in 1994. It is reprinted at the end of this chapter as a reference.

ETHICS

When you read the Code of Ethics you will see that it can serve as a source of the answers to many of the vexing problems you will encounter in your day-to-day work.

Under Principles of Ethics I is a statement that says, "Individuals shall honor their responsibility to hold paramount the welfare of persons served professionally." There is hardly a professional problem that cannot be solved by asking yourself, "What is best for the client?" versus "What is best for me?" or "What is best for the school?" Your role as a speech-language pathologist puts you in the position of a child advocate. In other words, you are on the side of the child. His or her best interests are your professional responsibility and it is that person for whom you speak.

Deciding what is best means that you will have to look at the needs of the whole person. A communication problem cannot be separated from the rest of the individual. The educational, health, psychological, and social aspects will have to be taken into consideration. Fortunately you do not have to make decisions by yourself because in a school system you will be working closely with the parent, classroom teacher, school administrator, psychologist, school nurse, physician, social worker, educational audiologist, and other professionals. The decision concerning what is best for the student is therefore a consensus of those persons in the child's life, who hold paramount the best interests of that individual.

Another important ethical consideration is confidentiality. You will have access to much information about the student with whom you are working and the child's family. This information is given in trust and should be regarded as confidential. The only other persons with whom you might share this information are other professionals in the school who may be working with the child. Within a school system the school policies usually state that pertinent information may be shared among interested professionals, whereas information that may be conveyed to professionals or agencies outside the school system must have the written consent of the parents or guardians. "Shared information" does not mean idle gossip. A conference with a classroom teacher is not to be carried on in the hallways, over lunch in the teachers' lunchroom, or in the teachers' lounge.

PERSONAL AND PROFESSIONAL QUALIFICATIONS

The communication disorders profession is a multifaceted one. Some members teach at the university level, some supervise in universities, some supervise in clinics, some administer programs, some provide treatment, some do research, and some are diagnosticians. The SLP who chooses to work in the education setting has the responsibility of preventing, removing, and alleviating communication barriers that may hinder a student from receiving the maximum benefit from the instruction offered in the classroom. In addition, the school clinician is a resource person to others in the school system. Another role of the school clinician is counselor to the family of the student who has the communication disorder or counselor to that individual.

In addition to the appropriate education and specialized knowledge and skills, what personality traits are desirable for the school SLP, who must wear so many hats? Among the most frequently mentioned are patience, understanding, honesty, adaptability, flexibility, sense of humor, warm and friendly nature, respect for others, acceptance of others, dependability, resourcefulness, and creativity.

Sadly, some speech-language pathologists view themselves as having no skills beyond their current functions. This simply is not true. SLPs are well prepared to pursue many careers. Examples of alternative career opportunities are provided in Chapter 12. Becoming aware of your unique skills and identifying career and life goals is very important to individuals who wish to function successfully in a complicated school system. In addition to the traditional clinical and research skills acquired through training and experience, there are many skills that can be applied to other professions including:

Detail/Follow-Through Skills: Speech-language pathologists must present organized and thorough work habits, be detail-oriented, and explicit in communication. These skills are evidenced through daily case management and leadership practices.

Financial Management Skills: Budget planning and responsible use of funds is a responsibility of many speech-language pathologists, especially in school districts where funding is severely limited.

Persuasion and Advocacy Skills: Speech-language pathologists and audiologists influence clients, parents, professionals in related areas, physicians, state legislators, and the public about the needs of individuals with communication disorders.

Mentoring Skills: Demonstrating intervention techniques to parents, teachers, and related professionals is an integral part of a speech-language pathologist's typical work week regardless of work setting.

Leadership: Speech-language pathologists demonstrate leadership skills by serving on committees and participating in activities in their place of employment, in the community, in their state association, and in their national association.

Communication: Speech-language pathologists are excellent communicators with clients, in the classroom, and with the public.

Human Relations: Speech-language pathologists interact with coworkers, employees, students and their families in many different interactive situations.

Educational Skills: Speech-language pathologists often teach undergraduate and graduate courses, give lectures at state association meetings and annual conventions, give in-service presentations to parents, teachers, physicians, and other professionals, and provide other continuing education opportunities.

Resource Designer and Developer: In addition to their other skills, speech-language pathologists frequently design, plan, market, and implement special programs.

Program Reviewer and Writer: They evaluate papers for conferences or state association meetings, publish articles in professional journals and newsletters. Some energetic clinicians work with the media to improve public understanding of the profession.

Fundraiser: SLPs raise funds to purchase materials for their facility or provide assistance to children in need.

BECOMING A "PROFESSIONAL"

Following graduation, you, the student, will become a professional person with all the rights and privileges as well as all the challenges that go along with being a speech-language pathologist. What does it mean to be a "professional"? Well, for one thing, you earn money for doing the things you did for free as a student clinician in the university clinic. During that time, your hours, your intervention plans, and your clinical decisions were subject to possible revision by your supervisor. When you turn that corner and become a professional, you become the decision maker in all these areas. Knowing who you are and what you are and where you fit in, together with your values and your attitudes, will provide the basis from which you will make decisions and plans in your professional life.

Guidelines for behavior as a professional speech-language pathologist have been set forth in the Code of Ethics. Please note that these are only guidelines. They can only assist you in making ethical, moral, and legal decisions. There are no clear-cut answers to many of the vexing problems that arise.

There are numerous behaviors that contribute to professionalism. What sort of message do your mannerisms convey? Are they distracting, annoying, or demeaning? Do you give the appearance of aloofness? Or do you present yourself as being a competent person who shows both friendliness and helpfulness?

Your general appearance also contributes to professionalism. You may be more comfortable in what you wear when relaxing with friends, but on the job this same style of dress may convey an unintended message to parents, to coworkers, and to the individuals who are your clients. It goes without saying that cleanliness, careful grooming, and good hygiene are at the top of the list.

By dressing appropriately and conservatively you underscore respect for your client and the seriousness of your purpose. No matter what your personal preferences are, you should take into consideration the impression you are making on others. Clothing that is comfortable, clean, and appropriate to your setting is another part of your professional self.

CERTIFICATION, LICENSURE, AND ACCREDITATION

Understanding the various forms of credentials that are required in speech-language pathology and education are part of each person's professional responsibility. To the neophyte clinician the task may seem formidable; however, some basic information may help clarify the situation.

The Voluntary Agency

Voluntary agencies have developed in countries with a democratic form of government. The voluntary agency is more clearly identified in the United States than in any other nation and has usually evolved out of an unmet need and a concern for one's fellows. The unmet need may be related to social issues, to leisure time and recreation, or to health. Voluntary health agencies may be related to specific diseases or disabling conditions. Usually the membership of voluntary agencies is made up of both lay persons (in many cases, parents) and professionals. Examples of voluntary health agencies are the United Way, the Brain Injury Association, and the Easter Seal Society. Voluntary agencies are not certifying agencies in the usual sense of the word; however, they perform extremely vital functions for individuals with disabilities.

The Official Agency

The official agency is tax-supported and may be on the city, county, regional, state, or federal level. Some agencies bridge two governmental jurisdictions. Official agencies cover a myriad of categories, including health, education, welfare, vocational, and recreational services. They are interested in the prevention of problems, in research, and in specific disease categories. Examples of official agencies are the city or county health department and the offices that offer vocational rehabilitation services. Some official agencies may be certifying bodies, such as a state department of education.

The Professional Organization

In addition to official and voluntary agencies there are also professional organizations. These, as the name implies, are made up of individuals sharing the same profession. Their goals are the establishment and maintenance of high professional standards, research, recruitment of others into the field, and the sharing of professional information. Examples are the American Speech-Language Hearing Association, the American Medical Association, and the National Education Association.

These various types of agencies often work together in a unique fashion, sometimes motivating each other to carry out specific tasks, often supporting each other financially and in other ways, frequently exchanging services and information and preventing duplication of services. The official agencies and the professional organizations are often accrediting and certifying bodies in addition to the other functions.

TYPES OF CERTIFICATION AND LICENSURE

There are different types of certification and accreditation that directly affect the individual speech-language pathologist. Certification in one type does not preclude holding certification in any or all of the other three. In fact, most professionals hold more than one type.

In looking at the academic, clinical, and experience requirements of all certifying and licensing bodies, you will note that they are almost, if not completely, identical. The academic requirements follow the same pattern. Specific courses can be used to fulfill requirements of several agencies. For example, a course in language development can fulfill the requirements for ASHA's Certificate of Clinical Competence, for public school certification from the state's department of education, and for a state license.

Certification by the American Speech-Language-Hearing Association

One type of credential is that issued by the American Speech-Language-Hearing Association (ASHA). Unlike licensing and state certification, it has no legal status, but nevertheless it is recognized by various states and by other professions as authenticating the holder as a qualified practitioner or supervisor. ASHA certification is known as the Certificate of Clinical Competence (CCC) and can be obtained by persons who meet specific requirements in academic preparation and supervised clinical experiences and who pass a national comprehensive examination. ASHA grants certification in speech- pathology or audiology. Some individuals have chosen to obtain certification in both areas. The certificate permits the holder to provide services in the appropriate area and also to supervise the clinical practice of trainees and clinicians that do not hold certification. Since 1977, persons who were not members of the Association were permitted to obtain the certificate by complying with the requirements.

At least a master's degree is required for certification as a speech-language pathologist (CCC-SLP) by the American Speech-Language-Hearing Association. Furthermore, the graduate coursework and the graduate clinical experience must be obtained at an institution whose program is accredited by the Council on Academic Accreditation (CAA) of the American Speech-Language-Hearing Association (ASHA).

The CCC is held by individuals who provide services in schools, universities, speech and hearing centers, clinics, private practice, and other programs throughout the United States, Canada, and many foreign countries. Information on how to apply may be obtained from the American Speech-Language-Hearing Association, 10801 Rockville Pike, Rockville, Maryland 20852 <http://www.asha.org>.

State Licensure and Certification

The speech-language pathologist who wishes to be employed in the public schools of a specific state must obtain a certificate or license issued by that state's department of education. Some states with licensure also grant approval for work in the schools. The qualifying standards are set by each state and include following a prescribed course of study and fulfilling the clinical requirements. They include both clinical practice in the university clinic or one of its satellite clinics, experience at an extern site, and student teaching. These experiences must be under the supervision of licensed and/or certified qualified professionals, including the clinic supervisor, the cooperating school SLP, and the university supervisor.

The recent passage of federal legislation regarding special education service delivery has resulted in activities in many states to improve speech and language services in schools by upgrading certification standards and requirements. The laws call for personnel standards to be based on the highest requirements in the state applicable to a specific profession or discipline. This is referred to in the law as the highest qualified provider. The majority of states in the United States require the master's degree or master's degree equivalent for state education agency certification. Information on the certification requirements of each state can be obtained by writing to the state department of education or its equivalent. Addresses of the various state departments of education are routinely published in ASHA materials or listed on state government websites.

Licensing

A license to practice a business or profession within the geographical bounds of a specific state is issued by that state's legislature, usually through an appointed autonomous board or council. Licensing came about originally to protect the consumer from unqualified and unscrupulous persons. It is also viewed by some as a way to control growth and income of professional interest groups. Obviously, the laws to create licensure are unique to each state.

In the speech, language, and hearing profession, the licensure board may establish rules for obtaining and retaining a license, continuing one's education, and setting standards for ethical conduct. The Board may also administer examinations for applicants and enforce the license law. Usually a fee is charged for the license, which may be renewed yearly.

Another aspect of licensing is the "sunset law," which means that periodically the legislature may review the licensing agency (and other regulating agencies) and recommend whether or not it should be terminated.

ACCREDITATION OF AGENCIES AND PROGRAMS

Relevant to the administration of speech-language pathology and audiology programs, the American Speech-Language-Hearing Association has established the Council on Academic Accreditation (formerly the Educational Standards Board). Accreditation by CAA assures that institutions offering educational programs in speech-language pathology and audiology at the master's level meet minimal standards. ASHA committees and boards continually review the standards to ensure that they reflect the profession's current needs and trends. Revised standards for the accreditation of programs will be implemented after 2005. Complete instructions for fulfilling CAA and PSB requirements are available from the national office of the American Speech-Language-Hearing Association.

PROFESSIONAL ORGANIZATIONS

The school SLP has a professional responsibility to keep abreast of new ideas, research, recent developments, materials, publications, and professional affairs. This is a lifelong commitment, and it is part and parcel of what being "professional" means. One way of keeping current and informed is through professional organizations. Organizations have meetings with reputable speakers, publish journals and newsletters, and provide an excellent way to get to know fellow professionals. Speech-language pathologists in schools often feel isolated even though they are in daily contact with clients and school personnel. This sense of isolation comes from not having enough contact with other speech-language specialists, with whom they can share ideas, information, frustrations, and triumphs.

The oldest professional organization in the field of speech-language pathology and audiology is the American Speech-Language-Hearing Association. The membership of ASHA is approaching 100,000 members. This organization has been one of the chief agents for growth and development in the profession.

Students are encouraged to affiliate with the National Student Speech-Language-Hearing Association (NSSLHA), which offers many opportunities not otherwise available to individuals in training. It is an affiliate of ASHA, with chapters in colleges and universities.

Within the ASHA structure there are currently 16 Special Interest Divisions:

Division 1: Language, Learning, and Education

Division 2: Neurophysiology and Neurogenic Speech and Language Disorders

Division 3: Voice and Voice Disorders

Division 4: Fluency and Fluency Disorders

Division 5: Speech Science and Orofacial Disorders

Division 6: Hearing and Hearing Disorders: Research and Diagnostics

Division 7: Aural Rehabilitation and its Instrumentation

Division 8: Hearing Conservation and Occupational Audiology

Division 9: Hearing and Hearing Disorders in Childhood

Division 10: Issues in Higher Education

Division 11: Administration and Supervision

Division 12: Augmentative and Alternative Communication

Division 13: Swallowing and Swallowing Disorders

Division 14: Communication Disorders and Sciences in Culturally and Linguistically Diverse Populations (CLD)

Division 15: Gerontology

Division 16: School Based Issues

In addition, a number of committees and task forces are formed on an ongoing basis to provide information and support for individuals who work in private and public school settings. These groups hold membership meetings annually at the national convention. They appoint liaisons to keep information and communication flowing between professionals and local or national organizations. Clinicians who are interested in developing their skills in a specific area or advocating for clients with a particular type of disability will benefit from membership in a special interest division.

Another organization with which the school speech-language pathologist may want to affiliate is the Division for Children with Communication Disorders, a division of the Council for Exceptional Children. This organization publishes the Journal of Childhood Communication Disorders, holds state and national meetings, and is organized as a state group in many states.

Every state has its professional speech-language pathology and audiology organizations that hold conventions, publish journals, and sponsor continuing education programs. The state organizations also publish directories of members' names and professional addresses. Many organizations lobby the state legislature for support of professionally related issues.

There may also be regional organizations in addition to the state professional organizations. Affiliation with the regional group provides an invaluable opportunity for exchange of information and offers support to individual members. Involvement in such groups is both rewarding and enjoyable. The national as well as state and local speech, language, and hearing professional organizations are concerned with such activities as research, the study of human communication and its disorders, the investigation of intervention and diagnostic procedures, and the maintenance of high standards of performance. The professional organizations are also interested in the dissemination of information among its members and the upholding of high ethical standards to protect the consumer. There are other benefits to be derived from affiliating oneself with a professional organization. Such a group can provide a forum for discussion of issues and can speak with a concerted voice on matters of professional interest and concern. If the professional individual wishes to have a voice in decisions and opinions, the best way to do so is through a professional organization on the state, local, or national level.

There are a number of other related professional organizations with which the school clinician may wish to become affiliated. Membership in other professional groups provides opportunities for valuable exchanges of information and enhances cooperation and understanding. You will learn about other organizational opportunities as you read the professional literature and interact with colleagues throughout your career. Most charge membership dues but the benefits are worth it.

DISCUSSION QUESTIONS AND PROJECTS

1. You are the school SLP. What do you do in these situations:
   - A parent asks you to continue therapy with a child even though the child has reached optimum improvement. The parent says that the child enjoys therapy and it would be traumatic to terminate the therapy. The parent offers to pay you for continuing to see the child.
   - A local hearing-aid dealer asks you to supply a list of the students in the school with hearing losses.
   - An elementary teacher asks if she may see the records and reports of a middle-school student enrolled in therapy. She asks your opinion concerning whether or not the student is mentally retarded. (Test results showed that the child isn't retarded.)
   - You are asked to do private after-school therapy with a child enrolled in a school in which you are working. The parents are willing to pay you for providing the service and you are interested in developing a private practice. The child is already receiving therapy and is on your caseload.
   - The parents of a student referred for medical evaluation ask you to recommend a doctor.
   - You are asked to do therapy in the school with a student who is currently receiving therapy at a nearby private speech, language, and hearing center. You are aware of this, but the parents did not provide you with this information.

2. Find out the requirements for licensure or certification in your state.

3. Find out what speech, language and hearing organizations are active in your region. Learn about their membership requirements, purposes, goals, and meeting schedule. Invite an officer of a local organization to speak to your class. Plan to attend one of their meetings. Obtain a copy of their newsletter or journal.

4. What are the advantages in joining the National Student Speech-Language-Hearing Association?

5. Investigate ASHA's Special Interest Divisions. Join one that interests you.

6. Review the program from a recent state or national convention. Which sessions are of interest to you and why?

7. Contact the president of your state speech-language-hearing association. Ask if they need volunteers for any committees or projects.

BOX 1.1

CODE OF ETHICS

Last Revised January 1, 1994

PREAMBLE

The preservation of the highest standards of integrity and ethical principles is vital to the responsible discharge of obligations in the professions of speech-language pathology and audiology. This Code of Ethics sets forth the fundamental principles and rules considered essential to this purpose.

Every individual who is (a) a member of the American Speech-Language-Hearing, Association, whether certified or not, (b) a nonmember holding the Certificate of Clinical Competence from the Association, (c) an applicant for membership or certification, or (d) a Clinical Fellow seeking to fulfill standards for certification shall abide by this Code of Ethics.

Any action that violates the spirit and purpose of this Code shall be considered unethical. Failure to specify any particular responsibility or practice in this Code of Ethics shall not be construed as denial of the existence of such responsibilities or practices.

The fundamentals of ethical conduct are described by Principles of Ethics and by Rules of Ethics as they relate to responsibility to persons served, to the public, and to the professions of speech-language pathology and audiology.

Principles of Ethics, aspirational and inspirational in nature, form the underlying moral basis for the Code of Ethics. Individuals shall observe these principles as affirmative obligations under all conditions of professional activity.

Rules of Ethics are specific statements of minimally acceptable professional conduct or of prohibitions and are applicable to all individuals.

PRINCIPLE OF ETHICS I

Individuals shall honor their responsibility to hold paramount the welfare of persons they serve professionally.

RULES OF ETHICS

A. Individuals shall provide all services competently.
B. Individuals shall use every resource, including referral when appropriate, to ensure that high-quality service is provided.
C. Individuals shall not discriminate in the delivery of professional services on the basis of race or ethnicity, gender, age, religion, national origin, sexual orientation, or disability.
D. Individuals shall fully inform the persons they serve of the nature and possible effects of services rendered and products dispensed.
E. Individuals shall evaluate the effectiveness of services rendered and of products dispensed and shall provide services or dispense products only when benefit can reasonably be expected.
F. Individuals shall not guarantee the results of any treatment or procedure, directly or by implication; however, they may make a reasonable statement of prognosis.
G. Individuals shall not evaluate or treat speech, language, or hearing disorders solely by correspondence.

(continued)

BOX 1.1   CONTINUED

   H. Individuals shall maintain adequate records of professional services rendered and products dispensed and shall allow access to these records when appropriately authorized.

   I. Individuals shall not reveal, without authorization, any professional or personal information about the person served professionally, unless required by law to do so, or unless doing so is necessary to protect the welfare of the person or of the community.

   J. Individuals shall not charge for services not rendered, nor shall they misrepresent, in any fashion, services rendered or products dispensed.

   K. Individuals shall use persons in research or as subjects of teaching demonstrations only with their informed consent.

   L. Individuals whose professional services are adversely affected by substance abuse or other health-related conditions shall seek professional assistance and, where appropriate, withdraw from the affected areas of practice.

For purposes of this Code of Ethics, misrepresentation includes any untrue statements or statements that are likely to mislead. Misrepresentation also includes the failure to state any information that is material and that ought, in fairness, to be considered.

PRINCIPLE OF ETHICS II
Individuals shall honor their responsibility to achieve and maintain the highest level of professional competence.

RULES OF ETHICS

   A. Individuals shall engage in the provision of clinical services only when they hold the appropriate Certificate of Clinical Competence or when they are in the certification process and are supervised by an individual who holds the appropriate Certificate of Clinical Competence.

   B. Individuals shall engage in only those aspects of the professions that are within the scope of their competence, considering their level of education, training, and experience.

   C. Individuals shall continue their professional development throughout their careers.

   D. Individuals shall delegate the provision of clinical services only to persons who are certified or to persons in the education or certification process who are appropriately supervised. The provision of support services may be delegated to persons who are neither certified nor in the certification process only when a certificate holder provides appropriate supervision.

   E. Individuals shall prohibit any of their professional staff from providing services that exceed the staff member's competence, considering the staff member's level of education, training, and experience.

   F. Individuals shall ensure that all equipment used in the provision of services is in proper working order and is properly calibrated.

PRINCIPLE OF ETHICS III
Individuals shall honor their responsibility to the public by promoting public understanding of the professions, by supporting the development of services designed to fulfill the unmet needs of the public, and by providing accurate information in all communications involving any aspect of the professions.

RULES OF ETHICS

A. Individuals shall not misrepresent their credentials, competence, education, training, or experience.

B. Individuals shall not participate in professional activities that constitute a conflict of interest.

C. Individuals shall not misrepresent diagnostic information, services rendered, or products dispensed or engage in any scheme or artifice to defraud in connection with obtaining payment or reimbursement for such services or products.

D. Individuals' statements to the public shall provide accurate information about the nature and management of communication disorders, about the professions, and about professional services.

E. Individuals' statements to the public—advertising, announcing, and marketing their professional services, reporting research results, and promoting product—shall adhere to prevailing professional standards and shall not contain misrepresentations.

PRINCIPLE OF ETHICS IV

Individuals shall honor their responsibilities to the professions and their relationships with colleagues, students, and members of allied professions. Individuals shall uphold the dignity and autonomy of the professions, maintain harmonious interprofessional and intraprofessional relationships, and accept the professions' self-imposed standards.

RULES OF ETHICS

A. Individuals shall prohibit anyone under their supervision from engaging in any practice that violates the Code of Ethics.

B. Individuals shall not engage in dishonesty, fraud, deceit, misrepresentation, or any form of conduct that adversely reflects on the professions or on the individual's fitness to serve persons professionally.

C. Individuals shall assign credit only to those who have contributed to a publication, presentation, or product. Credit shall be assigned in proportion to the contribution and only with the contributor's consent.

D. Individuals' statements to colleagues about professional services, research results, and products shall adhere to prevailing professional standards and shall contain no misrepresentations.

E. Individuals shall not provide professional services without exercising independent professional judgment, regardless of referral source or prescription.

F. Individuals shall not discriminate in their relationships with colleagues, students, and members of allied professions on the basis of race or ethnicity, gender, age, religion, national origin, sexual orientation, or disability.

G. Individuals who have reason to believe that the Code of Ethics has been violated shall inform the Ethical Practice Board.

H. Individuals shall cooperate fully with the Ethical Practice Board in its investigation and adjudication of matters related to this Code of Ethics.

American Speech-Language-Hearing Association (1994). Code of ethics. *Asha, 36* (March, Suppl.), pp. 1–2. Reprinted by permission.

CHAPTER THREE

FOUNDATIONS OF THE PROGRAM

This chapter contains basic information about the factors that need to be considered in planning and organizing a school speech-language program. It should be understood that the information about the structure of the school system is general. You, as the school speech-language pathologist, should acquaint yourself with the structure of the educational system in the state in which you live and work. The same is true about the city, county, or district school system in which you are employed. In fact, if you are considering a specific site for future employment it is a good idea to learn as much as possible before you sign a contract; then continue to increase your knowledge as you go along.

Federal legislation has had tremendous effect on public school special education and speech-language programming. As you read through this book you will find frequent references to several key laws. Your task will be to keep abreast of the changes and requirements of federal and state laws affecting your school speech-language intervention program.

Public schools are supported by state and local taxes as well as by federal flow-through funds. It is important to be knowledgeable about how your program is supported, how budgets are determined, and the process by which funds are allocated. In some cases the input of the SLP is required or expected and in some instances you may wish to request to have input. Without knowledge of how schools and programs are financed, the SLP is at a serious disadvantage. Another factor in planning a speech and language program is the number of students with whom you will be dealing. It would be nice if these figures were conveniently available, but unfortunately determining prevalence figures is a complex matter. The best we can do is to rely on all the current information at hand and make generalizations that apply to individual school systems. Much more attention is given to determining prevalence figures at the present time than in the past, and the developments in this area are promising.

THE ORGANIZATIONAL STRUCTURE
OF THE SCHOOL SYSTEM

The Program on the State Level

Because of our democratic philosophy of education, we are committed to the concept of education for all. The major responsibility for education rests with each state rather than with the federal government. Through a state board of education, all policies, regulations, rules, and guidelines are set. The laws for education in each state are enacted through the state legislatures, and money is appropriated through this body. A state superintendent of instruction is the chief education officer in each state. A state department of education is responsible for carrying out and developing policies, regulations, and standards related to schools.

State departments of education provide state consultants in various areas of special education. The responsibilities of the consultants in speech-language pathology may vary slightly from state to state, but in general the tasks are similar throughout the nation. A major task of the professional staff on the state level is to monitor and enforce *minimum* standards of practice in local programs that are partially or fully reimbursed from state money. Along with this, local programs are encouraged to approach optimal goals in serving the needs of students with disabilities. The state staff may provide leadership and assistance in identifying, developing, and maintaining optimal standards. Some examples of ways in which state and local consultants demonstrate their professional leadership to assist school districts, speech-language programs, and clinicians as they try to comply with established standards include the following:

Providing access to relevant professional resources and materials.   Busy SLPs sometimes find it difficult to stay abreast of the changing practices and trends in the profession. Consultants often assist by establishing procedures for exchange of resources and materials, providing bibliographies of significant materials, and developing abstracts or summaries of articles that describe important issues.

Organizing and conducting in-service education programs.   In today's climate, the practice of speech-language pathology is constantly changing. To best serve students needs, the SLP must keep up with changes in diagnostic methods, technology, and intervention procedures. In addition, they must be able to understand and implement new legislation. Consultants assist with this process by organizing and/or conducting meetings and conferences that SLPs can attend to continually improve their skills and qualifications. Ongoing education such as this will help practitioners in the field develop relationships with other professionals and provides a framework for ensuring effectiveness.

Promoting professional relationships with state agencies and other related professional disciplines.   Speech-language pathology is not practiced in isolation. By working with consultants in other disciplines, the state consultant can help facilitate understanding of how the disciplines can work in collaboration to provide the optimal services for youngsters. In addition, collaboration at that level can help facilitate greater efficiency and reduce the amount of duplication of effort that sometimes occurs.

Encouraging research studies, experimental projects, and grant proposals.   School-based programs offer excellent opportunities for collecting data and conducting research into the effectiveness of evaluation and treatment methods. In addition, there are numerous opportunities for experimental projects and pilot studies. Consultants can provide direction about the type of data that is needed; they can identify research partners and potential sources of funding. Clinicians who engage in research discover many new perspectives about children with communication disorders and options for treating those disorders. Such efforts can be rewarding and lead to professional growth opportunities. Findings of research efforts often lead to modifications in existing laws and standards.

Identifying underserved populations and unmet needs.   As the demographics of communities continue to change, so will the children who are enrolled in school programs. School-based clinicians sometimes feel frustrated because they experience difficulties fitting new groups of youngsters or different types of communication problems into existing caseloads and service delivery models. Consultants can help identify new needs and broaden the awareness of others so that they begin to understand the types of changes that will enable the program to be more responsive to those who are served.

Conducting preservice education programs.   Oftentimes, speech-language pathology consultants are asked to contribute to the preparation of future school-based SLPs. They do so by helping universities identify the qualifications SLPs will need to meet the needs of youngsters. They present lectures that help students understand realistic aspects of practice in the school setting. Some individuals are asked to advise university faculty on changes in the federal and state legislation that affect practice in the school setting and assist with review of the professional curriculum to ensure that key aspects are incorporated so that students will be well prepared for their roles.

Compliance with Legislative Mandates

Each state is required to submit annual plans confirming that they are in compliance with the mandates specified by the federal legislation. As the laws change at the federal level, states must undergo review of their rules and regulations to determine the types of changes that are necessary so that they can assure the government and citizens that all requirements will be met. One of the responsibilities of the state education agency is to monitor and evaluate the activities of the local education agency to assure compliance with the federal statutes.

Local boards of education are responsible for ensuring proper implementation of mandates at the local level. Funds flow from the federal and state levels to the local level. Districts must verify that they are in compliance with the legislative mandates. There is variation throughout the country on how the mandates are interpreted. This is the result of local philosophy as well as funding availability. There are different rules and regulations for public and private schools. It is incumbent upon the administration and teachers in each school to follow the rules and procedures that are expected. If the rules are not followed, funding can be discontinued, reduced, or withheld.

Regional Resource Centers

Regional resource centers have been established in states as a mechanism for providing the support school districts need in order to develop the programs and processes that are required to ensure that they are in compliance with the federal and state standards. Such centers provide an important link between the state and the local school district. They may be referred to by different names in different states but their goals are fairly common. The centers are generally staffed with special education professionals representing a wide variety of disciplines including speech-language pathology, audiology, occupational therapy, physical therapy, psychology, behavioral disorders, special education teachers, health care specialists, social workers, and educational administrators to name a few. Their roles are to provide school systems with the assistance they need to interpret, implement, and comply with legislative mandates, rules, and regulations. Having all of these disciplines working closely with one another permits a truly collaborative approach to identifying and planning for the educational needs of children with communication disabilities. Not all districts can afford to hire such a wide variety of specialists, therefore the concept of making a central pool of experts available to a region through a central agency has been valuable and cost effective.

Centers provide assistance to school systems in the initiation and expansion of programs and services for children with disabilities. This is accomplished through joint planning and collaboration among school systems within a specific region. As a result, many more youngsters can be served than if each district tried to provide educational and support services on its own.

The centers serve as the mechanism by which school systems can plan, organize, and implement strategies for identifying, evaluating, and teaching youngsters with disabilities. This is the first important step in providing appropriate programs and services for children and their families. In addition, many centers also serve as clearing houses and distribution sources for information pertaining to special education. Speech-language pathologists and other special educators can visit the regional resource center to attend in-service training seminars, learn about newly developed instructional materials and methodologies, or borrow materials. Many centers will even deliver materials to the school system.

By combining resources and personnel, regional resource centers can provide comprehensive services to school districts, education specialists, teachers, and families that might not otherwise be available or accessible.

The Program on the Local Level

On the local level, school systems are organized into school districts. In some states, these are known as intermediate units. The district, or intermediate unit, is a geographical area and may cross county lines. In school terminology, these are referred to as local education agencies (LEAs).

The board of education members are elected by the people of the district and are responsible for governance and for developing and establishing policies. The basic responsibility for each school system rests with the citizens of that community inasmuch as they elect the school board. The school board selects the superintendent, who recommends the needed staff to operate the schools.

The superintendent is the chief administrative officer and chief personnel officer for the school system in that he or she makes recommendations to the board concerning the hiring, promotion, and dismissal of staff members. The superintendent is responsible for the total operation and maintenance of the school system; leadership of the professional staff; and administration of the clerical, secretarial, transportation, and custodial staffs.

Depending on the size of the school system, there may be assistant superintendents who have specific areas of responsibility, such as finance or buildings and grounds.

The structure of individual school systems may vary from state to state and from community to community. Usually there are curriculum directors as well as directors of elementary education and of secondary education. There may be directors of pupil personnel service, instructional program services, special education services, child accounting and attendance, guidance and health services, and others.

Each principal is responsible for supervising the professional and support services staff assigned to that building. The role and function of the elementary school principal will differ from that of the middle school and secondary school principal. In addition, roles and functions of principals will vary according to the unique characteristics of the community and will reflect the various cultural backgrounds of the students and their parents. The principal is responsible for managing the school's instructional program, pupil personnel services, support services, and community relations.

An understanding of the structure of the school system is necessary for the speech-language pathologist to function effectively. Obviously there will be variations in organizational structures throughout the country; thus in addition to having a general knowledge of the school system, you, as the SLP, will need to be familiar with the educational facility in which you are employed. Figure 3.1 illustrates a partial organizational chart for the special education programs of a school district. Schools are organized in many different ways depending on the size and administrative philosophy of the district.

PUBLIC LAWS AFFECTING SPEECH-LANGUAGE SERVICE DELIVERY

Public Law 94-142, The Education for all Handicapped Children Act of 1975, was the original legislation that mandated a free, appropriate public education for all children and youth with disabilities. The law has since been reauthorized three times by the federal government. Following is a discussion of the major mandates included in each of the laws and the subsequent reauthorizations. (Table 3.1 summarizes the federal laws that affect special education.) There are several key aspects of Public Law 94-142 that have had remarkable impact on the delivery of all services to youngsters with disabilities, including those with communication impairments. Some of the most significant mandates are:

- Special education and related services must be provided at no cost to the child or parents.
- All children with disabilities and their parents are guaranteed due process with regard to identification, evaluation, and placement.
- A written individualized education program (IEP) must be developed and implemented for each child receiving special services. Individualized family service plans (IFSPs) are required for preschoolers and individualized transition plans (ITPs) are required for students age 14 and over.
- To the greatest extent possible, children with disabilities should be educated with children who are nondisabled. In addition, the education must take place in the least restrictive environment appropriate to the child's needs.

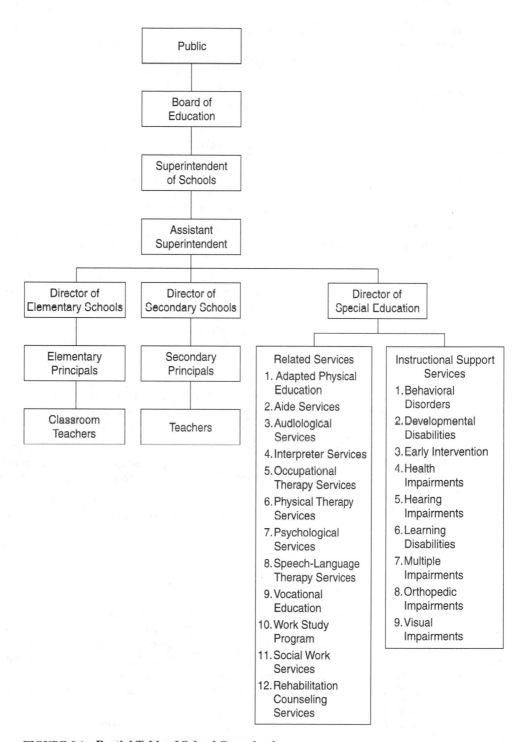

FIGURE 3.1   Partial Table of School Organization

TABLE 3.1 Federal Legislation Affecting Special Education

YEAR	LAW	KEY ASPECTS OF THE LAW
1973	PL 93-112 Section 504 of the Rehabilitation Act	Civil Rights law. Eliminates discrimination against individuals with disabilities by agencies that receive federal financial assistance.
1975	PL 94-142: Education for All Handicapped Children Act of 1975 (EHA)	Mandates a free, appropriate education for all handicapped students between the ages of 3 and 21. Provides for Individualized Education Programs (IEPs), due process, protection in evaluation procedures, and education in the least-restrictive environment.
1986	PL 99-457 Education for All Handicapped Children Act (Part H)	Extends protections of the PL 94-142 to infants and toddlers (birth to age 2) through the establishment of a formula grant program. Includes a mandate for a comprehensive Individualized Family Service Plan (IFSP) as part of the early intervention process.
1990	PL 101-476: Individuals with Disabilities Education Act of 1990 (IDEA)	Includes the additional categories of autism and traumatic brain injury as separate disability categories. Adds definitions of assistive technology device and service. Expands transition requirements.
1993	PL 103-85: Goals 2000: Educate America Act of 1993 (Goals 2000)	Describes inclusion of children with disabilities in school reform efforts. Develops eight National Education Goals.
1994	PL 103-382: Improving America's Schools Act	Provides for professional development for educators. Lists qualifications and competencies for individuals providing services, including related services and special education.
1997	PL 105-17: IDEA Amendments	Focuses on incorporating the general education curriculum into IEPs. Stresses involvement of parents in eligibility and placement decisions.

- The laws identify two groups of children as priorities among children with disabilities: (1) those not currently receiving any education and (2) those with the most severe handicaps within each disability who are receiving an inadequate education.
- The federal government is committed to assuming a percentage of the costs incurred in providing the programs for children with disabilities. Several different types of funding initiatives have been established by various states.
- The local education agencies are responsible for providing the appropriate educational programs.
- The local education agencies are responsible for periodic review and monitoring of such programs.

- Local education agencies must file a written plan clearly stating the procedures involved in meeting the provisions of the mandatory law. These include: (1) a child-find process; (2) nondiscriminatory testing and evaluation; (3) the goals and timetable of the plans; (4) guarantee of complete due process procedures; and (5) a guarantee to protect the confidentiality of data and information.
- Not only are children with disabilities eligible for appropriate educational programs but they are also eligible for all extracurricular activities such as music, art, and debate. The costs of educating children are borne by the school system. When the child's school cannot provide the appropriate educational placement, the local school system must pay for transportation, tuition, and room and board if the child is enrolled in a residential or tuition-based program.
- The legislation also states that the child with disabilities has the right to a nondiscriminatory evaluation of educational needs. Tests and evaluation materials must not be culturally discriminatory and must be administered in the predominate language spoken in the home. The evaluation is to be administered by a team of professionals and must include the child's parents and/or guardians.

The heart of the special education laws is the Individualized Education Program, or as it is more familiarly known, the IEP. Essentially the law requires that an IEP be developed for each child with a disability and reviewed jointly by a qualified school official, the student's teacher or teachers, the parents or guardians, and when appropriate, the student. The components of the IEP are explained in Chapter 9.

The special education public laws require each state to submit an annual plan, which is to be approved by the U.S. Department of Education. Each of the components of the act is addressed in the state's plan and the process by which specified requirements will be met is described. One of the responsibilities of the state education agency is to monitor and evaluate the activities of the local education agency to assure compliance with the federal statutes.

In addition, the state education agency is responsible for the proper use of federal funds in the administration of local programming for children with disabilities. The state education agency is also responsible for the following activities with regard to services for children with special needs: (1) the adoption of complaint procedures; (2) the disbursement of federal funds; (3) an annual report on the number of children served and the criteria for counting them; (4) the establishment of a state advisory committee on the education of children with disabilities; (5) a comprehensive system of personnel development; and (6) records on all the activities related to the public law.

Public Law 99-457

In 1986, Public Law 94-142 was amended to authorize early intervention programs for infants, toddlers, and preschool children who are at either biological or environmental risk for developmental delays. The amendment, known as PL 99-457, expanded the age ranges for receipt of services down to birth and increased the diversity of populations to be served by public school programs. It provided funding incentives for states to facilitate development and implementation of programs and services to children aged three to six years with handicaps. By the school year 1990–1991, states had to implement programs that ensured that the rights and protections of PL 94-142 were available to children ages three to five. State and local education agencies were to supervise the programs. To receive federal funding, school districts needed to include this population in their state education plan submitted annually.

PL 99-457 also established a discretionary program for provision of services to children birth to three years of age. States had to designate "lead agencies" to oversee the implementation of programs for infants and toddlers. In some states, schools accepted the responsibility for these programs. In other states, agencies such as the Department of Health or the Department of Maternal Care accepted the responsibility.

Because PL 99-457 is an amendment to PL 94-142, there are many similarities in the mandates of the two laws. All rights and protections of PL 94-142 are extended to infants, toddlers, preschoolers, and their families. Like PL 94-142, PL 99-457 mandated due process, services provided at no cost to families, interdisciplinary interaction and the team process, a comprehensive system of personnel development, and a comprehensive child-find and child-count system.

PL 99-457, like PL 94-142 had great impact upon the role of the SLP practicing in the schools. Since the target populations are infants, toddlers, and young preschoolers, the focus of programming necessarily shifted to the family unit. Family services began to play an important role in preschool programs. New partnerships between parents and professionals were forged. Changes were made in service delivery models and intervention procedures employed by speech-language pathologists working in preschool settings. Clinicians searched for infant and family assessment tools and interventions. They began to work with numerous agencies outside of the school system. Services to preschoolers can be provided by private practitioners, community-based programs, local education agencies, or in the family's home because appropriate services are not always available in the child's local school district. To make this happen, public education agencies were required to develop procedures for interfacing with other types of institutions.

Public Law 101-476: The Individuals with Disabilities Act (IDEA)

As professionals increase their understanding of the needs of persons with disabilities, the federal mandates regulating the provision of education and services continue to change. In 1990, The Education of the Handicapped Act was further amended. Reflecting sensitivity to the negative effects labels often carry for individuals, the title of the law was changed to the "Individuals with Disabilities Education Act (IDEA)." It reinforced the use of "person first" language, changing all references in the law to handicapped children to "children with disabilities."

Two new categories of disability were added: "autism" and "traumatic brain injury." Another change mandated that schools provide transition services for students, promoting movement from school to post-school activities. These include post-secondary education, vocational training, integrated employment, continuing and adult education, adult services, independent living, and community participation. The law also assured that students needing assistive technology services would receive them from trained personnel. The addition of these categories and services influenced the types of students carried on public school clinicians' caseloads. The changes supported developing therapy objectives and procedures that are *functionally based*. IDEA also required the inclusion of a statement of transition services in the IEP for students when they reach the age of 16. Suddenly speech language pathologists and special educators were expected to collaborate with other educators and agency representatives to plan school-to-work transition services and recommend strategies for meeting transition objectives.

Public Law 105-17: Reauthorization of IDEA

IDEA was again reauthorized in 1997 (Public Law 105-17). The changes further expanded and changed the role of the school-based speech-language pathologist. Montgomery describes the change as the logical next step in what SLPs have been doing to assist learners in school settings (Montgomery, 2000). The law stipulates the SLP's connection to the education process. It mandates the use of different service delivery models, the consideration of students' educational performance in the treatment plan and approach, and the SLP's close relationship with other educators. In other words, educators and SLPs have a common purpose—to educate the child. The reauthorized version of IDEA (Public Law 105-17) maintained and refined most of the basic requirements that were in the original Public Law 94-142. IDEA '97 added new provisions for discipline. Highlights of the IDEA '97 were explained to practitioners through special education publications such as newsletters and journals of ASHA and the Council on Education. A summary of highlights of the reauthorized law is presented in the following sections and in discussions throughout the book.

The definition of disabilities was clarified. A child with a disability who presents a need for a related service (such as counseling) is not considered to be disabled unless the related service is defined under law as special education. Family counseling, for example, is considered a related service not a special education service.

Developmental delays for children age three through nine may be defined as a disability. This change will positively effect speech-language pathology caseloads. Prior to this interpretation, children with developmental delays could not be served unless they were labeled as disabled and eligible to receive special education services.

Attention deficit disorder and attention deficit hyperactive disorder may lead to eligibility for special education under the "other health impairment" category. This is a change from previous versions of the law that limited the other health impairment category to physical conditions. The list of related services was expanded to include orientation and mobility services.

Supplementary aids and supports were added to the list of aids, services, and supports that could be provided to children within the context of the general education setting. This important addition enables more children with special needs to be educated with nondisabled children to the maximum extent possible. Prior to this change, funding that was allocated for children with special needs could not be used in settings where nondisabled children might also benefit.

One of the most complex changes is regarding the quality of instruction. A child shall not be determined to have a disability if the reason for the child's learning difficulty is lack of instruction in reading or math. This ruling will have a profound effect on educators. They will have to obtain training in order to ensure that they have the skills necessary to provide quality instruction to students.

Evaluations must be comprehensive. All areas of the suspected disability, including cognitive and behavioral factors in addition to physical or developmental factors must be evaluated. A variety of assessment tools and strategies for gathering functional and developmental information must be used. The assessment strategies must also help determine the student's educational needs. The child must be able to be involved and show progress in the general education curriculum. As in previous versions, the parents must consent to the evaluation prior to initiation.

States must establish goals for the performance of children with disabilities. They must develop indicators to evaluate progress. This means that children with disabilities must be included in state and district assessment programs. They may have accommodations as determined by their IEP. If children cannot participate in the assessments, states must develop alternative assessment options. The speech-language clinician can contribute much to the discussion of alternative assessments because many will involve the need to provide alternative methods for communication.

The law attempts to help schools develop programming for students with behavioral disorders. It mandates that a behavioral intervention plan must be developed for students who demonstrate behavioral disability and/or who are removed from school due to situations that occur as a result of poor behavior. Consider the fact that many youngsters who exhibit behavioral disabilities have difficulty understanding communication and being understood. The changes in the law are leading clinicians to gain a better understanding of the general education curriculum and what students have to learn at various grade levels (Ehren, 2000). SLPs must reconsider the testing they do to determine students' eligibility for speech and language services. Testing should be performance based and conducted in authentic settings. SLPs must change the design and goals of intervention. In addition, the treatment materials and criteria for success must be based on the requirements for performance in the school setting. The most significant result of the change is that SLPs are beginning to rethink the eligibility criteria, size, and composition of the caseload. They are striving to define functional goals. They are exploring and expanding alternative service delivery approaches. School systems are requiring teachers to improve their qualifications and skills so they can provide appropriate educational services to children. This will lead to increased use of collaborative service delivery and in-service education. SLPs must themselves become prepared for these changing roles.

INCLUSIVE EDUCATION

Instructing children with disabilities has always been very difficult. The practice of mainstreaming children with disabilities into regular class situations on a full-time or part-time basis was mandated in Public Law 94-142. The intent was to provide students with learning opportunities they would not have if they spent their entire day in the special class setting interacting only with other children who also have disabilities. Mainstreaming worked well in some school systems and not so well in others. Some educators and family members did not feel that mainstreaming went far enough in meeting the full needs of children.

Consequently, leaders in special education advocated meeting the challenge to provide improved programming for children with special needs by embracing the concept of the *inclusive education.* Also referred to by some as *integration,* the philosophy of inclusion is founded in the belief that children should be educated and completely involved in the activities of their neighborhood schools and within their communities regardless of the severity of their disability. Thus, with the implementation of IDEA, educators began to consider strategies for accomplishing effective inclusion when developing the educational plan. Inclusion involves bringing support services to the student rather than taking the student to the services. Full inclusion means that students will be in regular classrooms full time regardless of their disability and that all services will be brought to them.

Inclusion is a very controversial subject. Placing children with special needs into the same classroom as children who do not have special needs makes some people very uncomfortable. The alternative, segregating children with disabilities from those who are not disabled, makes others equally uncomfortable. The concept of inclusion relates to educational values, personal beliefs, and social values. Inclusion implies that all children are valued equally and that everyone is valuable. Accomplishing inclusion presents educators with many difficult challenges. In order for inclusion to work successfully, a great amount of support, communication, and interaction among teaching personnel is needed. Proponents of inclusion favor alternative forms of education service delivery; they are willing to try more creative, flexible methods for educating students.

To effect such wide reaching changes, the entire education system has to rethink its structure and organization. Watching educational programs spring into action and work toward the goal of implementing more effective programs for children with disabilities is very exciting. What you see are regular education and special education teachers forming partnerships and working closely together, *collaborating* to plan the best teaching strategies, materials, and techniques for individual children. The objective is for educators, regardless of their discipline, to combine their knowledge and expertise to jointly develop better solutions to problems than each could have done alone. The classroom teacher maintains the primary responsibility for the student's instructional program. Specialists, including speech-language pathologists and audiologists, provide support in designing and implementing special programs to meet the students' needs.

PARENTS AS TEAM MEMBERS

The public laws over the past 25 years have clearly given parents a major role in making decisions regarding the education and services provided to their children.

The rights and responsibilities of the parents and school district are described under the *due process* section of the laws for children with disabilities. Due process provides a procedure for reaching resolution when either party is in disagreement regarding the educational program for a child. Both the school district and parents have equal status at meetings. Parents have a right to question why any one procedure is necessary, why one may be selected over another, how a procedure is carried out, and whether or not there are alternative procedures. If parents disagree with the recommended procedures they have the right of review with an impartial judge. The purpose of due process is to give parents the right to have the school system explain to them and defend the recommended procedures. It does not necessarily make the parents adversaries to the system.

On the other side of the coin, the parents have the responsibility of dealing openly and honestly with the school system, accurately describing their child's behavior and reasonably and realistically requesting services. The school district has the right to disagree with the parents. Under due process the parents are entitled to the following procedures:

- A written notice before any action is taken or recommended that may change the child's school program
- A right to examine all records related to the identification, evaluation, or placement of the child
- A chance to voice any complaints regarding any matters related to the educational services the child is receiving
- An impartial hearing before a hearing officer or a judge in the event that the school and the parents cannot agree on the type of school program for the child
- An adequate procedure for appealing decisions. If parents are not satisfied with the due process procedure, the case may be taken to the state department of education or finally to a court of law.

PUBLIC SCHOOL REFORM: ISSUES AND TRENDS

Public schools are the concern of educators as well as parents, taxpayers, politicians, students, professional organizations, employers, and many other constituent groups. Citizens are concerned about literacy, discipline, drugs, cultural diversity in the curriculum, standardized methods for assessment, and safety in schools. These issues reflect the problems in society (Public Agenda Online, 1999). In recent years, calls for education reform have focused on several major issues including: setting higher standards for students; holding schools accountable for students' learning and performance; redefining what type of information is important for learning; improving teaching methods; altering funding streams to permit parents increased choices about how their school-related tax dollars are spent; and responding to calls for changes in the curriculum based on employer needs and/or religious convictions.

Even though problems such as these seem far removed from the therapy room, they do affect how well the clinician does his or her job, which goals are set for the program, the type of students who will receive services, and the funding that is provided for intervention. The national education reform debate is conducted in many arenas and about many topics. The arguments by each side are very compelling. Speech-language pathologists who work within the school setting may be asked to comment about their beliefs and stance on particular issues. The wise clinician will prepare to discuss the pros and cons of national, state, and local issues by following current events in the news media and school district publications.

GOALS FOR SCHOOLS

In the past decade there has been increased interest in reforming the way public schools operate and the curriculum that is taught. Schools are beginning to rethink their curriculum, instructional practices, and organizational structure. The driving forces have been to increase student achievement, to prepare students for the world after graduation, and to keep children safe.

In the Goals 2000: Education America Act (1996), eight major goals were set forth by the National Education Goals for American Education Institutions. These goals had profound impact on the direction for schools in the late 1990s. At the beginning of the new century they had not yet been achieved. In fact, in many cases schools fell short of the goals. Yet, one cannot deny the attention they brought to the challenges that schools faced and the potential positive results if the goals are achieved. Perhaps they have not yet been realized because schools continue to lack resources, educators continue to need better preparation for their teaching responsibilities, and viable partnerships have not yet been forged with families. The goals that were determined are as follows:

Goal 1.   By the year 2000, all children in America will start school ready to learn.

Goal 2.   By the year 2000, the high school graduation rate will increase to at least 90 percent.

Goal 3.   By the year 2000, all children will leave grades 4, 8, and 12 having demonstrated competency over challenging matter including English, Mathematics, Science, Foreign Languages, Civics and Government, Economics, Arts, History, and Geography, and every school in America will ensure that all students learn to use their minds well, so that they may be prepared for responsible citizenship, further learning, and productive employment in our nation's modern economy.

Goal 4.   By the year 2000, the nation's teaching force will have access to programs for the continued improvement of their professional skills and the opportunity to acquire the knowledge and skills needed to instruct and prepare all American students for the next century.

Goal 5.   By the year 2000, United States students will be first in the world in Mathematics and Science Achievement.

Goal 6.   By the year 2000, every adult American will be literate and will possess the knowledge and skills necessary to compete in global economy and exercise the rights and responsibilities of citizenship.

Goal 7.   By the year 2000, every school in the United States will be free of drugs, violence, and the unauthorized presence of firearms and alcohol and will offer a disciplined environment conducive to learning.

Goal 8.   By the year 2000, every school will promote partnerships that will increase parental involvement and participation in promoting the social, emotional, and academic growth of children.

What do these goals mean for speech-language pathologists and other educators across the country? And, what role can SLPs play in their success? As youngsters enter the school setting, they must present basic communication skills that will enable them to learn to participate in the classroom setting and learn to read and interact with their peers. Competency in specific subject matter will depend upon their ability to read, comprehend, and respond to materials that are in their texts or presented by their teachers. Speech-language pathologists, like teachers, will have to maintain their qualifications so they can provide appropriate services to children. To be successful adults and contributors to society, school graduates will need to communicate with their peers and at their jobs. They will have to arrive ready to follow instructions and to participate in complex tasks. Clinicians will be expected to involve parents in all aspects of the service delivery program so they can gain a meaningful understanding of their child's communication problems and know how to provide assistance when needed. Professionals cannot do their jobs and students cannot benefit from the school situation when they are afraid for their safety. All will have to demonstrate that violence and other forms of inappropriate behavior will not be tolerated.

ELEMENTARY AND SECONDARY EDUCATION ACT (ESEA)

In July of 1999, the United States House of Representatives passed a bill referred to as HR 1995, The Teacher Empowerment Act. Representatives then referred the bill to the Senate Committee on Health, Education, Labor, and Pensions. HR 1995 amends the Elementary and Secondary Education Act of 1965. The bill supports grants to improve the quality of teaching and learning. As a result of the bill, efforts to change teacher training and certification will be inevitable. Schools, universities, and state boards of education will work together to determine ways to promote improvements in teacher preparation including mentoring, measuring educators' performance in the classroom, development of cost-effective and easily accessible professional development opportunities, and changes in tenure and retention of teachers.

HIGH SCHOOL EXIT TESTS

Across the country, parents, educators, and citizens are calling for verification that students are prepared for work and post-secondary education after they graduate from high school. Over one third of the states require that students pass a high school exit test as one mechanism to document that students meet high educational standards. Opponents argue that minority students may have less chance to succeed because of problems that may exist in educational settings that have high numbers of minority students. Similarly, many special educators believe that students with disabilities are at a disadvantage when they take these types of tests. SLPs should be able to discuss the key issues surrounding a debate such as this. In addition, they should be able to provide data-based information about problems youngsters with communication disabilities may encounter on high school exit tests. They should be able to pose alternative methods of evaluating the level of learning students have achieved and students' preparation for employment or post-secondary education. If students experience difficulty with the tests, they must receive support and assistance. Tests that are used should be designed to promote success, not failure, for the student.

PREVALENCE AND INCIDENCE: HOW MANY CHILDREN ARE WE TALKING ABOUT?

The *prevalence* figures of speech, language, and auditory problems, or the *existing* number of persons affected at a *specified* time, are difficult to obtain. *Incidence* figures, the number of *new* cases occurring during a given time period, are usually not available. When reading or interpreting statistical reports, care should be taken not to confuse these two terms. Why is it important for prevalence figures to be known? One of the most crucial reasons is that programs and funding for services for children to 21 years of age are based on the number presently being served and those to be served in the future. The infusion of money into states by the federal government is based on prevalence figures. Therefore, these figures should be available and as accurate as possible.

Not only is it important for national and state educational planners to have prevalence information, but it is important on the local level as well. The school speech-language pathologist needs to know approximately how many students in a given school population can be expected to be eligible for speech-language services. The principal needs to know because of space requirements and because it will be important to plan for the coordination of other educational services. The superintendent needs to know so that an adequate number of speech-language pathologists may be hired and that the budget will accommodate personnel and equipment needs.

Unfortunately, determining the number of individuals with communication impairment is not simply a matter of taking a head count. Reports on incidence and prevalence of speech, language, and hearing problems among preschool and school age pupils have been difficult to complete, for several reasons. Definitions and terminology regarding disabling conditions may vary from state to state and from person to person so that the reporting of various conditions is not consistent. There is not yet a universally accepted, comprehensive classification system for speech and language disorders. Sometimes the data reported are based on too few children, and sometimes survey results are based on reports completed by persons with little or no training in identifying speech, language, or hearing problems. Often children who are nonverbal, non-English speaking, institutionalized, school dropouts, preschool age, or in special classes are not considered in the survey collection. Many children who might have died at birth or who survived accidents such as traumatic brain injury are now enrolled in public schools with the expectation that services will be available. Years ago youngsters with severe mental retardation were placed in mental health institutions. Due to changes in treatment philosophies and funding mandates, it is not unusual for school systems to be responsible for educating youngsters who may not have been served previously. Factors such as these have led to an increase in the numbers of youngsters reported with communication problems.

Very few comprehensive prevalence and incidence studies have been completed in recent years. Therefore, a reliable database has not yet been established. Much of the information reported in the literature is still based on studies and surveys that were completed several decades ago. While this is not ideal, it does provide us with some insights into data available about prevalence and incidence. In addition, some understanding of the prevalence and incidence of communication disorders can be gleaned from data submitted by state departments of education.

Based on research conducted over the past 30 years, it is probably safe to judge that between 8 and 10 percent of the children now enrolled in school exhibit some kind of oral communications disorder (Hull, 1964; Phillips, 1975).

There may even be indications that the figure of 10 percent is a conservative one. There are possible reasons for this. In reporting it is often common practice to report the presence of only one disability condition. For example, a child with learning disabilities may also have accompanying speech, language, or hearing problems, but in a survey that child is reported as being learning-disabled only.

The issue of identifying students with language disabilities has become even more complicated as the definition of language disorders has expanded to include pragmatics, literacy (problems related to reading and written language), cognition, emotionally-based disorders, and nonverbal communication.

The difficulty in ascertaining the incidence of children with language delay and language deviations continues to be a problem, not only for speech-language clinicians but also for all professionals in the field of special education. The number is actually larger than we suspect. Beitchman, Nair, Clegg, and Patel (1986) conducted a study to determine the prevalence of speech and language disorders in five-year-old kindergarten children in the Ottawa-Carlton region of Canada. Their results indicated that 6.4 percent of the children exhibited a speech impairment without concomitant language disorder, 8.04 percent presented language disorders only, and 4.56 percent showed a combined speech and language disorder. They identified differences between boys and girls in that age group, with the prevalence of disorders being higher among boys than girls. The authors suggested that these results be interpreted cautiously due to the many variables surrounding prevalence research. Their study also did not suggest whether the children identified would benefit from therapy. They recommended further study of these issues.

Recent research in the area of prevalence and incidence remains scant. The American Speech-Language-Hearing Association maintains reports on the prevalence and incidence of communication disorders. In recent years they have increased their efforts to gather and disseminate data due to increased demand for that data for decision making and reimbursement. ASHA's information is derived from a variety of sources including omnibus surveys, census statistics, the National Center for Health Statistics, National Institute on Deafness and Other Communication Disorders (NIDCD), and annual reports to Congress from the U.S. Department of Education Office of Special Education. Based on sources such as these, staff in the ASHA Research Division reported the following statements that have been made about the prevalence and incidence of communication disorders in children in recent years (ASHA, 2000; U.S. Department of Education, 1998):

- Approximately 46 million individuals in the United States experience or live with some type of communication disorder. Of these, approximately 14 million have a speech, voice, or language disorder.
- More than one of every 25 preschoolers exhibits some type of communication disorder.

- Phonological disorders affect approximately 10 percent of the preschool and school-age population. For 80 percent of the children with phonological disorders, the disorders are sufficiently severe to require clinical treatment. In addition, children with phonological disorders often require other remedial services.
- Sixty to 70 percent of the preschool children identified as having disabilities exhibit speech or language impairments.
- Over 3 million Americans stutter, most frequently between the ages of 2 and 6 years when language is developing.
- Vocal nodules are responsible for 38 percent to 78 percent of chronic hoarseness in children.
- In 1988, over 2 million school-age children received speech-language services; over 57,000 children were classified as hard of hearing or deaf.
- Of the approximately 5.2 million children (ages 6 to 21) with disabilities served in 1996–1997, 20 percent received services for speech and language disorders. Approximately 1.3 percent (68,766) children received services for hearing impairment.
- Seventy-five percent of children experience at least one episode of otitis media by their third birthday.
- Eight to 12 percent of preschool children have some form of language impairment.
- The overall prevalence of specific language impairment in kindergarten children is estimated to be 7.4 percent.
- It is estimated that the incidence of strokes in children is 2.5 per 100,000 children. Other causes such as brain injury are estimated to be approximately 200 per 100,000 children.
- The number of children ages 6 to 21 with disabilities receiving services in the 1996–1997 school year was 5,235,952 children. Of these, 20 percent received services for speech and language disorders.

The exact numbers of children who demonstrate communication disorders may be difficult to obtain due to several factors including improved and more discriminating identification procedures, provision of speech and language services outside of the special education delivery system (such as within the regular education classroom), and a current trend to identify students with language disorders as having specific learning disabilities rather than having speech and language impairments.

NUMBER OF STUDENTS REPORTED AS RECEIVING SLP SERVICES

Each year, the Office of Special Education Programs of the U.S. Office of Special Education and Rehabilitative Services in the Department of Education reports the progress on United States schools are making in the provision of a free appropriate public education for all children with disabilities. The report includes statistical information on the number and percentage of children who received special education and related services in a given time period. It also indicates the implementation of particular sections of the law and the provision of financial assistance to state and local education agencies through formula and grant funding to support the delivery of services.

The system for determining the amount of funds schools receive for providing services for children with disabilities necessitates categorizing and counting children according to the disabilities they present. The data presented in the reports concerning the numbers of children served are referred to as "child count" data. States collect the information annually and these numbers are used as the basis for allocating funds to states in order to provide necessary services. Counts are nonduplicative, representing the number of children served rather than the prevalence of disability conditions. Unfortunately the statistics are often interpreted as prevalence or incidence data resulting in inadequate funding and limited services. Services provided for the primary disability are referred to as "special education" and are included in the count. Services provided for concomitant conditions are designated as "related services" and are not included in the child count. Thus, only those children whose primary handicap is speech or language can be counted as receiving speech-language services. Children with other handicaps who receive speech-language services as related services have to be counted in the category which represents their primary disability (mental retardation, specific learning disability, serious emotional disturbance, multiple disabilities, hearing impairment, and so on). Therefore, the numbers reported in the "speech-language impairment" category are not representative of the total number of children actually served by speech-language pathologists in schools. This procedure for counting has made it difficult to determine how many children in the nation have actually been receiving speech-language services and may have resulted in unreasonably low funding for speech-language and hearing services over the past several years.

CASELOAD COMPOSITION

Speech-language pathologists in the schools provide services to students with a wide variety of communication impairments. Results of a 1985 ASHA Omnibus survey showed the following caseload composition in the school setting: language (52.2%), articulation (34.8%), fluency (4.1%), hearing (4.5%), voice (2.4%), and other conditions (2.0%). These findings were supported by the results of a 1988 ASHA Omnibus survey indicating that the largest portions of speech-language pathologists' caseload were language disorders (median 50.2%) and articulation disorders (median 39.7%). Informal reports by practitioners indicate that at least 45 percent of their school caseload was comprised of students who had primary disabilities other than speech-language and were receiving therapy as a related service.

Data collected over the years by the Department of Education reveal that the percentage of children served for communication disorders ranges from .9 percent to 4.1 percent of the total school age population. The variance is due to the procedures used for identifying, classifying, and reporting students with speech-language impairments.

The educational placement (environment) for the majority of students with speech and language impairments has been documented as being the regular class versus special education classes.

PUBLIC SCHOOL FUNDING

Public education has been the responsibility of government in America for hundreds of years. Education in most states is funded through a combination of local taxes, state funding, and money from other sources such as federal grants, interest on investments, rent, and tuition. Those funds that school districts do receive are allocated to many aspects of the education process including salaries, building maintenance, transportation, educational materials, and special education.

Thomas Jefferson was one of the first proponents of a free, universal education for all children, benefiting not only themselves, but society as a whole. Jefferson believed that education was necessary for democracy to flourish and sustain itself. (Ohio Coalition for Equity and Adequacy of School Funding, 1998). This was referred to as the "common school movement." Horace Mann, who became known as the "Father of the American School" wrote the following about the philosophy behind the common school movement:

> The cardinal principle, which lies at the foundation of our educational system is, that all children of the State shall be educated by the State. As our republican government was founded upon the virtue and intelligence of the people, it was rightly concluded by the framers, that, without a wise educational system, the government itself could not exist, and in ordaining that the expenses of educating the people, should be defrayed by the people at large, without reference to the particular benefit of individuals, it was considered by those, who, perhaps without children of their own, nevertheless would still be compelled to pay a large tax, would receive an ample equivalent in the protection of their persons, and the security of their property.

There is great debate in the United States currently about funding schools. The debate will certainly continue for years to come. Speech-language pathologists must be aware of the key issues and how changes in funding will impact on the types of services they can provide, their salaries, and the environment in which they work. It is not wise to ignore these issues and leave advocacy for better school funding to others. Most state speech-language pathology and audiology professional associations have established committees or employ lobbyists to stay on top of school funding issues.

FUNDING FOR SCHOOL
SPEECH-LANGUAGE SERVICES

Who pays for speech-language intervention services in the schools? Not surprisingly the answer is everyone who pays taxes pays for the schools and their many services. Special education is paid for by local, state, and federal education dollars. Local education agencies are supported in part from local taxes, with reimbursement from state foundation programs. In recent years the federal government through the Public Laws have reimbursed states for a portion of the expenditures for special education. National statistics show that special education programs are claiming an increasing share of school budgets (Rothstein, 1998). Special education costs include instructors, materials, administrative costs of programs, structural modifications, and transportation. In 1998 federal regulations took effect that allowed local education agencies (LEAs) to combine IDEA Part B funds with other state, local, and federal funds to carry out school-wide program activities.

States have set minimal standards for speech education programs including speech and language services. The standards may cover such areas as personnel qualifications, housing, facilities, equipment, materials, transportation, caseload, and case size. Failure to comply with state standards may result in the loss of foundation money to the school district.

There are three basic types of reimbursement to the local education agency: unit reimbursement, per pupil reimbursement, and special. Each state has its unique features in funding patterns, but generally they fall within these three categories.

In unit funding, states define a specific number of students or a special class as the basis for allocating funds. For example, a unit for a speech-language pathologist may be approved on the basis of 2,000 children in average daily membership. Therefore, a school system with a total population of 6,000 students would be eligible for three full-time SLPs. Or a school system with a population of 5,000 students would be eligible for two and one-half units, which would be two full-time and one half-time SLP. There may be stipulations such as class size, numbers of children with particular types of disabilities, or number of regular class units.

The per pupil reimbursement model means that the local education agency is compensated for each student receiving special education services. This could be based on average daily attendance (ADA) or average daily membership (ADM). School attendance is generally determined on a given day in the fall and spring of the school year.

A special reimbursement plan usually supplements a unit or per-pupil reimbursement. For example in Ohio a special unit for speech-language pathology may be approved on the basis of 50 children with multiple impairments, hearing impairment, orthopedic and/or other health impairments in special class or learning center units. Many of these reimbursement formulas encourage high caseloads because the amount of funds generated for a local education agency increases as numbers of students served increases. These reimbursement procedures fail to account for the total number of students with communication disorders or the frequency and intensity of services needed. The special reimbursement model may provide funds for instructional materials and equipment, transportation, facilities, personnel training, pupil assessment, residential care, specific professionals or ancillary services (physicians, audiologists, psychologists, social workers, physical therapists, occupational therapists, and so on).

The various funding models employed by school districts do not always have a system of accountability built in. Recent recommendations at the national level have encouraged states to consider systems for funding special education that are linked to standards such as pupil/teacher ratios and type of services. For example, funding would be allocated specifically for related services such as speech-language pathology so that funding would be allocated for services provided to youngsters who are classified as "speech only" (without other types of special education needs). A similar recommendation supports establishing some means of "equalization" of funding. This means that local and state funds pay equal amounts for special education.

While the intent of the laws which enable government supported education to children with disabilities is noble, the reality is that Congress has never adequately provided the needed level of funding to support services and programs. Only about 15 percent of the total costs are paid for by the government sources of funding. This has created financial difficulty for local school districts. Out of need, schools have had to seek alternative methods of funding programs to help defray expenses for providing education and services to students with disabilities. The regulations interpreting the federal laws indicated that states could use any sources available to pay for services included on the child's Individualized Education Program. The regulations implementing IDEA indicated that "nothing in IDEA relieves an insurer or similar third party payer from an otherwise valid obligation to provide or pay for services provided to a child receiving special education" (deFur, 1999). This included state, local, federal, and private funding sources such as insurers or third party payers such as Medicaid (Kreb, 1991; Power-deFur, 1999). According to Peters-Johnson (1990), school districts in some states started billing private insurance companies, health maintenance organizations (HMOs), and Medicaid for services provided. Reimbursable services included audiology services, case management, mental health services, allied diagnostic services, and treatment for physical therapy, occupational therapy, and speech-language therapy. Specific terminology must be used to describe the student's disorder and recommended treatment protocols in order to be considered for payment by third party payers. See Appendix A, The American Speech-Language-Hearing Association Classification of Procedural and Communication Disorders.

Medicaid billing is limited to children eligible for special education and related services under IDEA. This is an important interpretation for speech-language pathology services because it means that students who receive speech-language services but not special education and related services are ineligible for payment for services by Medicaid and other third party payers (Power-deFur, 1999).

In order to receive Medicaid funding, providers (SLPs and educators) must meet licensing and certification requirements. In addition, they must maintain records and submit documentation according to standards established by the third party payers. This can lead to additional paperwork and duplication of effort when the district requires one type of paperwork and the payer requires a different type. It is especially frustrating when different entities ask the same questions in different ways and on different forms.

School districts had difficulty trying to collect funds from private and third party funding sources until Public Law 94-142 was amended in 1986. At that time, Public Law 99-457 required interagency cooperation and coordination of resources. This requirement is still necessary; there must be coordination when a school-age student is receiving services from multiple sources.

DISCUSSION QUESTIONS AND PROJECTS

1. Why is it necessary for the school speech-language pathologist to know the administrative and organizational structure of the school system on the local level?

2. What questions would you ask about the structure of the school system if you were being interviewed for a position as SLP?

3. What relationship do you see between the prevalence figures for students with speech-language impairments and program planning?

4. Why are most prevalence figures for children with language disabilities difficult to obtain?

5. Public laws state that test and evaluation materials must be nondiscriminatory. Give examples of what this means. How will you know if the tests and evaluation materials you select are discriminatory?

6. Find out the minimum standards for speech-language programs in your state. Who will you call?

7. Find out if there is a regional resource center in your area. What services does it provide? Visit the center.

8. Interview a school SLP to find out to whom this individual is directly responsible in the school structure. What is their role and relationship to you?

9. Invite your state's Department of Education consultant in speech-language pathology to speak to your class. Prepare a list of questions to ask.

10. How would you explain the parents' rights and role in program planning to the parents of a child if they do not speak fluent English?

11. Why is it important to use "person first" language when referring to individuals with disabilities? Discuss some of the ramifications of referring to individuals by labels such as "mentally retarded," "learning disabled," "emotionally disturbed," "deaf," and the like.

12. What type of documentation is required in order to receive reimbursement from third party pay sources?

13. Briefly describe the impact of three key federal laws on the practice of speech-language pathology in the school setting.

■ ■ ■ ■ ■

CHAPTER FOUR

THE SPEECH-LANGUAGE PATHOLOGIST AS A MANAGER

When school speech-language clinicians are asked about their programs, services, and job performances, they are quite likely to make the following responses: "We need more time to plan." "There are too many children on my caseload." "We need more staff members." "I have trouble scheduling students because of all the other school activities." "My budget isn't large enough for me to purchase all of the equipment I need." "It's too hard to keep up with all of the types of disorders I have on my caseload." Interestingly enough, the school clinician is generally pleased with the progress of the children in the program, and the teachers and school administration are pleased with the program. Why, then, the complaints? Very possibly the reason is that each school speech-language pathologist is constantly faced with the challenge of providing the highest caliber of services with the most efficient expenditure of time, money, and resources, including physical, technical, and human resources.

In this chapter we will examine how the school SLP, in the role of manager, may utilize time more efficiently and expand human resources more effectively to provide optimal services to students. Topics covered include planning ahead, establishing goals, managing time and paperwork, utilizing supportive personnel, assessing teachers' impressions of and satisfaction with the program, and using computers to carry out administrative functions.

MANAGEMENT: BASIC PRINCIPLES

Perhaps the best place to start is to admit to ourselves that in the field of management we need to acquire new skills, new techniques, and new instruments, as well as an understanding of the principles of the management process: planning, organizing, staffing, directing, and controlling. The goal of comprehensive services for all children with disabilities points out the need for appropriate managerial skills at the local level as well as at the state and national levels.

Presently, there is a trend in health care and educational settings toward implementation of formal systems for program planning, development, management, and evaluation. Strategic planning and continuous quality improvement (CQI) principles are gaining acceptance in business, government, and educational settings at the national, state, and local levels. By adhering to the philosophy and processes associated with strategic planning and continuous quality improvement, professionals can identify their program's strengths and weaknesses and work toward better development of programmatic goals and objectives. The basic tenet of CQI is consumer satisfaction. Speech-language pathology programs serve many consumers including students with communication impairments, teachers and other specialists, parents and family members, school administrators, and the community. Efforts to provide quality services should be supported through all aspects of the program including planning and managing time, developing program goals and objectives, scheduling, implementing assessment and treatment, report writing, and so on.

The need to examine closely the school programs, what they are attempting to do, how they are doing it, and how effective they are is vital. The school speech-language clinician today and in the future will need to be acquainted with sophisticated tools and systems for evaluation and measurement of programs and personnel. A "cookbook" approach is not the answer because there is no single "recipe" for a good program.

THE MANAGEMENT ROLES OF THE SCHOOL SPEECH-LANGUAGE PATHOLOGIST

There was a time when most speech-language pathologists entering the job market had to start from scratch in organizing the speech-language therapy program in a school system. Fortunately for you, speech-language pathology programs are already in place in most school systems thanks to federal and state legislation mandating help for children with communication impairments. And thanks, too, to far-sighted school boards and administrators who realized that children needed to communicate effectively in order to benefit from what the educational system had to offer. Last, but not least, thanks to our founding fathers (and mothers) whose foresight and concern established the professions of speech-language pathology and audiology.

Today, however, the picture is different. You, in all probability, will take a position in an already established program. But this condition has its own set of challenges and problems. What are some of the possible roles you may fill in a school system?

The role of the speech-language pathologist is a dynamic one with many different areas of responsibility. Following is a list of some of the possible roles you may fulfill when you are employed as a speech-language pathologist in a school system. This list is by no means complete and it should be pointed out that you could be fulfilling a combination of any of these roles simultaneously. You may be:

- The only SLP in a small school district and would be working in several school buildings within the district
- One of a large staff of SLPs serving a large city system
- One of many SLPs in a rural school district covering a large geographic area
- Assigned to a self-contained special classroom in one building
- Assigned as a specialist in one specialty area of communication disorders (for example, severely disabled), and providing assessment and treatment
- A consultant in one area of specialization (such as autism) providing consultant services to classroom teachers and other SLPs

- Serving only preschool and special education classes
- Providing consultative services through in-class intervention in regular classrooms
- Offering consultative services through in-class intervention in self-contained special education classrooms (for example, a modified learning disabilities classroom)
- Supervising paraprofessionals or aides
- Supervising student teachers or students completing field experiences
- Coordinating the speech-language services in a school district, or an entire school system
- Managing a department of pupil personnel services and special education
- Offering speech-language services in a geographical area encompassing several counties or school districts

You may sometimes find yourself as an administrator. In examining all of the professional roles of a school speech-language pathologist, as we will do in this textbook, you will see that all of them require administrative and managerial skills. Your very first position out of college as an SLP will require that you have a firm grasp of the administrative hierarchy of a public school system and your place in it. You will gain managerial skills as you carry out your own program in concert with others.

THE MANY FACES OF MANAGEMENT

What is management? It has been said that management is the art of getting things done through people. The major function of management is to see that people function effectively to accomplish what needs to be done. The skills necessary for good management include the following: communicating effectively; managing time; understanding the job of supervision; understanding leadership and developing a leadership style; and planning, setting goals, and measuring results.

Many colleges and universities offer credit and noncredit courses in management and supervision through their colleges of business, continuing education, or education. Professional organizations such as the American Speech-Language-Hearing Association and the Council for Exceptional Children offer seminars in management and supervision. In addition, there are many publications and resources available on the topic.

The school speech-language pathologist's job is a very complex one consisting of many responsibilities. Let us look at some of the responsibilities the school clinician's job entails:

Program Organization and Management. Much of the clinician's time is spent organizing, planning, implementing, and analyzing various aspects of the school program. Clinicians who meet with their administrators on a frequent basis have a greater opportunity to educate them about the goals and purpose of the speech-language pathology program. SLPs who take time to develop and disseminate information about their programs are doing what is necessary to help others learn about communication disorders and see the role they can play in the success of the speech-language pathology program. These marketing efforts will pay off in the end.

Screening and Case Finding.   In this activity the clinician works with others to identify children with speech, language, and hearing problems who might be eligible to receive speech and language intervention services.

Diagnosis and Assessment.   This task includes administering formal and informal instruments to determine the communication characteristics the youngster presents. Recommendations for treatment are based on the findings of these activities. In most school districts testing is carried on throughout the school year. However, during the first few months and last few months of the school year most SLPs engage in more assessment activities than at other times. Assessment activities may include any or all of the following: administering tests, observing the youngster in various settings, interviewing parents and teachers, or reviewing portfolios of the students' classroom materials.

Determining Eligibility, Case Staffing, and Decision Making.   The SLP is a member of the school special education placement team. Along with other team members, she discusses the student's communication problems and needs, and provides and reviews data for individual students to jointly develop the individualized educational program for each student. The SLP participates in multifactored team meetings to develop plans or discuss children's needs.

Providing Intervention Including Collaborating with Other Professionals.   The heart of the speech-language pathologist's role lies in the delivery of intervention services for youngsters with communication disabilities, including direct intervention and collaboration with others to ensure that treatment is carried out in a broad varied of contexts. When collaborating, the SLP exchanges information and jointly shares responsibility with parents, teachers, psychologists, health care professionals and others in regard to individual students. Providing intervention does not always mean meeting face-to-face with the student. In service delivery models that employ collaboration, the SLP may actually provide instruction for others to carry out.

Preparing Materials.   SLPs often need to prepare materials for use in their program or for use by others. Materials do not always have to be constructed or designed by the SLP. They must, however, be suited to the students' age, interests, and communication needs. SLPs who work with students with severe disabilities must prepare technological equipment for students' use in the classroom. This includes programming computers and installing assistive listening devices.

Record Keeping.   This task includes all activities involved in maintaining information on the delivery of services to each student and other important programmatic aspects such as the demographics of the caseload, annual activity report, treatment outcome data, program statistics, and so on.

Consultation.   Other services, not directly related to students with communication disorders, enable the clinician to maintain, promote, and enhance the speech-language pathology intervention program. These activities are essential to the program. Examples include providing in-service training programs for staff, parents, and colleagues. SLPs must also meet with administrators to discuss program goals and needs and to report outcomes of treatment.

Participating on Curriculum Selection Committees. Speech-language pathologists have a unique contribution to make regarding the selection of curricular materials. Many are not asked to do so because their colleagues in education do not realize the knowledge base that SLPs possess. To really begin articulating the SLP program with the rest of the educational goals for youngsters, SLPs must willingly exchange information with others about how the selected curriculum will positively or negatively impact on a student's performance because of communication requirements and demands within the curriculum.

Other Activities. Many specialists are engaged in research related to the school programs. To maintain professional currency, SLPs attend professionals meetings and conferences. Some school specialists spend time supervising student teachers in speech pathology. Conservation and prevention programs may be carried out by the school clinicians. In addition, clinicians participate in public information activities such as talks to various groups, radio and television programs, and newspaper articles.

School-based speech-language pathologists are a part of the educational organization. Consequently, they must take every opportunity to ensure that their program fits into that organizational structure. This means interacting with all educational colleagues during important school-related activities such as curriculum design, program planning, and social events.

The roles and responsibilities of speech-language pathologists have expanded and changed in recent years. The many types of service delivery models employed along with the increasing numbers of children with severe disabling conditions served demand more time and greater expertise of the school clinicians. This means that there must be careful planning and careful allocation of time by the speech-language pathologists in order to get the job done by the end of the day. While the clinician is responsible for the list of duties presented above, this doesn't mean that they must "do" each and every one alone. This is where SLP assistants can be very useful. The SLP can maintain responsibility while delegating the actual execution of many of these activities to others.

MANAGING PROGRAM DEVELOPMENT AND CHANGE

Strategic planning is a program planning process that many school districts and organizations are using to define their goals and resolve their problems. The strategic planning process incorporates several steps: it involves analyzing the program's strengths, weaknesses, opportunities, and potential problems. After analyzing these factors, reasonable goals and actions are determined that will lead to the fulfillment of the program's mission. This planning method sensitizes you to the school culture and environment. You learn about situations that pose barriers to accomplishing the goals you would like to achieve. The planning process becomes ongoing and never ending. Thus, you stay aware of situations that may change and you can alter your plans accordingly.

Through strategic planning, a staff can be more forward thinking about what they want to do or be in the future. It can be useful as a tool for addressing problems. During the strategic planning process, the expertise of many people is utilized and teamwork is reinforced. The strategic planning process can help an educational staff develop plans for decreasing high caseloads, offering services to a new population, implementing a new intervention program, or acquiring additional resources.

The following sections will demonstrate how the strategic planning process could be used to make a change in the program service delivery model.

Determine the Mission.   Effective planning requires that an organization very clearly express its mission, or purpose for existing. The mission statement provides direction to program development efforts. When the mission is clear, the decision-making process becomes easier.

Those staff members who will need to embrace and implement the mission must participate directly in its creation. This enables all participants to approach initiation of new goals and actions from the same perspective and with the same philosophical understanding.

To develop the mission statement, a multidisciplinary planning group should determine specifically what is to be accomplished. For our example, let's assume that the team wants to implement a collaborative service delivery model in the school building. The mission should be clear and understandable to all individuals who are associated with the program. To increase the chances that this will occur, administrators and educational staff members should participate directly in formulating the program and designing the plan for implementation. The sample mission statement in Figure 4.1 is the type of statement that could be used to guide the planning for a collaborative model. Note that it is stated in general terms.

Scan and Analyze the Environment.   In formulating the statement, team members would discuss information obtained from an environment or situational analysis. The team would review those situations that pose problems or barriers to effective collaboration. They would also identify those situations or persons that present opportunities for success. During meeting, the team should identify what has been successful or unsuccessful with regard to current intervention methods or approaches. Following are the types of questions that the team should answer. What kinds of problems can be better solved via a new approach or program model? What resources can be used to solve the problems or eliminate the barriers? Why will such a model be more responsive to meeting the needs of students with communication disorders? A sample environmental scan to determine challenges and opportunities for implementing a collaborative service delivery model is briefly outlined in Figure 4.1.

State the Program Concept.   After the mission statement is developed, the team must clearly and accurately describe the type of program they ideally want to establish and what they want it to accomplish. Discussions should lead to descriptions of the population to be served, the type of personnel who will represent the program, equipment to be used, operating procedures to be initiated, tasks and activities to be accomplished, and differences

FIGURE 4.1   Sample Strategic Plan for Developing a Collaborative Model of Service Delivery

MISSION STATEMENT FOR A COLLABORATIVE MODEL

"Our mission is to provide quality, ongoing, and comprehensive speech-language assessment and intervention services that interface effectively with the educational program."

ENVIRONMENTAL SCAN

Strengths

SLPs on staff have expertise in specific areas (integrating technology into therapy, parent training, classroom-based intervention).

Networks have been established among various teachers and clinicians within the school district.

Weaknesses

Personnel and funding for the speech-language program are limited.

School district personnel and administrators are resistant to adopting the collaborative/consultative model.

School personnel do not understand the impact of communication disorders on academic success.

Parents have expressed a desire for more direct services.

Opportunities

The school district has just determined that inclusion should be a priority for the coming school year.

Educators have requested more information about strategies for working with students with communication disorders.

Potential Problems

Administrators believe that direct service is the best mode of cooperation for the SLP program.

A principal who was easy to work with just retired.

Funding is limited.

Data supporting benefits of the collaborative/consultative model is lacking.

Administrators and education professionals do not understand how SLPs can contribute to the education process.

SAMPLE PROGRAM CONCEPT POPULATION TO BE SERVED

Infants and toddlers, ages 0–3.

CURRENT SERVICES PROVIDED

Assessment by individual specialists and referral to community agencies dependent on presenting disabilities.

PERSONNEL TO BE INVOLVED

SLPs with experience in working with infants, toddlers, and preschool educator; psychologist; building principal; representative form a local pediatric hospital; kindergarten teacher; physical education teacher; district curriculum consultant; primary special educator.

(continued)

FIGURE 4.1 **Continued**

EQUIPMENT TO BE USED
Assessment instruments appropriate for infants, toddlers, and preschoolers; early childhood toys; augmentative devices.

OBJECTIVES TO BE ACCOMPLISHED BY THE CONSULTATIVE/ COLLABORATIVE TEAM
Observe and assess the child, formulate expectations and goals, interact with family members, review and select curricular objectives and materials, develop lesson plans focusing on identified target skill areas, in-service educators.

BENEFITS OF COLLABORATION/CONSULTATION FOR THIS POPULATION
Language intervention and teaching techniques can be identified and integrated into the child's natural environment including preschool program, home, and community; intervention services can be offered to an increased number of children; time will be more efficiently used; professionals' expertise will be shared.

SAMPLE GOALS FOR IMPLEMENTING A COLLABORATIVE SERVICE DELIVERY MODEL

1. Conduct a prevalence and incidence study of two school buildings to determine groups of students and types of disorders that would benefit from this type of service delivery model. Actions: Conduct a screening program. Distribute teacher surveys. Conduct a needs assessment.
2. Determine two specific content areas of the school curriculum where the SLP program and education program can best be articulated. Actions: Review courses of study, curriculum objectives, and teaching materials for key target grade levels.
3. Develop and disseminate written materials explaining the collaborative service delivery model to five key administrators and school personnel. Actions: Review literature on collaborative programs. Develop descriptive materials. Make a presentation at an upcoming administrators' meeting.
4. Develop resource materials for use when working with classroom teachers. Actions: Outline the type of materials needed. Review materials currently available commercially and in your resource library. Determine applicable materials. Compile in usable, retrievable formats.

TIMES TO COMMUNICATE WITH OTHERS

Conferences	Annual Reports
Progress reports	Newsletters
Parent training programs	Written notes
Observation days	E-mail messages
Budget requests	In-service meetings
Lunch and coffee breaks	Social activities

from current practices. Ideas can be generated by viewing model programs, reading professional literature, and talking with colleagues who have initiated similar (collaborative) programs. While examples can be drawn from these sources, the mission statement and program concept that are generated should be unique to the specific school district and responsive to its specific needs. It should reflect the resources and expertise available in the district. Figure 4.1 shows a sample program concept for a collaborative model.

The implementation of a new program does not need to be an all-or-nothing approach. After reviewing your environment, present situation, and resources, you may realize that a collaborative model might be most effective in only a few aspects of the SLP program. For example, you might decide to launch the new model with only high risk infants and toddlers, with students needing augmentative communication systems, or with students from diverse cultural populations. You may decide to implement a particular model in one school building rather than another because the teachers are more willing to work with you. In such a case, you would determine one or two specific areas of concentration on which to focus the collaborative services for the first year. You would then make a plan for the second and later years. Team members should decide how to phase in the new model so resistance to change is reduced. A key factor in the successful initiation of any new program will be the way it is introduced and explained to others in the building or school district.

Formulate Goals or Objectives. Goals, objectives, and an action plan are developed after the challenges are identified, the mission statement is written, and the program concept is developed. The goals and strategies for achieving those goals need to be formulated using "operational terms." This means the goals should be *feasible, acceptable to colleagues and administrators, valuable,* and *achievable.* They should be either *quantifiable or observable.* Goals should be designed to take you in the direction of your mission. Write goals that tell administrators and colleagues what they can expect from the new model and how they will benefit from it. A goal statement such as "to increase accuracy of teacher referrals by 15 percent" indicates clearly what is to be accomplished by adopting the new service delivery model. Care should be taken to be realistic when developing goals. If they are not realistic, the chances are slight that they will be realized or that you will yield the results you want. Sample goals are illustrated in Figure 4.1.

Your mission and strategic goals are achievable only when they are based on accurate information and developed in a systematic manner with input from a variety of sources, including those professionals who will be charged with implementing them. There are a number of interactive planning techniques that can be used when formulating your mission and goals, including developing storyboards, creating scenarios, brainstorming, and using consensus-building techniques. You may even want to invite a consultant in to work with the staff by facilitating an open discussion about what they want and what would work for them.

Develop an Action Plan for Accomplishing Goals. Through discussion with the team, prioritize your goals and then develop an action plan indicating major activities for accomplishing each goal. A number of activities will be required for accomplishment of each goal. This is where the team effort is important. Encouraging participation in the planning process will engender teamwork and ownership in the program when it is up and running. Work with people to identify tasks they wish to pursue and skills they can bring to the project. To keep participants on task, list deadlines, persons to be involved, individuals responsible for overseeing each action step, potential obstacles to completion, and enabling steps. Be realistic in establishing deadlines. You want these activities to be an enjoyable, doable task. Monitor progress by reviewing actions taken on each objective periodically. Take corrective action when it appears that efforts are off-track. Figure 4.1 provides examples of actions that can be taken. Of course there will be objectives, steps, timelines, and assigned responsibilities for completing each of the actions.

Evaluate the Organizational Structure to Determine Support for Implementation.   The organizational structure has to be conducive to adopting a new model if implementation is to be successful. Therefore, during the planning process, the organizational structure should be examined. The organization needs to be designed so the mission and goals can be accomplished. For example, in order to collaborate with educators about ways to improve students' academic abilities, a professional must be available who understands what specific needs are important for classroom success, the subject content that is taught at various grade levels, and what classroom techniques need to be enhanced or adapted. Administrators must be supportive of the change.

Administrators will need to be convinced with concrete data and evidence that the new program or model is going to have a positive impact on the treatment practices and educational methods used with students. Only then will they provide the support that is needed and create a school environment that is conducive to ensuring success. The potential for this occurring is increased in districts where organizational management is participatory, where there are well-developed communication systems, where administration is responsive to staff members' ideas, and where there is a willingness to be creative and innovative. Recognize that it may be impossible to change the organizational structure of the school or district. However, analyzing the existing structure with respect to the model you want to implement will give you the advantage of knowing the forces you will confront.

If top-level management embraces the program change and goals, top-down changes can be initiated to support it. School building and caseload assignments can also be adjusted accordingly. Financial resources can be allocated to support its development.

Develop Systems for Sharing Information.   To implement your program effectively, there must be an organized flow of information to professionals involved in the program and to consumers of the services. With clear exchanges of information, individuals can function responsibly to carry out goals, understand priorities, and form effective relationships. Examine the communication style, needs, and opportunities in your organization (school district). Ask yourself and your team, "Who in this school district needs to know and understand what we are trying to do?" In order to create an information-based system, there needs to be mutual understanding, shared values, and mutual respect. As part of your strategic plan, develop a plan for communicating with your various colleagues and consumers to make them aware of your new program and get them involved in it. Figure 4.1 lists numerous methods for communicating with colleagues and consumers about our sample case. Communication strategies will be discussed more thoroughly throughout the book.

Conduct Ongoing Planning and Evaluation.   If the new model was given life by a small group of individuals, efforts need to be made to integrate the new program into the comprehensive plan of the whole organization (e.g., special education program, related services division, pupil personnel department). Duplication of services and efforts must be avoided or eliminated. Already-scarce resources will need to be shared. For example, for a new service delivery model to succeed, there will need to be frequent and systematic interactions with individuals involved and periodic review to see if modifications are needed.

After the planning team has taken a good look at what actions the strategic plan entails, he or she must determine priorities. Inexperienced clinicians in a new situation sometimes try to do everything the first year. This is not only unreasonable, but also unwise even to attempt. The result may be that of spreading oneself too thin and not accomplishing anything satisfactorily. For example, the team may have to decide whether a teacher in-service program or a parent in-service program is more important during the first year. The clinician may then rationalize that the teachers are more readily available and need to understand the program more immediately than do the parents, so the in-service program for teachers would take precedence. During the following year, however, the clinician may decide to devote more time and energy to the parent in-service program, and that program would be given top priority.

The goals for the year should indicate the time (or times) of the year that the goals would be implemented and accomplished as well as the amount of time involved. Goals may be written for an entire school year or for one semester at a time.

Monitoring and evaluating the evolution and development of the program are important aspects of the strategic planning process. There are many mechanisms for evaluating and maintaining control over the program. Evaluation can be achieved by means of periodic staff meetings, reports of activities, periodic progress reports, and feedback from colleagues. Since planning is a cyclical process, results should be reviewed on an ongoing basis and corrective actions are taken in light of new situations. The program change should be evaluated periodically to determine if modifications are needed. During each review period, strengths, weaknesses, opportunities, and potential problems ought to be reconsidered. The following questions could guide a discussion of changes that might affect the program. Have there been major changes in personnel or school policies that will impact the program? Has anything new emerged? Future direction and ideas for expanding the program to other grade levels, school buildings, and disorder populations should be reviewed. All staff should participate in the review process. Major changes should be reviewed and/or approved by administration.

Program goals should not be confused with goals that individual clinicians establish for themselves. These clinician's goals and the program goals may not necessarily be at odds, but it should be kept in mind that although clinicians may come and go, programs, it is hoped, go on forever. Setting goals for the program, with the clinicians as the implementers, will allow smooth, continuous functioning of a program despite changes in personnel. There is probably nothing more frustrating for a school clinician who is stepping into a job than to learn that the previous clinician left no records concerning what was planned, what was accomplished, when it was accomplished, how long it took, and what remains to be done.

In addition to establishing yearly or semester program goals based on a priority list of the tasks involved in the clinician's job, other information would have to be available, including:

- Number of speech-language pathologists on the staff
- Number of schools to be served
- Amount of travel time between schools
- Enrollment figures for each school building (enrollment by grade level and enrollment of special education classes, including hearing impaired, physically impaired, developmentally delayed, emotionally disturbed, and so on)
- Number of preschool children in the school district

The school clinician can use this information to decide on the appropriate methods of delivery-of-service and scheduling systems.

MORE ABOUT WRITING PROGRAM GOALS AND OBJECTIVES

The school SLP, although responsible to another person in the hierarchy of the administration, is responsible for the management of the school's speech-language pathology program. The school system may be a large urban system, a small community system, or a sprawling countywide system, and the school SLP must assess the needs in light of the local situation and plan accordingly.

If the school system employs more than one SLP, there must be coordination of their activities. If it is a large or moderately large system, one SLP may be designated as the coordinator of the program. But even the school SLP who is working alone in a small school system needs to have a plan of action.

Planning ahead is the key to a successful program. Setting goals and objectives is one of the most critical elements of the planning process. Once the goals and objectives have been determined, the next step is writing them down in such a form that they clearly communicate their intent to all the persons concerned and involved in the program.

The utilization of written goals and objectives has many potential advantages in the school speech-language program. First, it allows for change, because through the system of periodic review, objectives will need to be revised and rewritten. Also, it creates a positive pressure to get things done. Communication among professionals will be improved. There will be more precise definitions of the roles and responsibilities of the school speech-language clinician. A system for evaluating and assessing the overall program is inherent in the written goals and objectives. Better utilization of each staff member's time and capabilities will be encouraged. And finally, there will be a better basis for understanding the program both within the school system and in the community.

When trying to determine goals and objectives, it is helpful to view the program and your responsibilities in terms of a problem that needs to be solved. First, there is a need to establish major goals, objectives, and policies that guide decision-making. In the larger context, it is helpful to ask yourself some questions:

1. What is the purpose of the (speech-language pathology or education) program?
2. What are the major goals, objectives, and policies that guide the program's decision making?
3. What is the structure that is in place to assign responsibilities for the various tasks that must be achieved in order for accomplishing the objectives?
4. What resources (space, equipment, furniture, staff, and supporting services, to mention only a few) are available to support the program so the purpose can be accomplished?

Goals are long-term and short-term, tangible, measurable, and verifiable. They are not nebulous statements but specific statements of a desired future condition. Ideally, goals should be set by all persons involved in the structure so there is a commitment on their part. Once the goals have been determined it is crucial to get them down in writing. The language must be clear and concise and must communicate the intent to all relevant parties. Let us look at some examples of goals and objectives. We will first consider writing long-range program goals, assuming that you have already evaluated the existing situation and have determined the overall needs of the program. Keep in mind that although these are long-range and broad in focus, they still need to be stated specifically and concretely. The examples are listed below:

- One year from (date) the clinician will have developed and written a language curriculum guide for special education teachers in the county.
- By (date) the clinician will have completed a research project related to determining criteria for case selection at the kindergarten level.
- By (date) 90 percent of the pupils in Butler Elementary School identified as having communication problems and needing intervention will be receiving services.

Some goals and objectives may be narrower in focus and have a shorter time frame.

- By (date) the clinician will have obtained referrals from 75 percent of the K–6 teachers.
- By (date) the clinician will have conducted group parent meetings for parents of all children enrolled at Lakeside School.
- During the second week of school in September, the clinician will acquaint teachers at Jefferson School with referral procedures through an in-service meeting.
- By (date) the clinician will write an article for the local newspaper and prepare items for the local radio and television stations announcing the prekindergarten communication evaluation program to be held during the first week in May.

A *criterion,* or *standard of performance,* is the description of the results of a job well done. It represents the desired outcome or benchmark for success. Using numbers or another indication of quantity such as *how much* and by *when* provides a framework for determining if the goal has been achieved. The outcome should be realistic and high quality enough so that when the task is completed it will have been of value to the program. Some examples follow:

- Dismiss 30 percent of the pupils enrolled as functionally corrected and 50 percent as greatly improved by the end of the school year.
- By (date) the clinician will provide three demonstration language-development sessions in 50 percent of the kindergarten classrooms of Revere School, and receive written positive feedback from 90 percent of the teachers involved.

The *evaluation* is the method used to determine if the goal or objective has been accomplished. An indication of the evaluation may be a report sent to the coordinator of speech-language and hearing services. Or it may be a list of post-test scores, a list of referrals made, or a chart indicating that change has occurred as the following example shows:

- By (date) the clinician will have completed speech-language screening tests of 95 percent of the first-grade pupils in Marblehead School, and a report will be submitted to the school principal and the director of speech-language and hearing services.

Occasionally, objectives are difficult to measure or confirm, even though they are activities or events that when accomplished lead to the overall improvement of a situation or condition. The following example demonstrates this:

- The clinician will attempt to improve communication with the classroom teachers by eating lunch with the teachers at least two times per week; inviting teachers to observe therapy sessions and attending as many school meetings and social functions as time permits.

School SLPs are familiar with the process of writing goals and objectives for the students with whom they work. Program goals are also important so that there is a clear understanding of *where* the program is going, *how* it will get there, and *how* to know when the objectives and goals are achieved. The manager of the program should be sure everyone understands the goals and, ideally, each participant should have a part in formulating them.

THE MANAGEMENT OF TIME

The management of time is an important factor in considering the role of the school SLP. Due to mandates within the state and federal laws, SLPs are confronted with great amounts of paperwork in the implementation of procedures. Although this has undoubtedly accounted for an increased expenditure of time, there are ways of managing time that can lead to increased productivity.

Planning for the Week

In planning for the week the key word is *flexibility.* The school clinician will have to decide how much time during the week will be spent working directly with students, providing guidance to teachers, supervising assistants, or traveling from school to school. Specific blocks of time can be allocated for each of these categories of activities. An activity such as parent training may be carried out in a block of time. The school clinician may want to reserve blocks of time at certain times of the year or the semester for various aspects of the program.

Such activities as diagnosis and assessment, staffing and placement, and consultation are necessary parts of the program, and time for these activities may be set aside in daily or weekly blocks. For example, the staffing and placement team may not meet every week, so the block of time set aside weekly could be used on alternate weeks for meetings to discuss placement recommendations or for conducting diagnostics or providing consultation.

Record keeping and time spent in organizing, planning, implementing, analyzing, and evaluating the program could be scheduled at times of the day when staff members are in the school but children are not present. For example, mornings before children arrive at school and afternoons after they are dismissed could be utilized for these activities. Many school systems set aside a time usually referred to as *coordination time* for tasks of this nature.

Two very important activities are consulting and collaborating with the classroom teacher and other educators. This may be done on an informal one-to-one basis or as part of an in-service training presentation for teachers, school administrators, other school personnel, and parents. Because communication is the keystone of the education process and because even the most skilled classroom teacher cannot teach a child who has not developed adequate communication skills, the school speech-language pathologist has much to offer in helping to improve communication abilities. The school SLP needs to plan for time for consulting and collaborating with others.

Over the last decade, an increasing number of SLPs began to expand the types of service delivery models they use to meet the needs of youngsters on their caseload. For example, it has become commonplace to provide intervention within youngsters' classrooms or to teach critical communication skills alongside of the classroom teacher. Each of these service delivery models requires time to plan and execute. Others clinicians have hired assistants to work side-by-side with them. If assistants and aides are assigned to the program, time must be planned to train them and time must be allocated for the supervision of such personnel.

For many of the activities mentioned, time is not planned on a regularly scheduled basis but certainly must be set aside to include these important facets of the program.

Planning for the Day

In planning time for the day, the school clinician will have to know how many hours per day the children are in school. What is their arrival time and what is their dismissal time? How much time is allowed for lunch and recess?

The time that the teachers are required to be in school and the time they may leave in the afternoon is set by school policy, and school clinicians should follow the same rules that teachers are required to follow. This sometimes poses a problem for the school clinician who is scheduled in School A in the morning and School B in the afternoon, but who must return to School A for a parent conference or staff meeting after school is dismissed. The problem arises when the teachers in School B think the clinician is leaving school early. Difficult situations such as these can usually be alleviated by following the rule of always informing the principals of School A and School B of any deviation from the regular schedule.

The school clinician will have to decide the length of the therapy sessions and amount of time devoted to diagnostics and other services. There does not have to be a predetermined length of time. Sessions may range from 15 minutes to an hour or more. The length of treatment depends on a number of factors including the student's unique needs, the composition of the caseload and resulting demands, and the school schedule for classes, recess, lunch, dismissal time, and so on.

Future chapters will include an in-depth discussion of factors that must be considered when constructing a caseload and schedule. Among the considerations are the total number of children to be seen, range of disorders to be served, extent of services to be provided, composition of caseload, and structure of therapy sessions (group versus individualized sessions versus classroom-based intervention). Also, children will inevitably progress at different rates. Some may be in the final phase of therapy and won't require as much time as children who are just beginning. The caseload and schedule should be "fluid" to accommodate children moving into and out of treatment as their communication skills and needs change.

It is wise to schedule the sessions a few minutes apart to allow for children to arrive on time or to allow time for the clinician to locate a child whose teacher has forgotten to send a child to therapy. In planning the daily schedule the school clinician will need to retain as much flexibility as possible. Children change and their needs change. The child who once required 30 minutes of individual therapy per day may later need only 15 minutes twice a week. Or the child who once needed individual therapy may need the experience of a group or in-class activity to continue making progress. The principal and the teachers must also understand the benefits of offering a flexible program. It is the responsibility of the clinician to interpret the rationale involved in making changes in schedules.

As a result of inclusion and the influx of more children with serious disabilities into the public schools, the school clinician must allow time for working with classroom teachers of youngsters who are mentally retarded, emotionally disturbed, hearing impaired, learning disabled, autistic, and multihandicapped. In fact, any child with communication disabilities may require direct as well as indirect intervention by the speech-language pathologist.

Allocate Time for Planning

In most school systems, the SLP sets aside a specific time which is allotted to the numerous activities that must be carried on in addition to the time spent in therapy. This is usually referred to as "planning time" or "coordination time." This may be a block of time allocated during the week or it may be several periods of time during the week that are not scheduled for therapy. Or it may be a combination of the two. Planning time is not a "right" and should be used wisely or others may interpret that it is not needed.

SLPs spend their planning time accomplishing a broad range of tasks and activities. These might include conducting screening programs, administering diagnostic tests, completing re-evaluations, participating in teacher conferences, attending administrative conferences, contacting parent, making phone calls, writing individualized education plans, completing summary reports, attending professional meetings, making referrals, observing youngsters in class or other settings, volunteering for state professional associations, attending in-service meetings, reviewing and ordering materials, organizing resources, gathering data, and reading professional literature.

Successful service delivery requires administrative support. You will quickly lose that support if others perceive that you are wasting time and not meeting the goals and objectives of the educational organization. The best way to gain the support you need is to demonstrate that you are engaged in your program and accomplishing what you are expected to do.

Personal Time Management

The school clinician who is the sole speech-language specialist will have much greater responsibility than a person stepping into a job where there is an ongoing program with other school clinicians already involved. In the latter situation, the new clinician fits into the program that has already been set up. In the former, the clinician may be the key planner and organizer. The school clinician must take into consideration two factors in overall time management. The first is the need to plan time on a long-term, yearly, semester, weekly, and daily basis; the second is the need for the clinician to manage his or her time within the larger framework. With respect to both factors, planning is an essential first step. The next important step is setting priorities and sticking with them.

Use of time is a matter of personal preference but time efficiency experts make some useful recommendations. Timesaving techniques are not necessarily new. Most people think they are too busy to implement them or perhaps do not know how to implement them. One technique is to make a list of things to be done today, then to set priorities on that list and follow them. Long "To Do" lists become more manageable if you first prepare a list and work from your list throughout the time period, checking off tasks as they are accomplished. Group together similar tasks. For example, make all phone calls, prepare written reports, administer tests to children, or conduct conferences within given time periods. Delegate tasks to others if support staff is available. Organize materials so they are easily retrieved and accessed.

Keep a file containing alphabetized names and telephone numbers of persons and agencies necessary to the work. A record of incoming and outgoing telephone calls might be recorded in a notebook or computer file, providing a record and synopsis of those conversations.

Another important factor in personal time management is not to let paper work or E-mail messages pile up. One efficiency suggestion often heard is, "Handle each piece of paper (or E-mail message) only once." A period of time each day or each week should be devoted entirely to this task. It is also important to look at habits or practices that may be wasting time, for example, attending too many meetings, spending too much time on phone calls, allowing too many interruptions, or attempting to do multiple tasks in a short time. Most school clinicians would like to add an extra hour to a day now and then or think in terms of an occasional eight-day week. Because time is scarce it must be managed with maximum effectiveness. Experts in time management tell us that selecting the best task from all the possibilities available and then doing it in the best way is more important than doing efficiently whatever job happens to be around.

No matter how one looks at it, we are dealing with that precious and fleeting commodity—time. It is scarce, inelastic, does not have a two-way stretch, cannot be stored or frozen for future use, and cannot be retrieved. It can, however, be managed with effectiveness.

PROFESSIONAL DEVELOPMENT PLANS

Administrators in some school districts require educators, including speech-language pathologists, to submit a Professional Development Plan (or Professional Growth Plan). There are important reasons for such a document. First, it enables administrators and practitioners to mutually agree upon issues such as the workload, responsibilities, and duties. Second, the plan makes a statement of competencies and skills the clinician needs to have to effectively provide services to youngsters. To ensure accountability, the Professional Development Plan often specifies how training for those competencies and skills will be accomplished, including when, where, and who will pay for the training. This is especially necessary when new competencies are needed to serve a child with a particular type of disorder or to implement a new service delivery model. The use of professional development plans demonstrates the necessary and expected link between treatment outcomes for the student, competencies needed by the SLP, program development goals, and accountability.

In 1999, the state of Florida mandated that educators must have a Professional Growth Plan tied to student learning. The plan must be teacher directed and must focus on the state education standards, subject content, teaching methods, technology, assessment and data analysis, classroom management, and school safety (Ehren, 1999). In the plan, staff development efforts are aligned with student and instructional personnel needs. If the school principal identifies a teacher's performance as deficient, then a Professional Development Plan must be constructed. Different needs assessment instruments can be used to determine the skills and competencies the educator must learn including inventories, classroom observations, interviews, self assessments, student achievement data, and the like. Educators may engage in a wide range of learning activities as part of their Professional Growth (or Development) Plan including: study groups, action research, journal reading groups, in-service training programs, self-guided study, peer coaching, workshops, college courses, and independent studies. Figure 4.2 shows excerpts of key elements from the professional development plans of a classroom teacher and a speech-language pathologist (Ribbler, 1999).

QUALITY IMPROVEMENT

Another aspect of the management of school speech-language pathology programs must be taken into consideration. This aspect is *quality*. The profession's commitment to quality began as early as 1959 when the American Speech-Language-Hearing Association established its accreditation program with the founding of the American Boards of Examiners in Speech Pathology and Audiology (ABESPA). Later, the name of the accrediting body was changed to the Professional Services Board (PSB). At the present time, standards and guidelines are established by ASHA for the accreditation of educational programs, certification

FIGURE 4.2   Key Elements of a Professional Growth Plan for a Teacher

Student Outcomes—This is a statement of what the student will be able to do as a result of the teaching or intervention.

- Student will increase reading level by one grade level
- Student's journal will reflect appropriate organization

Staff Outcomes—After completing an assessment of skills and competencies that the staff member needs, a statement is made indicating what the staff member must learn.

- Teacher will understand the impact of students' communication impairments on the learning process.
- SLPs will determine how to assist children with oral reading exercises during speech-language intervention activities.

Student Performance Evaluation—This is the verification that the student's expected achievement gains have been met.

- Student will take turns during informal classroom conversations as measured by observations on a teacher observation checklist.
- Student will use recall of pertinent information as measured by her job coach during a mock interview.

Staff Development Activities—Staff members indicate those learning activities they will do during a given time period.

- Teacher will attend training seminar on assessing reading levels offered by the school system.
- SLP will review the school district's course of study for reading.

Staff Development Impact—This is a presentation of data indicating the activities the staff completed and verifying that they contributed to the student's achievement gains.

- Teacher incorporated comprehension-building strategies into daily instruction.
- SLP learned to recognize different types of reading characteristics and make appropriate referrals.

standards for professionals, and standards for professional services. These standards and guidelines are continually reviewed and, when necessary, changed to meet current needs.

Quality Improvement of Professional Practices

The communication disorders profession is continually evolving. Our understanding of the nature and impact of disorders is improving as are our techniques and approaches to diagnosis and treatment. Consequently, it is important to monitor and review professional practices on an ongoing basis to assess the quality of service delivery and to determine adjustments needed to make improvements.

Speech-language pathologists in various settings have begun to develop and use continuous quality improvement (CQI) approaches to improve performance and service delivery in order to better meet consumer expectations and needs (Frattali, 1991). State and local education agencies, third party payers, government regulators, and accreditation agencies have supported these efforts. School clinicians should establish a comprehensive quality improvement plan which is appropriate to the school setting. The plan should reflect a commitment to ongoing program assessment and continual improvement. It should focus on all activities of the program. It should include a process for monitoring, assessing, and evaluating various aspects of the program's work process and service delivery such as the program *structure* (facility and staff characteristics), the *process* (methods of treatment and care), and the *outcome* (end result) (Frattali, 1990). The plan should also state the specific elements (e.g., criteria, indicators, standards, or protocols) against which aspects of quality are compared. The intent is to use performance-based and outcome-oriented measures to identify areas in service delivery in need of improvement. If deficiencies are noted, then actions or steps must be taken to make improvements.

It is important that staff members work as a team in developing and implementing the quality improvement plan. This means jointly assuming responsibility for identifying problem areas and implementing change. Therefore, to be effective, the plan should incorporate procedures for peer interaction and review. In this way, problems can be discovered and resolved before they interfere with the quality of services. It should encourage collaboration among staff and administration in joint planning efforts to improve areas where problems are noted. The concept of continuous quality improvement crosses all health and education settings. It is a professional and ethical responsibility. Frattali (1990) recommends the following ten steps for designing a quality assurance process:

1. Select a structure, process and/or outcome approach (e.g., *structure* (clinician qualifications, condition of test equipment, adequacy of test environment), *process* (treatment methods, selection of diagnostic measures, appropriateness of goals), *outcome* (client satisfaction, functional communication, goal attainment).
2. Define a target client population (e.g., age group, diagnosis, disorder severity).
3. Choose a method of assessment (e.g., retrospective, concurrent, prospective).
4. Select a data source (e.g., clinical records, interview, observation, survey questions).
5. Select or develop standards against which to measure the quality of care provided.
6. Set the level of compliance.
7. Specify expectations.
8. Collect and analyze data. Evaluate the quality of services.
9. Formulate corrective action if deficiencies are found.
10. Monitor the service until deficiencies are corrected.

Lastohkein, Moon, and Blosser (1992) developed a sample quality improvement plan appropriate for the school setting. As a process for review, they selected the implementation of a collaborative service delivery model within a local school district. Following is an explanation illustrating how each of the ten steps described by Frattali would be applied to evaluate and improve collaborative efforts. (See Table 4.1, Quality Improvement Plan.)

Step One (Assign Responsibility).   The first step in Frattali's model is to determine who will be responsible for monitoring the speech-language pathology program's collaborative

TABLE 4.1 Quality Improvement Plan

ASPECT OF CARE	QUALITY INDICATOR AND THRESHOLD EVALUATION (TE)	DATA SOURCE	COLLECTION METHOD	TIME FRAME
Administrative Issues: Time Constraints and Scheduling Conflicts	Establish regular meeting times. A) Full Team TE: 90% attendance at scheduled meetings	Records of meeting dates & attendance at meetings	100% review; Concurrent	Quarterly
	B) 2–3 Person Collaborative Partner Teams TE: 90% attendance at scheduled meetings	Records of meeting dates & attendance at meetings	100% review; Concurrent	Monthly
Long-Term Plan	All team members (as listed in Step 1) will participate in setting long term goals (e.g., goals to be met in 5 years). TE: 90% actual participation	Staff minutes and reports	100% review; Concurrent	March 2002
	All team members will participate in setting short term goals used to achieve above long term goals. TE: 90% actual participation	Staff minutes and reports	100% review; Concurrent	June 2002
Participants' Responsibilities	Specific responsibilities will be assigned to each team member for completion during a specific period of time (e.g., 3 month increments over a 2 year period). TE: 85% completion of all task assigned	List of assigned tasks, activity reports, summary reports	100% review; Concurrent	Quarterly
Team Members' Expertise and Competence	Team members identify areas of knowledge necessary for collaborative model to be successful (e.g., knowledge of each others' disciplines, knowledge of speech and language development, impact of communication on academic success, school curriculum, process of collaborative model). TE: 85% agreement on topics selected	Topics for discussion identified by team members at staff meetings or via questionnaire	100% review; Concurrent	Ongoing

(continued)

TABLE 4.1 Continued

ASPECT OF CARE	QUALITY INDICATOR AND THRESHOLD EVALUATION (TE)	DATA SOURCE	COLLECTION METHOD	TIME FRAME
	Team members obtain information on specified topics necessary for the collaborative model to be successful. TE: 80% participate in learning activities	Agendas and brochures from inservice programs, continued education credits, academic records, summaries of literature reviews, information received from other professionals	Periodic review; Retrospective	Ongoing
Case Selection Criterion	Accurate identification of language-learning disabled children to be served under the collaborative model. TE: 90% agreement of team members regarding eligibility criteria and case selection	Test scores of students placed in learning disability classes	50% of caseload; Concurrent	Semi-annually

efforts. The following individuals will most likely be involved in collaboration: the speech-language pathologist, audiologist, parents/caregivers, special education director, principal, superintendent, classroom teacher, social worker, school nurse, psychologist, and other professionals in special education.

Any of these professionals could function as the quality improvement coordinator responsible for assigning each individual with specific responsibilities and establishing a formal reporting mechanism. For the purpose of this discussion, the SLP on the team is designated as the quality improvement coordinator.

In order to determine the effectiveness of collaborative efforts and areas where improvement is needed, it was necessary to narrow the focus of the quality improvement plan by delineating the scope of care in the following ways.

Step Two (Delineate Scope of Care).   The second step, delineating the scope of care, determines the who, what, when, where, and how aspects of the QI process. In our school collaborative program, the following guidelines are specified:

- *Who*—Individuals needing services in schools who may be served under a collaborative model include elementary children who have language-learning disabilities with class placement in a program designated for children with learning disabilities.
- *What*—Services provided under a collaborative model include but are not limited to the following: consulting with other professionals, in-servicing the caregivers and other professionals, establishing goals and treatment plans, cotreating, maintaining and exchanging reports, teaching other individuals to implement intervention strategies, counseling caregivers/individuals regarding student's communication disorders and the impact on education.
- *When*—Collaboration should continuously be occurring among professionals. This may take place throughout the school day, at weekly staff meetings, or at IEP meetings.
- *Where*—Collaboration can occur in the students' learning environment, at staff meetings, at IEP meetings, or via other forms of communication exchange.
- *How*—Collaboration can be achieved by communicating face-to-face (e.g., at staff meetings, IEP meetings, in the classroom), via written communication (e.g., exchange written reports, memos, newsletters), or via telephone.

Steps Three Through Six (Identify important aspects of care, identify quality indicators, establish thresholds for evaluation and collect and organize data, respectively).   Important aspects of care must be identified to provide a focus for the quality improvement efforts. Aspects of care required for effective collaboration include: long-term planning, assigning responsibilities, improving participant's competence in specified areas, identifying case selection criteria, and addressing administrative issues such as scheduling conflicts and time constraints. For each aspect of care identified, a quality indicator, threshold evaluation, data source, collection method, and time frame are established. To complete the process, Frattali indicates that the following four steps are necessary.

Step Seven (Evaluation of Care).   If a predetermined threshold is not met, the data should be analyzed to determine if opportunities for improvement exist.

Step Eight (Action Plan to Improve Care).   If improvements can be made, an action plan to improve care should be established. Because this step provides an opportunity to make revisions (i.e., review plan, change indicators, identify new indicators), this is a critical step in the model.

Step Nine (Assess the Actions and Document Improvement).   Procedures should be established for continuous monitoring, evaluation, and documentation of revisions specified in Step Eight.

Step Ten (Communicate Findings).   Finally, a report to communicate findings is distributed to all team members involved.

This chapter has focused on the management and planning aspects of the speech-language pathologist's role. Most students never anticipated that they would find themselves in the position of working on a district-wide planning team or thinking of ways to solve problems such as school violence, curriculum selection, or service delivery models. Yet, this is the nature of the job in today's school environment. The most important benefit for professionals who use this planning process is that the result will be a systematic process for making serious, important decisions that affect children's lives. Hopefully, it will inhibit the urge to just jump in to implement a new service delivery or approach without careful review and advance planning. Without such efforts, new programs are likely to fail or have less impact than is possible.

DISCUSSION QUESTIONS AND PROJECTS

1. Describe the mission of the program in which you are currently participating at the university, a local hospital, or school district. Is the mission in writing in any of the marketing materials?

2. Obtain a copy of the strategic plan for your local school district. Request to meet with administrators who oversee implementation of the strategic plan.

3. What are some yearly program goals you, as the SLP, might develop?

4. What are the advantages of written program plans and goals?

5. What are various ways of quantifying or measuring the success of a speech-language pathology program?

6. Develop a quality improvement plan for initiating a parent or teacher training program in your local school district.

7. Identify three program goals that will improve service delivery to children in your school districts.

8. Write a personal professional development plan that includes statements of how to improve your clinical skills in a particular area.

CHAPTER FIVE

TOOLS OF THE TRADE: SPACE, FACILITIES, EQUIPMENT, AND MATERIALS

It is important that adequate facilities and equipment are available to school speech-language pathologists so that students are appropriately served. Additionally, comprehensive accountability procedures and efficient record keeping practices can assist the clinician in documenting responsible service delivery. Space, facilities, equipment, materials, and reports may be considered the tools of the trade. Just as a carpenter needs good tools, so does the SLP. In this chapter, we will consider those basic needs and how they can be met.

PHYSICAL FACILITIES

There is at the present time a wide variation in the quality of workspace and work environment available to school-based SLPs. The reasons for this are not always clear. Some schools are overcrowded, and the school clinician is in competition with other school personnel for the available space. Many school districts are financially strapped and can't provide the space. School buildings, new as well as old, have not been planned with the speech-language services taken into account. In some cases the school administration is either unaware or apathetic about the issue of adequate working space. On the other hand, increasing numbers of school systems provide excellent facilities.

MINIMAL STANDARDS FOR FACILITIES AND SPACE

Appropriate facilities are necessary to provide an adequate atmosphere for performing responsibilities and implementing program goals. State and federal guidelines stipulate that the workspace for the delivery of speech-language intervention services be suitable and appropriate. The Professional Services Board (PSB) of ASHA has recommended minimal standards of operation for programs offering speech-language and hearing services. As a general guideline, the standards suggest that the physical facility should be barrier-free, in compliance with all applicable safety and health codes, and suitable for the conduct of those activities required to meet the objectives of the program.

In many states, minimal standards for facilities are established by the state board of education. These do not necessarily describe superior facilities, but they do provide a standard below which schools may not go. There is sometimes confusion about this issue, and the school clinician needs to be aware of exactly how the standards are worded. Some local school districts and professional organizations have also developed recommendations for physical facilities and equipment necessary for operating programs effectively. This can be determined by visiting the organization's website, reviewing operational manuals, or interviewing program administrators.

The beginning school clinician needs some sort of yardstick by which to evaluate and define adequate facilities. The checklist presented in Table 5.1 can be used as a reference when observing a school speech-language pathology program, selecting a site for your student teaching experience, or interviewing for a job. If several elements are inadequate, don't be afraid to discuss them with program administrators. While it is not wise to engage in confrontations, questioning an administrator based on sound information and a desire to provide the best services possible can result in improved understanding of the speech-language program and an improved environment for service delivery.

PLEASANT, COMFORTABLE, AND FUNCTIONAL SPACE

In establishing criteria for evaluating physical facilities, the factors of realism and idealism must be taken into account. Although it might be ideal for the speech-language clinician to have a room used exclusively for the speech language intervention program, it may not be realistic. The speech-language pathologist may be following an itinerant schedule. Other educators could utilize that space on the alternate days.

Another factor to consider is the existing facilities (things as they are today) and the potential facilities (things as they might be with some modifications), particularly in setting up a new program. It is important to establish a set of criteria that indicates how the existing facilities could and should be modified in the future. In assessing this aspect of the program the policies of the school must be known. For example, is the supervisor of the speech-language pathology program involved in the planning of new facilities or the modification of existing ones? Will staff members be included in future planning? Are alternative plans considered, such as the use of mobile units, remodeling of areas of buildings, or rental of additional space? What are the budgetary allowances and constraints?

In addition to evaluating the room itself, there are other considerations. First, the room must be accessible to pupils who are disabled and located in an area of the building convenient to others who use it. It should not be too far from the youngest students in the building because these children sometimes have difficulty finding their way to and from the room.

Space is often at a premium in school buildings, and many buildings are old and not well planned for present-day needs. With a little imagination and resourcefulness, however, some simple remodeling and rejuvenation can transform unused space into completely adequate facilities for the school pathologist. In buildings where space is limited, SLPs can work with administrators, teachers, and plant maintenance personnel to identify space that could be partitioned and utilized for the SLP program.

TABLE 5.1 Program Environment Observation Checklist

ROOM

Location

_____ Quiet, private enough to permit confidentiality; free from distractions

_____ Easy to locate; accessible for individuals who are nonambulatory or exhibit severe learning disabilities

_____ Near students' classroom and restrooms

_____ Designated for exclusive use by the SLP program during all times when the speech-language pathologist is on site

_____ Easy access to emergency exits

_____ Secured for storage of equipment and materials

Lighting

_____ Suitable for reading and manipulating pictures and objects

Power

_____ Adequate number of electrical outlets for operating program equipment (e.g., tape recorders, computers, amplification systems, augmentative devices, typewriters, and the like)

Size

_____ Adequate to meet safety standards for the maximum number of persons who will be in the room at a given time

Temperature

_____ Adequate ventilation, heating, and cooling; thermostatic control available

Safety Devices

_____ Audible as well as visual safety devices (fire and smoke alarms)

FURNITURE

Chairs

_____ Appropriate size and number to accommodate clinician, students, and observers; matched to the table size and space

Desk

_____ Office style with lockable drawers

File Cabinet

_____ Lockable

_____ Appropriate size for number and type of files used for the program

Tables

_____ Appropriate height and number to accommodate a broad range of students' sizes and ages

_____ Adequate support for equipment (typewriters, computers, and the like)

Shelves

_____ Adequate number and structure for storage of books and therapy materials

ASSESSMENT AND INSTRUCTION MATERIALS

_____ Age appropriate

_____ All parts and pieces available and in working order

_____ Sanitary and in good condition

_____ Appropriate mix of standardized and non-standardized instruments

EQUIPMENT AND MATERIALS

Audiometers

_____ Appropriate for testing pure-tones and immittance

_____ Properly calibrated

(continued)

TABLE 5.1   Continued

Amplification Devices

_____   Appropriate to meet individual and group needs

Augmentative Communication Systems

_____   Appropriate for various age and functional communication levels

Computers

_____   Available according to need

_____   Suitable for word processing, and data storage

_____   Appropriate software for program management and intervention

_____   Accessories necessary to operate uniquely designed programs

Expendable materials

_____   Conveniently located

_____   Easily accessed

Mirror

_____   Appropriate size for viewing faces and bodies

_____   Constructed of safety glass

Tape Recorder

_____   Designated for exclusive use by the speech-language program

_____   Ample supply of tapes

Telecommunications display device

_____   Available if needed to meet the needs of students who are hearing impaired

Telephone

_____   Available when needed;

_____   Located in a private area where confidentiality can be maintained

Typewriter

_____   Available and easily accessed

Video recording and viewing equipment

_____   Available and easily accessed

If a new building a being contemplated, the speech-language clinician will need to be in on the planning stages to ensure adequate space allotment. School architects are not always well informed about the space and facility needs of the program, and the school pathologist can be of invaluable assistance in providing needed information.

The policies of the school with regard to space must also be known when planning physical facilities. For example, the school pathologist should know how space is assigned in a building and whether or not staff members are consulted when the assignments are made. The school pathologist should also know whether or not there are provisions for modifying the room. If space is to be shared, staff members should know the procedures for obtaining input from all the persons sharing the room.

Most people feel better and do better in surroundings that are attractive, comfortable, and pleasant. Children are no exception. Color, adequate lighting, and comfortable furniture are conducive to good results in therapy. A child who is seated on a chair that is too big is going to be very uncomfortable. In a short time the child will begin to squirm and wriggle and will be unable to focus on whatever the clinician is presenting. The child may seem like a discipline problem to the unseeing clinician, but in reality the child may simply be attempting to find a comfortable position.

One of the most attractive therapy rooms I have seen was in an old school building in a rural area. The whole building sparkled with cleanliness—wooden floors were polished, walls were painted in soft colors, and furniture was in good repair and arranged harmoniously. The therapy room was pleasant, with a carpeted floor and colorful draperies. A bulletin board served both a useful and decorative purpose. The obvious pride in the surroundings was reflected by the way that the children treated the therapy room and its furnishings. The clinician reported that everyone in the school, including the custodian, the principal, the teachers, and the children were proud of their attractive building and worked to keep it that way.

SPACE ALLOCATIONS

The space allocations in schools have been improving in recent years, perhaps because SLPs now spend more time in each school and more schools have full time or nearly full-time speech-language intervention programs. Also, school administrators are becoming more aware of the importance of speech-language pathology programs, and the needs of the programs are receiving more attention. Nonetheless, it is of vital importance that the school SLP assumes the responsibility of making the needs of the program known to the principal, director of special services, and superintendent. The school pathologist must be assertive and forthright in this endeavor. The student with a hearing loss, language-learning disability, fluency problem, voice disorder, or phonological problem cannot benefit from therapy in a room where there are constant interruptions, exposure to illnesses, noise from band practice, or a storage room that is inadequately lighted, ventilated, and heated or cooled.

Overcrowded schools and substandard space within school buildings have prompted some pathologists to look elsewhere for the solution to the problem. Mobile units and stationary trailers located on the school grounds have provided solutions for many clinicians. There may be a number of advantages in using mobile units. They contain everything necessary for the program, thus eliminating gathering up and storing items every day. Equipment will not be broken when it remains stationary and doesn't have to be transported in the trunk of a car. Mobile units provide quiet facilities for testing. They may also represent a savings in tax dollars in comparison to the cost of building permanent facilities.

SPECIAL CONSIDERATIONS
FOR SPECIAL POPULATIONS

Careful thought and planning should go into designing, organizing and decorating your therapy room. Keep your students' special needs, ages, learning capabilities, and interest levels in mind. Decor should be attractive and motivating. Care should be taken to avoid arranging the room in a way that is distracting or condescending to students' ages or intelligence. Certain groups require special considerations.

Infants, Toddlers, and Preschoolers.   After Public Law 99-457 was enacted, school districts became responsible for providing services to a younger group of children than they had accommodated previously. Many school buildings are not designed for such a young group. Room location, furniture size, and equipment selection is of utmost importance. The environment must be bright and stimulating. Children in this age group do not learn by sitting quietly at a table and taking turns talking. Learning quite often takes place on the floor or while the child is in motion during play. Therefore, the atmosphere and materials should invite manipulation, creativity, movement, and interaction. Toys are appropriate, especially if they can be used to encourage investigation, experimentation, imitation, and questioning. Because of the way in which children play with toys, they will need to be cleansed frequently and maintained in proper working order.

Adolescents.   Obviously, facilities for intermediate and high school students will be different from those for elementary and preschool students. The size and type of furniture as well as the arrangement of the classroom and decorations should facilitate group discussions and lessons. The typical classroom or rows of desks is not conducive to the type of learning that takes place in a typical situation. The use of carrels and learning centers provides the opportunity for independent work. Activity centers related to specific learning skills could incorporate vocabulary cards, work sheets, and learning games. Learning centers might include tape recorders, objects that can be manipulated, and computers. A library center might have reading materials, books used for book reports, story wheels, and writing materials. A career education center might contain materials related to various occupations, job application requirements, and forms.

Children with Severe and Multiple Impairments.   There is likely to be wide variation in skill levels, capabilities, mobility, sizes, and intervention needs for children with severe and multiple impairments. Consequently, facilities for this group of children need to be designed so that easy adaptation is permitted throughout the day. Furniture should be of sturdy construction, adjustable, and easily moved to meet positioning requirements. Treatment materials should be selected to permit teaching important concepts and skills while still being motivating. Augmentative and alternative communication systems are valuable assets to children whose communication skills are severely restricted.

Some children with severe and multiple impairments become easily distracted by auditory or visual stimuli. Children with sensory problems, brain dysfunction, or developmental delays may have difficulty functioning in a room that is too stimulating or distracting because of garish colors or busy patterns. To accommodate these youngsters' needs while still providing a bright, stimulating environment for other children on the caseload, the clinician may wish to arrange one section of the therapy room in such a way that all potentially distracting materials are out of the child's range of vision.

FACILITIES FOR OBSERVATION

The school clinician may want to invite parents, educators, and school administrators to observe diagnostic and intervention services. This would provide opportunities for involving valuable members of the child's world in the therapy program, teaching others about the profession, and promoting collaboration.

One way to facilitate observation is to invite persons to join you during the session. If the presence of others would distract the students, one-way mirrors and intercom systems can be used to enable observation without interruption. Through observational experiences such as these, parents and teachers can learn important speech and language stimulation and correction techniques. Team members such as school psychologists can observe the child's communication skills under optimum conditions to obtain valuable diagnostic information. Administrators can learn about the scope and services of the speech-language program.

Often school clinicians hear the comment from others, "But what do you actually do in a therapy session?" Having people observe would take some of the mystery out of therapy and would make vividly clear the role they can play in the therapy process in the home or classroom. This would ultimately help the child generalize what he or she has learned. Observers will be able to follow the flow of the session better if they are provided with a brief explanation of the goals of the session and the intent of activities they are about to observe. One effective method is to write those goals on a blackboard or sheet of paper.

DEMONSTRATION CENTERS

Some large school districts and regional resource centers house demonstration centers where parents, students, and teachers may go to learn about communication devices including assistive listening devices and alternative/augmentative communication systems. By displaying devices, potential users are able to gain an understanding of assistive technology that is available. They can learn about how the technology works or how the device might help in adapting the classroom environment. In addition, visitors can gain a sense of the possibilities that are available for enhancing the communication experience. Children with hearing impairments can be exposed to alerting, listening, and telephone devices. Youngsters with limited verbal skills can sample various types of voice synthesizers and response options.

EQUIPMENT AND MATERIALS

In addition to the therapy room and its furnishings, several types of equipment, materials, and supplies are needed for a successful program. Equipment and materials should be appropriately selected to meet the needs of the students and types of disorders being served. Appropriate schedules of maintenance and calibration should be followed to ensure that equipment remains in proper working order.

Equipment is an item that is not expendable; retains its original shape, appearance, and use; usually costs a substantial amount of money; and is more feasible to repair than to replace when damaged or worn out. Materials and supplies, on the other hand, are considered expendable. They are used up, usually inexpensive, and are more feasible to replace than to repair when damaged or worn out.

INTEGRATING TECHNOLOGY INTO ALL ASPECTS
OF THE PROGRAM

The growing use of the computer in education, business, and everyday life has become a reality on the American scene. School SLPs who use computers have discovered that they are able to save time, conserve energy, increase benefits to students, and cut down on that greatest of all time thieves: paperwork. School clinicians are finding that computers can be invaluable tools for managing program information and as an integral adjunct to intervention. SLPs use computers to record students' screening and test results, track case management information; develop and catalog therapy materials; maintain therapy logs; and compile statistical data for accountability to school administrators, boards of education and state departments of education.

Much of the SLP's workload involves paperwork and reporting tasks. Computers can provide a number of advantages by helping the SLP save time, conserve energy, and increase benefits to clients. Software programs that permit word processing, data management, and spreadsheet functions enable SLPs to communicate with other professionals, store and manage important information, and prepare reports with efficiency.

Data can be stored for administrative and research purposes. An analysis of data can help identify trends such as increases in the caseload size, disorder type, or a population shift within the school district. Accurate caseload figures, demographic figures, and disorder and severity data can promote more efficient use of school personnel and program development. Required reports can be compiled more quickly, efficiently, and accurately. Computerization now permits clinicians to prepare reports which are comprehensive, easier to read, and more professional in appearance. In addition, the time saved can be used for an extension of direct therapy time.

A centralized information management system can store a large number of data. Test results, pertinent medical information, referral sources, treatment outcome data, and follow-up information unique to each student can be added at any time. Sorting options for producing printed reports are numerous. For example, a report that alphabetically lists student enrollment data by grade and room number for a given school can be printed for the school principal. Results may also be sorted according to those students enrolled in a special education program or as a compilation of students with a particular type of disorder. This flexibility for storage and maintenance of records eliminates time-consuming cross-checking tasks and provides accurate records for studying screening, testing, and intervention data.

Software programs have been developed that can save clinicians considerable time and effort in dealing with the deluge of paperwork involved in developing Individualized Education Programs. Computers can be used in the generation of IEPs and for documenting completion of steps necessary for compliance with due process. The memory capacity of the computer allows storage of a virtually unlimited number of items in the goal and objective bank. In addition, items may be added to the bank for students who are not adequately described by existing statements or whose team members request additional objectives.

The stumbling blocks to computer use in the schools include lack of familiarity with computers, financial restraints, fear of learning how to use a computer system, and a dearth of speech-language professionals who understand its potential applications. Computers may be purchased by a school system for use by the speech-language pathology staff. Before purchasing a computer system and software programs, identify your needs and the applications you plan to use. Take into account the types of service delivery model employed (pull-out, collaborative, consultative, resource room, or self-contained program).

There are many issues to be decided prior to investing in a computer system. Prior to spending valuable funds to purchase a computer, clinicians should determine how they plan to use it. Will it be used for program management and administration or for intervention? Who will be the primary user—the speech-language pathologist, a staff person, an assistant, or the students? What are the skill levels of the users? Will additional training be necessary? Where will the computer be located? Who will have access? Will security measures be necessary to protect data and equipment? Will the computer be networked with others to permit exchange of information and integration of school district records and information?

The school SLP contemplating the purchase of computer software is faced with a bewildering array of information and material. Many professionals review currently available computer software and accessories. Care should be taken before spending limited school funds on computers and software. They should offer broad use and flexibility.

TECHNOLOGY IN SERVICE DELIVERY

In the past, speech-language pathologists' equipment use was limited to audiometers, acoustic immittance instruments, tape recorders, and simple amplification devices. They used word processors only for preparing reports or organizing data. Many clinicians are now routinely integrating more advanced technology into their programs They are also recommending the incorporation of technology into the classroom setting to improve conditions for communication exchanges within that environment. It is not unusual to see students with communication disorders wearing assistive listening devices or the teacher speaking through a microphone. Children can be observed sitting at computers practicing language exercises or using a voice synthesizer to express their needs. Today's clinicians are using technology to manage program information as well as to develop their students' communication skills.

Computer technology presents a window of opportunity for people with disabilities. If software is selected properly, it can be used to facilitate drill practice, encourage transfer and generalization of learned skills, and permit individualized practice and self-correction. For example, treatment for students who are severely impaired can be enhanced through computer programs that use interactive learning and synthesized speech. The computer is also valuable to students as a means of access to information and visually oriented training and instruction. Computers won't replace competent clinicians but the use of computers by SLPs and audiologists in the schools can make a positive difference in the delivery of services to students with communication impairments.

AUGMENTATIVE AND ALTERNATIVE
COMMUNICATION SYSTEMS

Perhaps the most exciting result of advanced technology is the increased opportunity for persons with severe impairments to communicate with others in their world. Speech-language pathologists are teaching persons with disorders such as dysarthria, verbal apraxia, aphasia, glossectomy, dysphonia, mental retardation, autism, brain injury, tracheostomy, and deafness to interact with their families, peers, and teachers via augmented and assisted-communication systems (Silverman, 1989). Augumentative communication refers to communication systems that supplement speech. This can be accomplished through common techniques such as writing, gestures, and pictures or via more specialized techniques including electronic aids (Vanderheiden and Yoder, 1986).

Experts in augmentative communication believe that trying to "fix" the speech of a person with a severe motor disorder so that it is intelligible results in a sense of failure for the student as well as the SLP. One cannot fix a severely impaired neurological system, but you can offer the student alternative modes of communication. Even very young children become frustrated when they are unable to communicate. Early exposure to augmentative communication systems helps them understand how to communicate.

Today's clinician needs to know how to work with students' families and professionals representing a broad range of educational, medical, and technological disciplines to help select augmentative and alternative communication systems which will be optimally suited to the student's needs (Silverman, 1989; Yorkston & Karlan, 1986). Vanderheiden and Lloyd (1986) describe several dimensions professionals can use to determine the usefulness or advantages of particular augmentative communication system components for meeting functional communication requirements. They group these dimensions into three broad categories that include: functionality/ability to meet needs; availability/usability; and acceptability/compatibility with the environment.

When selecting and implementing augmentative and alternative communication systems, it is necessary to match the student's physical and cognitive skills with the devices that are to be used. This is not an easy goal to accomplish. Many experts who confront such decisions on a frequent basis generally base their selection on the knowledge they have about devices and the knowledge they gain about the student through comprehensive assessment. The student's potential ability to use the device to communicate should be the driving issue. Other aspects to consider when making a selection include: ease of use, growth potential, keyboard layout, rate of communication output, voice output, visual output, auditory output, structure for positioning and mobility, adaptability for rapidly changing needs, client response capabilities, and funding resources.

Experts in the field of alternative and augmentative communication believe that AAC-based intervention should be implemented as early as possible to help students effectively participate in their home and school activities. The benefit of increased understanding of interactive and pragmatic communication can make a great difference in the student's ultimate success in home, school, community, and work. Children must be able to proceed at their own pace. The clinician must be sensitive to frustrations and make the learning experience fun and rewarding.

Clinicians who are interested in learning more about alternative and augmentative communication intervention would benefit participating in ASHA's Special Interest Division 12: Augmentative and Alternative Communication. The manufacturers of augmentative and alternative communication products participate in a national not-for-profit organization, The Communication Aid Manufacturers Association (CAMA) in Evanston, IL. They conduct educational outreach projects such as workshops and in-service training. In addition, they provide helpful guidelines and suggestions to SLPs who provide AAC intervention. Efforts such as these help clinicians stay abreast of rapidly changing technologies.

After selecting the device, the clinician is then involved in instructing the student and incorporating the communication system into classroom and social communication activities. The school clinician interested in incorporating augmentative and alternative systems into the speech-language program is faced with an important decision-making task. There is great variability in capability and complexity in the devices available on the market. Cost can be high. Sometimes, it is necessary to help the student's family seek financial assistance. The Prentke Romich Company (a company that develops, manufactures, and distributes augmentative communication systems) suggests that there are numerous sources that can be sought for funding the purchase of devices including:

- insurance companies and Medicaid programs
- vocational rehabilitation programs
- school system equipment funds
- private corporations
- trust funds
- service clubs
- fundraising agencies
- organizations which grant wishes to people with specific disabilities

Training must be provided for teachers of students who use augmentative and alternative communication systems. Student success will be greater if teachers learn to integrate educational and functional activities with AAC intervention. This will help to merge the SLP and classroom goals. Training is most effective if the SLP and teacher attend training sessions jointly. This will facilitate a team approach encouraging them to collaborate in the selection and structuring of activities. Planning must first begin with identification of the students' needs and competencies. Teachers and others who engage in communication interactions with the student must learn to prompt student use of the communication device and to engage in conversation with the student.

As technology development continues to progress, it is essential that school-based SLPs gain the expertise they need to match students with the appropriate devices so they can develop communicative competence. One device cannot possibly meet the needs of the broad range of students in a school district. There are numerous device options that should be considered such as the type of voice output and accessories such as optical pointers. E-mail continues to offer students with severe disabilities opportunities to connect with others in their school, community, or the world at large. Most regional resource centers make augmentative communication devices available on loan to parents. They also offer regional training workshops and in-service programs.

INTERVENTION MATERIALS

During recent years, there has been an increase in commercial materials. Some of them are excellent and some of them are not useful for the purposes they claim to accomplish. On the other hand, there are many excellent homemade materials. These have the advantage of being inexpensive, and because many of them are designed for a specific purpose, they are useful. Without decrying the use of materials, homemade or commercial, the clinician would do well to evaluate them from another point of view. Do they accomplish a goal in therapy for the child, or do they serve as a prop or a "security blanket" for the clinician? This letter from a staff member at Shady Trails, a camp for children with communication disabilities, illustrates the point:

> Before I went to Shady Trails Speech Improvement Camp in Michigan they sent me a list of things to bring along. I didn't notice any mention of therapy materials. Should I take some along? I had been working as a school clinician and had therapy materials of my own. What should I do? Well, if they didn't tell me to bring any, perhaps they furnished staff with them after you got there. When I got to camp no materials in sight! What was I expected to do for therapy! I panicked.
>
> Within a very short time we were plunged into the camp program and things moved along at a fast clip. Suddenly, in the middle of the summer, I realized I had been doing therapy for several weeks and hadn't even missed my therapy materials. How could this be? In analyzing the situation I realized we had been using the life experience situations at camp, the activities, the surroundings, the educational programs and the other people in the camp as our "materials." The therapy grew naturally out of the environment.

EDUCATIONAL MATERIALS

We often overlook the most obvious source of materials—the school itself. If therapy in the schools is to be meaningful to the child it must be a part of the school program. The school clinician needs to know what is going on at various grade levels in the way of instruction and should then tie the therapy to the classroom activities. Looking at the books children read, talking with the teacher about the instructional program, becoming familiar with the school curriculum, and looking around the classroom itself will help the school clinician become more familiar with classroom instruction and will suggest ideas for intervention techniques and motivational devices. School districts develop curriculum guides that outline the objectives of the curriculum and activities that should be a part of the educational program. See Appendix B for a representative curriculum for Language Arts.

In most states there are regional resource centers that provide local school districts with resources designed to improve the quality of instruction for children with disabilities. Instructional and diagnostic materials are available on a loan basis to school clinicians. The instructional resource centers provide other services with which the school clinician will want to become familiar. Visiting the resource center gives the clinician an opportunity to examine a large number of tests, materials, and books before making a decision on which ones to purchase for the school. Personnel at the resource centers are also helpful in discussing the use of various items of material and equipment.

Regional, state, and national meetings of speech-language pathologists usually include displays by commercial companies of equipment, materials, and books. Company representatives provide demonstrations of equipment. This is also a good opportunity to get on the mailing lists of commercial companies. The school clinician may want to maintain a file of company brochures and current prices.

INTEGRATING MULTIMEDIA INTO TREATMENT

There are many multimedia computer systems and CD-ROM technology programs that feature language learning activities. These offer fun and effective intervention tools for children. Creative speech-language pathologists may want to consider incorporating software for music, artwork, and other creative forms into treatment sessions. Youngsters can progress at a rate comparable to what they achieved in traditional therapy if properly administered by qualified clinicians. The graphics, sound, text, and animation capabilities incorporated into computer programs may help to keep students focused on activities. Remember, however, the computer is an intervention tool. To be effective, a qualified professional must develop the goals and plans for use.

Computer programs can be located in catalogs from publishers of clinical materials. In addition, some commercial software programs that involve language use can be adapted for speech-language therapy. Care and attention should be given to the selection of computer-based products. As with other clinical materials, the programs should be relevant for the students' academic curriculum and communication needs. The cautious clinician will review articles in the professional literature to determine the potential efficacy of using various devices including software programs.

SURFING THE NET

The World Wide Web (WWW) offers students and practitioners many avenues for exploration. Speech-language pathologists can find information about a wide range of topics such as treatment protocols for specific disorders or interesting resource materials to suggest to parents by accessing the many commercial and free websites offered by businesses and organizations. Judith Maginnis Kuster (2000) has been a leading influence in the discipline by cataloging hundreds of the best speech-language pathology websites and links <http://www.mankato.msus.edu/dept/comdis/kuster2/welcome.html>. The site features a communication disorders library, a speech and language disorders section, an annotated bibliography of references, global links, an extensive list of interactive discussion forums, guidelines for designing and presenting research and much more. ASHA's website is also a good launching pad for professionals and consumers who want to investigate communication disorders.

ASSISTIVE LISTENING DEVICES

Students' success in the classroom and in therapy is often limited by their inability to monitor their own speech or to hear, attend to, and discriminate others' speech during conversations and classroom discussions (Flexer, 1999). Audiologists and speech-language pathologists are finding assistive listening devices (ALDs) to be very useful tools for working with students who have hearing impairments as well as students with other types of communication and learning impairments (Flexer, 1989). Assistive listening devices include various products that provide solutions to problems created by noise, distance from the speaker, or room reverberation or echo. These problems cannot be solved with hearing aids alone (Berg, 1987 and

Leavitt, 1987). ALDs offer effective means for sound amplification by improving the intelligibility of the speech signal by enhancing the signal-to-noise ratio (Flexer, 1992, 1991).

Two types of devices, personal FM units and hardwire assistive listening devices (ALDs), can be beneficial to individual children in the therapy situation or groups of children in the class-room setting (Flexer, 1989). To use these units, the teacher/clinician wears a microphone transmitter and the student wears a receiver unit equipped with insert earphones. The cost and design of this equipment varies, but inexpensive portable devices can be assembled without much difficulty (Sudler and Flexer, 1986). The amount of amplification needed depends on a number of factors and individual needs for amplification vary greatly. There is some risk of damaging a child's auditory system if an inappropriate sound level is used. Therefore, the advice of an educational audiologist familiar with the performance potential and benefits of various types of assistive listening devices should be sought when recommending units for particular children or classroom situations.

EVALUATION OF MATERIALS

At the present time there are numerous speech and language assessment and intervention products on the market. Unfortunately many of them have not been field tested on a variety of populations. The clinician that purchases them may have no information concerning their effectiveness, applicability, validity, or reliability. Clinicians should not purchase communication intervention products unless the information necessary to evaluate their usefulness is available from the company publishing them. New tests, in particular, should be evaluated carefully before they are purchased. Advertising brochures should not be the only criterion for selection, and the clinician should seek the pertinent information by querying the publishing company directly. Some school districts that are experiencing financial constraints limit the funds that can be spent on materials. Publishers will often provide free use of materials if SLPs offer to conduct and report field test data.

Prior to purchasing programs, tests, or equipment, clinicians should request to use the materials on a trial basis. This provides opportunity for clearly determining the applicability to specific populations, the capability for meeting your program objectives, and to predict the durability, frequency of use, and maintenance requirements.

Shared Purchasing of Equipment.   Another way to become familiar with materials and equipment is to discuss them with other clinicians in the area or with university staff members, if there is a university training program nearby. School clinicians in a geographical area may want to consider joint purchase of expensive pieces of equipment that could be shared. Or one school district may purchase one item which could be loaned to a neighboring district, while that district may purchase another item with the idea of setting up a reciprocal loan system. Time sharing policies and insurance considerations would have to be worked out in advance.

Portability.   The portability of materials should also be taken into consideration. The clinician on an itinerant schedule should keep in mind the bulk and the weight of the materials. Lugging materials and equipment in and out of buildings, not to mention up and down long flights of stairs, several times a day requires the stamina of a packhorse and has caused more than one school clinician to trim down the amount of materials used.

ORGANIZING MATERIALS
AND INTERVENTION ACTIVITIES

Usually students enrolled in clinical classes start to collect their own materials and ideas. Many students have found it useful to start files of various intervention and motivational ideas. If the file is well organized it can be expanded and ideas can be added for years to come. The file should be organized in such a way that material can be easily retrieved and replaced after sessions or at the end of the day. It is suggested that information be consistently placed in uniform size files or on uniform size file cards.

Some students have found it convenient to color code the file, whereas others have preferred to alphabetize the information under topical headings. Computers have offered a very dynamic way of producing, storing, and organizing activities for therapy.

Here are some suggestions for the ingredients of a file for treatment materials and motivational ideas:

- Various ways to teach a child to produce a consonant or a vowel
- Lists of words containing specific phonemes in different positions within words
- Words taken from the student's spelling, reading, mathematics and science books
- Sentences loaded with specific sounds
- Ideas for auditory discrimination and bombardment
- Poems, riddles, finger plays, and stories
- Flannel board ideas
- Barrier games
- Worksheets for home practice
- Exercises for tongue and lip mobility
- Unit topics (Native Americans, holidays, baseball, good nutrition)
- Role playing ideas
- Experiential activities for parents to try at home
- Progress sheets or charting methods
- Bulletin board ideas (these could be related to seasons or holidays or be of general interest)
- Word lists and pictures related to holidays
- Puppets for use in therapy and diagnostics
- Laminated picture cards illustrating nouns or verbs
- Lists of records and books for children
- Lists of suggestions for mentoring parents and teachers
- Movement activities
- Ideas for speech development and speech-improvement lessons in the classroom
- Teacher study guides and workbooks
- Careers and vocational information

The file can serve a number of useful purposes: It can be an inventory of available materials and publications; it can aid in lesson planning; and the materials can be easily removed from the file and used during the sessions. In addition, it can serve as an aid when consulting with classroom teachers in speech and language development and improvement, and serve as a source of ideas when working with parents. Plus, it is concise, easy to construct, convenient to use, and inexpensive.

EXPENDABLE MATERIALS

Supplies, such as paper, crayons, chalk, and some materials that can be used only one time, are usually supplied by the school; however, it does not necessarily follow that the school clinician has access to an unlimited supply. These items may be rationed or budgeted to the clinician on a yearly or semester basis. The clinician should be aware of the school's policy with regard to supplies. It should also be pointed out that because clinicians may function in several different schools within the same system, each school may have its own policy in regard to the availability of supplies.

Sometimes budget allowances are made on the basis of pupil enrollment. Both money and supplies may be determined in accordance with the total number of children enrolled or the number enrolled at any given time. Because budgets must be made out in advance, the figures may depend on last year's enrollment or on the estimated enrollment for the next year.

BUDGETING FOR MATERIALS, EQUIPMENT, AND SUPPLIES

Schools purchase materials, supplies, and equipment. In some schools the clinician is given a fixed sum of money each year to spend for these items. In considering the purchase of equipment, it should be kept in mind that although the initial expenditure may be great, the equipment may not have to be replaced for many years. There is, however, the matter of repair, maintenance, and general upkeep to be considered. For example, an audiometer needs yearly calibration. This should be taken into account before the purchase of the audiometer and discussed with the company representative.

Commercial therapy materials are subject to wear and tear if they are used frequently and may have to be budgeted for periodically. Considerations in the purchase of therapy materials might be whether or not they can be adapted for a variety of uses and occasions and whether or not they serve the purpose for which they are being purchased. They must be appropriate to the age, maturity, and interest of children.

Another matter to be considered is insurance on audiometers, computers, assistive devices, augmentative systems, and other items of electronic equipment—a figure that should be in the budget. Also, if equipment is to be leased, the rental costs will have to be included in the budget. When budgeting for a program, don't forget to account for ongoing material needs such as office supplies (disks, paper, pens, paper clips, and the like).

Budgeting for Professional Materials and Activities. Professional books may also be included as part of the school clinician's equipment and therefore would be justifiable budget items. The clinician may want to add to his or her own library of professional books, and these, of course, would not be a part of the school budget. The same is true for dues for professional organizations.

Budgeting for Travel.   Some school systems allow travel money and expenses for personnel who attend professional meetings. It is wise for the new clinician to check the policy regarding this matter. If a clinician must travel between schools as part of the job, a travel allowance is available. Some school clinicians are paid a flat amount for a specified period of time, whereas others receive reimbursement on a per-mile basis. Some school systems make up for this difference by paying the clinician a higher salary than the person whose job does not entail travel between schools during the working day (for example, the classroom teacher).

INVENTORY RECORDS

It is a good idea to maintain a systematic record or inventory of materials and equipment purchased for the program. This will facilitate sharing materials between several clinicians, locating articles when needed, and replacing articles should they become misplaced or damaged. The inventory record should include the name of the article, the manufacturer's name, address and phone number, the date purchased, the cost, serial numbers if applicable, the intended use, the storage location, and dates equipment was repaired or calibrated. Computerized data management systems often include software programs which can be used for developing inventory records and reports. The storage of equipment during the months when school is not in session, or equipment is not in use, is a matter to be determined by the SLP and the administration.

DISCUSSION QUESTIONS AND PROJECTS

1. Visit several school speech-language programs and rate their facilities using the Program Environment Observation Checklist in Table 5.1.

2. Are mobile units used in your state? What are their advantages and disadvantages? Under what conditions would you use one?

3. You are the school clinician. The principal has assigned you to a small former storage room with no windows but a convenient location. You are not satisfied with the room. Would you try to have another room assigned or would you modify the assigned room? Outline the steps you would follow, using either alternative.

4. Collect five advertisements from publishing companies of speech-language assessment and intervention materials and equipment. They can be brochures or advertisements in professional journals. Determine the strengths and weaknesses of the materials.

5. Start an activity file. Justify the method you have chosen to organize it.

6. Interview an SLP to find out how he or she budgets for equipment and materials and how the materials are procured through the school system. How are maintenance and insurance handled?

7. Draw a design plan for your ideal therapy room (a) for an elementary school and (b) for a high school.

8. Start a collection of record and report forms used in the schools. How would you organize report forms for a school system?

9. Technological assistance is needed to select appropriate ALDs and augmentative communication devices for intervention. Make a list of ten questions you might ask of persons who have technological expertise with these devices.

CHAPTER SIX

DOCUMENTATION AND ACCOUNTABILITY

The American public is demanding that school systems be accountable for the educational results of their students. This has come about because there are a number of problems in the schools that are troubling to the public. Problems that are most distressing with regard to students with disabilities are differential educational opportunities based on type of problem and location; high drop out rates; low graduation rates; high unemployment rates; and limited community integration of adults with disability (Blackstone, 1995). Research on effective schools and effective teaching has repeatedly proved that student achievement is not at the expected level. In addition, teachers are not adequately prepared for the challenges they face in the classroom. Leading education experts claim that models of special education programs that pull children away from the regular education classroom tend to compound problems and reduce the potential for student success.

Findings such as these have led to increased urgency for accountability and ways to determine student outcomes. Schools have initiated various options for documenting the performance of students with disabilities. Options include diplomas, certificates of attendance, or certificates of competency. Changes in methods of assessing performance have also evolved to include the use of performance-based assessments such as portfolios. Comprehensive accountability procedures and efficient record keeping practices can assist the clinician in documenting responsible service delivery.

The scope of practice and responsibilities of speech-language pathologists continue to broaden and change. In addition to changes in the educational world, speech-language pathologists are now providing more invasive, hands on procedures than in the past. This places clinicians at a greater risk of doing physical harm to students and clients in other types of settings. The chances are now greater that a practitioner may face or be involved in a lawsuit. Standards for our profession are not yet clearly defined. Problems can be decreased or avoided when SLPs document services properly.

DOCUMENTING TREATMENT EFFECTIVENESS

School-based SLPs continue to seek valid instruments that can be used for describing students' communication skills and measuring change in communication status following treatment in a school-based treatment program. A uniform methodology is needed to describe the populations served, report intervention models used, measure treatment outcomes and benefit, and ultimately make caseload and treatment decisions that are cost-effective.

Increasingly SLPs are faced with complex problems in the current school environment. These include: high caseloads; diverse student needs; inconsistent scheduling patterns among clinicians; financial constraints; limited personnel; and increasing demands for accountability; efficiency, and cost effectiveness. Recent trends in special education and speech-language pathology service delivery have encouraged greater consistency and accountability for service delivery decisions. Practitioners are seeking better methods of describing the populations they serve, selecting service delivery models for intervention, and determining the effectiveness of treatment.

THE RATIONALE FOR BETTER RECORD-KEEPING PROCEDURES

Typically, speech-language pathologists across the country do not have access to data collection instruments that promote or permit the following practices:

- Consistent practices across the entire school district identifying delivery practices among district SLPs
- Consistent descriptions of students' communication status at the time of admission and discharge
- Consistent documentation of treatment interventions provided
- Documentation of educators' perceptions of students' functional communication skills based on classroom performance
- Results of treatment (outcomes)
- Documentation and comparison of clinical decision making and service

Consequently, SLPs continue to express concerns about caseload management problems that occur due to inconsistent patterns of:

- Referring children for SLP services
- Describing communication skills and problems
- Communicating with one another meaningfully about students
- Determining priorities for treatment
- Selecting appropriate models for service delivery
- Determining progress in treatment
- Measuring the effect of communication disability on school performance
- Measuring and comparing treatment effectiveness of various intervention models
- Making decisions regarding referral for additional services or dismissal

This type of information has broad implications beyond the speech-language pathology program. The diversity of the population and number of students with communication disorders creates a number of service delivery challenges for SLPs and educators. SLPs struggle to accurately identify students who are most in need of speech-language pathology services. They try to determine the effect of students' communication disabilities on school performance and participation in other home and community activities. They strive to establish priorities for treatment and to select appropriate service delivery models to accomplish goals. They seek methods for documenting progress and effectiveness. In addition, SLPs want to provide quality services to students with diverse needs in spite of complex barriers such as financial constraints, limited personnel, increasing demands for accountability, efficiency, and cost effectiveness.

Records and Record Keeping

There are good reasons for maintaining a comprehensive record and report system on the language and speech program. Although it has always been done by clinicians, the reasons today are somewhat more compelling and the goals more inclusive.

Federal and state laws place tremendous emphasis on accountability in the school system. Accountability has made it urgent that special services in the schools develop a method of reliably and accurately reporting data on children with disabilities. Historically, the school clinician has maintained written records for many reasons:

- To inform others about the program
- To keep track of the services provided
- To provide continuity both to the program and to the child's progress in therapy
- To serve as a basis for research
- To coordinate the child's therapy with the child's school program
- To serve as a basis for program needs and development

These reasons remain valid; however, there are additional reasons why an accounting system is needed today. There are ethical, legal, and fiscal reasons. Parents occasionally question the nature and quality of the educational program their child is receiving. Their concerns may include special service programs such as speech and language intervention. As a result, they may request detailed information about the goals of therapy and techniques used. On rare occasions, there may be enough disagreement with placement decisions and the education professional's practices to pursue legal recourse in order to implement changes.

Several court decisions in the past few decades have ruled in favor of the parents' concerns about the school's failure to provide appropriate education or services. In these cases, the school districts have incurred large financial obligations. This can be financially detrimental to a school district and professionally damaging to the professional. The clinician that keeps detailed records of diagnostic findings, treatment procedures, and outcome of therapy will be in a better position to explain and defend the clinical decisions he or she has made.

Another legal issue relates to professional qualifications. Many states have licensing for speech-language pathologists and audiologists. This implies a legal responsibility for service delivery and the need for accountability. In recent years, laws have been passed which enable school districts to seek reimbursement for services from third party payers such as Medicaid (Peters-Johnson, 1990). In order to obtain funds, documentation of services must be provided including the diagnosis, rationale for therapy, treatment procedures, short- and long-term goals, and duration and frequency of treatment.

There is increasing competition for tax dollars. As a result, government agencies are requiring statements of accountability prior to awarding funds to programs. Local, federal, and state agencies want to know what results are being obtained for the tax money spent. Schools must demonstrate compliance with federal and state department of education rules and regulations. Appropriate records and documentation can provide the proof needed during the program review process.

O'Toole (1971, pp. 24–25) posed some questions for school speech-language pathologists in regard to accountability. With some slight variation, many of those questions are still relevant today: How appropriate is speech intervention for each student in your program? Does each one belong on the SLP caseload? Have you established goals that, if accomplished, will make a difference? Is therapy time so well used as to justify taking students away from their academic subjects? Do you know how much progress each of your students is making? Is that recorded? Are you aware of the rate of change? If progress is very slow or nonexistent, are you seeking additional help? How many cases have you followed through either to complete habilitation or rehabilitation or to the greatest degree of compensation that can be expected? If not very many, why not? Are you using treatment time as efficiently as possible? Can you account for all of your time? Is time that is not scheduled with students justifiable? Are you making use of all the knowledge and resources available? Are you moving children along as fast as they can progress, or only as fast as is comfortable for you? Are you adapting to student needs, or are they suiting yours? Does your immediate supervisor understand what you do and the type of students you can and should see in therapy? Does your supervisor understand the support that is necessary to ensure a quality program?

In addition, the federal mandates add impetus for appropriate record and report keeping. It makes good sense for the clinician to keep an account of a child's progress in therapy simply because the clinician is dealing with a large number of children and it would be impossible to remember all the facts and details pertinent to each of them.

Management of Student Records

In order to be useful, record and report systems should permit quick retrieval of information regarding the status, disposition, and intervention of individual students as well as the collective data that must be recorded to report program statistics. Many school districts have developed concise forms to help itinerant school clinicians who are responsible for managing caseloads of between 50 and 125 children throughout a school year. There is increasing demand for accurate record keeping, case management reporting, and statistical data for accountability to school administrators, boards of education, and state departments of education.

A school clinician going into an established program will probably find a record and report system already set up and in operation, whereas a clinician who starts a new program will have to develop his or her own. In both instances it will be necessary to evaluate and monitor the system continuously and make the necessary changes in the forms to be in compliance with state and federal regulations. The confidentiality of information makes it imperative that the storage of records and reports be a major consideration. The policies regarding security measures should be established and in writing. The same is true of the availability of such records and reports to other school personnel, administrators, referral sources, other clinicians on the staff, and parents. Policies and procedures for sharing information should be in writing and should be adhered to once agreed upon. For example, parents should be asked to give written permission for you to release or obtain information about their child to or from anyone.

The abundance of records and reports essential to a program should be taken into account on the clinician's weekly schedule. One of the most time-consuming tasks is filling out reports, keeping up to date on information recorded, and filing and retrieving material. The task is a daily one for much of the information. When weekly, monthly, or yearly reports are involved, a large chunk of time is needed. Some of the work can be assigned to an aide and some of it might be given to the school secretary; however, there are usually many demands on their time as well. A large program may need some secretarial help, either on a part-time or full-time basis, depending on the size and scope of the program. Most of it, however, will be up to the school clinician, and if this is the case, scheduled time should be allotted for it.

Most school systems provide a central office for the school clinicians and in this way a uniform filing, retrieval, recording, and security system can be utilized. A central office system has another advantage in that secretarial or SLP assistants can be pooled.

School clinicians will have to abide by the policies of the school system with regard to how long records and reports on individual children should be retained, which records should be retained, and how records are transferred from school to school as well as from school system to school system. Statistical information with relation to program management and incidence figures can be very useful to clinicians in planning future programs and serving as a basis for research. The school clinical staff might make decisions about retaining of this type of information. Provisions for the storage of such information would have to be made.

Table 6.1 is an outline suggesting the type of information that should be included in documentation of program and student records. The school speech-language clinician might consider this outline as a framework for developing the record and report forms necessary to the program. Such an outline also could be used as a framework for evaluating clinician behaviors in the clinical process as well as analyzing program data to effect changes in program design and practices. Paul-Brown (1995) prepared a comprehensive document recommending elements that should be incorporated into clinical record keeping. Her document would be an excellent resource for school clinicians interested in reviewing and/or improving their clinic record-keeping procedures.

Storing Records and Reports

Many individuals are likely to review the speech-language pathology records including parents, school administrators, teachers, attorneys, and fellow speech-language pathologists. Therefore, records should be written so that they are understandable and contain the type of information others will be able to use to better understand the student and determine the services that are required.

TABLE 6.1   Recommended Outline for Documenting Program and Case Management Records

I. SPEECH-LANGUAGE PROGRAM INFORMATION
   A. Schools served
      1. Names
      2. Locations
      3. Demographic information
         a. Composition of student body
         b. Number of students
         c. Economic/cultural status
      4. Travel time between buildings
      5. Schedule for servicing each building
      6. Student-clinician ratio
      7. Facilities
      8. Projected need for services
   B. Caseload size and composition
      1. Types of disabilities served
      2. Ages
      3. Severity levels
      4. Numbers of students served
      5. Number of continuing cases; number of new cases

II. SPEECH-LANGUAGE PATHOLOGIST INFORMATION
   A. Names of individuals providing speech-language services to students
   B. Licenses and/or certification held and numbers of each
   C. School designated as home-base or office location
   D. Schools assigned to serve
   E. Areas of specialization and/or interest

III. SERVICES PROVIDED
   A. Screening
   B. Assessment
   C. Treatment/Intervention Service Delivery Models
   D. Consultation
   E. Collaboration
   F. In-service programming

IV. CRITERIA OF CASE SELECTION
   A. Eligibility criteria
   B. Severity rating criteria
   C. Prioritization criteria

(continued)

TABLE 6.1   Continued

V. COMPONENTS FOR STUDENT RECORDS

   A. Identifying information

      1. Student's name and address, phone number, chronological age, social security number

      2. Caregiver's name and address

      3. School district; building; grade or placement; homeroom

      4. Identification number (if applicable)

      5. Referral source, date of referral

   B. Student History

      1. Medical history and/or diagnosis

      2. Educational history

      3. Communication disorder diagnosis (behaviors observed)

      4. Prior functional communication status

      5. Prior treatment for speech, language, hearing problems, and outcomes of that treatment

      6. Frequency, length, duration of treatment in prior settings

   C. Description of current status (communicative and educational)

      1. Date or multifactored evaluation

      2. Current functional status

         a. Baseline testing (standardized, nonstandardized procedures); observations

         b. Interpretation of test scores and results

         c. Other relevant clinical and educational findings (contributed by other specialists)

         d. Statement of potential for rehabilitation; estimate of student's abilities based on findings

   D. Treatment Plan

      1. Date treatment plan is established

      2. Long- and short-term functional communication goals

      3. Treatment objectives

      4. Recommended service delivery model, frequency, and duration of treatment

   E. Documentation of Treatment

      1. Date treatment is initiated

      2. Number of times treatment was provided to date

      3. Objective measures of communicative performance (use functional terminology; compare performance against original measures)

      4. Significant developments that might influence rehabilitation potential

      5. Changes in treatment plan

      6. Recommendations for follow-up treatment or continued service

      7. Record of consultation and/or collaboration with other individuals and outcomes

   F. Documentation of clinician and qualifications

      1. Signatures (including titles on all reports and records)

Critical information is generally incorporated into the student's master file held in a central location in the school district. The SLP, teachers, and other educators working with the student also keep pertinent materials in their locations. Materials might include physician reports, test results, work samples, observation notes, attendance logs, and much more. Much care should be placed in the development of written documents including the IEP, IFSP, and ITP. They should be located in a place that is secure, yet accessible since they should be referred to often to verify goals, document progress, and determine future steps.

There are numerous questions that school speech-language pathologists should consider as they develop and store records. First and foremost, the records should be available to provide the type of accountability others seek about the speech-language program. Soon after receiving an inquiry, the SLP should be able to provide responses to questions about the caseload, treatment goals, kinds of disabilities served, goals for treatment, impact on education, intervention schedule, and students' progress. Your immediate supervisor may visit periodically and must understand what you do and the type of students you serve in your program.

TREATMENT OUTCOME MEASURES

There is great pressure for speech-language pathologists, health care professionals, and other educators to demonstrate the efficiency and effectiveness of their services (Blosser, 1997; Eger, 1997). *Treatment efficacy* and *treatment outcomes* are both important elements for determining quality of services. Information can be gathered in a number of ways and results are used for multiple purposes. Treatment efficacy addresses the efficiency of treatment and the time and cost it takes to achieve optimal outcomes. It requires controlled conditions. Treatment outcomes assess the broad value of treatment. They include the clinician's and client's perceptions of change that has occurred. Outcomes are measured at the time of discharge from a program. They are based on the student's functional ability. Spady (1994) defines outcome as "clear learning results that we want students to demonstrate at the end of significant learning experiences." (p. 2). This means that educators at every level within the school district, including SLPs, must establish what it is that students will be able to master at given points in time as they progress through school. To accomplish the goals Spady outlines in his work, schools must establish systems for ensuring that students are equipped with the knowledge, competence, and qualities needed to be successful. Schools must be structured and operated in ways that enable the outcomes to be achieved and maximized for all students (1994). Outcomes must be measured and managed so that students can learn and succeed (Eger, 1997). To summarize, consumers are asking what they are getting for their education dollar. There is a shift of focus from process (what we do) to results (what we produce).

Outcome results can help clinicians demonstrate the effectiveness of services. They can also provide some insights about the prognosis for successful treatment. Parents, teachers, and students with communication disabilities often ask how long intervention will take. Administrators are interested in finding out how much the services will cost. Clinicians can use the information to determine if others perceive that the approaches they are using are effective. This information is especially valuable for planning budgets and resources, demonstrating accountability to administrators, and verifying that standards are being met. When results show that treatment efficiency is not quite as expected, the information can be used to identify clinical training needs and plan staff development opportunities.

Eger (1997) and Ehren (1999) suggest redefining how IEPs are written and used. The days of writing a "speech" IEP are gone. Rather, the IEP should be written for the student. Professional jargon must be eliminated so that others have the benefit of understanding the student's problems and needs as well as the role they can play in the treatment. Eger and Ehren suggest writing speech and language outcomes in the context of learning instead of writing the type of language goal we have seen in the past. As a beginning, education teams should determine what one communication skill, if improved, will have the most impact on the student's performance in the classroom.

Goals should be measureable. Ehren provides the following interpretation of measurable. *Measurable is observable.* Significant communicators in the student's life should learn to make observations of the student's communication in order to determine if changes are occurring as a result of treatment. *Measurable is repeatable.* The target behavior should be repeated in a variety of contexts. Evaluations of performance can be made over a regular period of time. *Measurable is functional.* The behavior should be observed in a variety of settings and authentic conditions. *Measurable is understandable.* Teachers and parents who are asked to be involved in observations and monitoring activities should understand the reason for collecting information. *Measurable is achievable.* Treatment should be altered on an as-needed basis to meet the student's current needs. Following are a few examples based on these principles:

- The student will apply problem-solving and decision-making skills in math and English class as measured by observations of classroom discussions recorded by the teacher.
- The student will follow written instructions on objective tests as measured by review of performance on tests in social studies.
- The student will employ effective fluency strategies when confronted with a stuttering episode during a classroom presentation as measured by an observation made by two peers using a checklist.
- The student's interview skills will be increased by recalling specific information when questioned as measured by an interview rubric completed by the job coach.
- The student will increase his or her ability to use complex sentences to tell about experiences as measured by a transcribed language sample collected by the speech-language pathologist.

Another indicator of learning outcome is the dismissal criteria employed. At this point, national standards for dismissal criteria have not yet been developed. Clinicians continue to wrestle with this issue. We must determine dismissal criteria for each communication disorder.

THE NATIONAL OUTCOMES MEASUREMENT SYSTEM (NOMS)

The American Speech-Language-Hearing Association is sponsoring a treatment outcomes project entitled the National Outcomes Measurement System (NOMS) (ASHA, 1993; 1998). The project has multiple purposes including providing an instrument that will enable professionals to create a national database, confirm and demonstrate the value of its services, provide tools for advocacy and negotiation, enhance opportunities for reimbursement, offer a mechanism for benchmarking clinical progress, and provide guidelines for determining staffing patterns. The National Outcomes Measurement System can provide valuable information about the speech-language pathology program including the number of treatment sessions the student attended, how much progress has been achieved, the cost of the treatment, the type of services delivered and if they were effective, and the level of satisfaction of the student, teacher, and/or parent. This is valuable information for decision making and program planning.

The overarching goals are to increase the amount and quality of efficacy research being completed in the profession and to systematize the way that data is collected, reported, and used. The instruments are designed to reflect changes in clients' functional skills from admission to discharge, provide information about the number of treatment sessions required, and solicit consumer satisfaction.

ASHA has taken a leadership role in the development of this measurement system and in facilitating research to determine the usefulness of such a system. The project has been underway since early 1993 when ASHA established the Task Force on Treatment Outcomes and Cost Effectiveness. The task force was charged with creating a national outcomes database for SLPs and audiologists. Health care professionals from many disciplines have encouraged this type of efficacy research for years.

Recently there have been increased calls for accountability and documentation of efficacy. Clinicians are being asked to prove their worth to external constituents. Supporters of the NOMS project hope that this system will provide an acceptable profession-wide, standardized method for documenting the effectiveness of treatment procedures. Data will enable clinicians to demonstrate functional changes following intervention. It is hoped that the data gathered will provide SLPs with opportunities for better decision making and communication with administrators, third party payers, legislators, other health care providers, consumers, and educators. In addition, trends in treatment will be documented.

School-based personnel, like their counterparts in health care settings, are under scrutiny by decision makers who are looking for ways to cut costs, stretch dollars, and reduce expenses. Unless practitioners provide credible data regarding the clients they serve and the procedures they use, service delivery will be greatly impacted. School-based SLPs need methods for documenting progress, measuring significant change, and identifying the service delivery models that are effective.

The NOMS instruments use a seven-point rating scale that has been developed to measure different aspects of a student's functional communication ability at the time of admission and discharge. There are fifteen possible FCMs: ten for speech-language pathology and five for audiology/aural rehabilitation. Each scale ranges from least functional (Level 1) to most functional or independent (Level 7). They are designed to collect the following:

- Demographic information
- Information on diagnoses
- Information on service delivery model used
- Financial information
- Customer satisfaction information
- Scores on functional communication measures

The data collection process has been ongoing since 1997. In Phase I of the collection process, national data was collected on adults receiving speech-language pathology services in healthcare settings (Johnson, 1997). Phase II began in 1997–1998. Projects were initiated to collect data on children in kindergarten–grade 12 (Iowa, 1997; Blosser, Subich, Ehren, & Ribbler, 1999).

The data collection instruments enable SLPs to gather descriptive information about the student at the beginning of the treatment period including date of birth, school, eligibility for special education, previous services, disorder codes, and functional communication measures. At the end of the treatment period, similar information can be obtained including the reason for discharge, the frequency and length of sessions, the hours of service, the service delivery model, and changes in functional communication status (changes in behavior). The Functional Status Measures (FSM) portion of the instrument enables persons who are significant in the child's life to observe behaviors, communication skills, social skills, and educational skills.

Prior to enrolling students on the caseload, the SLP should document the nature and extent of the disorder and the appropriateness of speech-language services to treat the disability. Children who do not clearly demonstrate communication impairment should not be included in the caseload. Goals that are established should make a difference in the student's educational performance. If students will be taken out of the classroom to participate in therapy, the team members should be convinced that it is justified to take students away from their academic subjects. Administrators, parents, and others will want to be assured that you are using therapy time as efficiently as possible.

Progress records for each student in the caseload must be maintained. If progress is very slow or nonexistent, what additional steps or alternative strategies can be taken? Are you moving children along as fast as they can go? Are you adapting to students' unique personality and needs? Very talented individuals from a large number of disciplines staff school systems. Students will benefit maximally if SLPs make use of all the knowledge and resources available.

Recently, federal legislation has mandated that special educators (including SLPs) provide parents with periodic report cards. Undoubtedly SLPs will be very creative in their design of a report card. It will be important to use terms that parents can understand to describe the student's speech and language characteristics, goals and objectives of intervention, progress to date, and how that progress is determined. The good news is that periodic records will provide a mechanism for ongoing communication with others.

Perhaps the most critical documents the educational team prepares are the individualized educational programs (IEP, IFSP, ITP). These will be discussed extensively in other chapters. It is important to note, however, that care should be taken to identify the students' learning problems and needs; expectations for performance; goals for classroom and all related services; the context and materials for learning; and the role each teacher is to take.

Even without demands made by federal mandates for record and report keeping, it makes good sense for the clinician to keep an account of a child's progress in therapy. Since most clinicians deal with a large number of children, it would be impossible to recall all the facts and details pertinent to each of them.

A sample of the forms used to inform parents, document test results, and plan for a student's individualized education and/or transition program can be found in Appendix C. These forms are discussed in greater detail in other sections of the text.

WRITING PROFESSIONAL REPORTS

The speech-language pathologist is responsible to many different people including students, parents, school administrators, teachers, attorneys, legislators, and fellow speech-language pathologists to name a few. Therefore, records and reports should be written so that they are understandable and contain the type of information others will be able to use to better understand the student and determine whether and what kind of services are required. As stated before, jargon should be eliminated or, at the very least, defined.

The ability to express ideas on paper as well as verbally is essential for the speech-language clinician. Some persons seem to be born with this knack, whereas others have to learn it. In any event, the techniques of writing professional reports and letters can be learned. Professional letters and reports must follow a specific framework. In addition, the basic essentials of good writing must be observed.

First, the writing must be clear and concise. Simple terms are much better than complex ones, and the simplest and easiest way of saying something is usually the best. The professional vocabulary and terminology must be accurate and appropriate. The beginner who is learning the skill of professional writing should keep in mind the person to whom the report is being written. This person may be another clinician, the teacher, the family doctor, or the parents. Appropriate word choices should be made in keeping with the understanding of the potential reader of the report and the purpose for writing it. Avoid professional jargon when writing to others and do not assume that they know the meanings of technical words.

Remember that you are one human being writing to another human being. Try not to sound like an institution writing to a human being. Imagine you are a parent who receives a letter from the school clinician stating: "Periodically during the therapeutic intervention the speech-language pathologist will attempt to assess Billy's receptive language abilities by the administration of norm-referenced and criterion-referenced instruments to determine his linguistic status in relation to his peers." Why not say, "During the time Billy is enrolled in therapy, I will give him several tests to help us find out how well he is progressing in the development of his language skills."

The Progress Report. The progress report covers a span of time, for example, a period of one month, two months, six weeks, six months, or a year. It may be written for the clinician's own information or at the request of the person responsible for the management of the students in that particular setting. The progress report could include such information as the specific dates of the therapy, the number of therapy sessions, the name of the clinician, an evaluation of the progress, a listing of the therapy goals and a statement concerning whether or not they are accomplished, the methods of therapy, and the overall results of the treatment to date. In a school the progress report may be written for the teacher's use and should be specific about what was done in therapy and what would be recommended for the teacher to follow up on. Progress reports are usually filed in the child's cumulative folder, and if the child moves from one school to another the reports may follow to the new school. Progress reports may also be sent to parents. The clinician must be sure the terminology is geared to the parents' understanding. The report card can function as a progress report.

Final Reports.   Final reports or closure reports may follow a checklist format or narrative style or a combination of the two. The factual information included in the closure summary may include name, date of birth, type of problem, date of the latest service, name of the clinician and the supervisor, date when student was first seen, starting date of the therapy, and the date and results of recheck. Information about the therapy and the number of sessions may also be included. In addition, statements of type of therapy—group or individual— can also be obtained. A rating of the progress during the time covered by the report could also be included. The rating may be on a continuum, such as "no progress, very slight, slight, moderate, good, excellent." Clarification of these categories should also be included. Federal and state legislation requires progress reports and final summary reports. The reports would contain information to help determine whether or not the student had achieved the short-term instructional objectives. The contents of the final reports are shared with the parents and, in some cases, with the student. The reports must be as accurate as humanly possible and written so that they will not be misconstrued.

If other services were utilized during this time it would be necessary to include a reference to them and, if available, a summary. Such services would include psychological, social, remedial reading, medical, vocational, educational, and psychiatric. In some cases it might be necessary to attach a copy of the report. The report should indicate whether the service was obtained within the school system or in a community agency.

General Information.   In writing professional reports the school clinician should keep in mind that opinions, rationalizations, hunches, and unsubstantiated ideas should not be included unless they are labeled as such. They may be included under clinical impressions or a similar category. As long as they are labeled it is permissible to include them.

Report writing, as the name implies, means a reporting of the facts without any editorializing by the writer. The reader of the report must be allowed to draw his or her own conclusions from the facts submitted.

RISK MANAGEMENT PLAN

Because speech-language pathologists and audiologists in educational settings work closely with children, they are at risk for contracting chronic, contagious diseases such as Acquired Immune Deficiency Syndrome (AIDS), Hepatitis B virus (HBV), herpes simplex, and cytomegalovirus (CMV). It is wise to take precautionary measures to manage these risks and prevent transmission of disease. School clinicians should have a risk management plan outlining infection control procedures.

The ASHA Committee on Quality Assurance (Kulpa et al., 1991) recommended several administrative considerations for clinicians interested in developing a risk management plan for their school. They also suggested supplies necessary for implementing a risk management plan and infection control procedures for decreasing the possibility of transmitting disease through treatment materials, skin contact, and contact with materials and body fluids. Tables 6.2, 6.3, and 6.4 provide an outline of a risk management plan, supplies needed, and procedures to be followed. These procedures are adapted from the Universal

TABLE 6.2   Risk Management Administrative Considerations: A Checklist

_____ School policy in place for risk management.

_____ Person designated responsible for implementation of policy.

_____ Committee established at the building level for identifying risk management policy and procedures, as follows:

    _____ Identifying risk management needs

    _____ Developing risk management procedures for implementing precautions

    _____ Implementing precautions

    _____ Assessing effectiveness of precautions

    _____ Modifying precaution policy, as indicated

_____ Mechanism established for purchase of required materials to implement infection control procedures.

TABLE 6.3   Infection Control Supply Checklists

A. The following materials are needed to implement proper infection control procedures.

_____ Latex gloves

_____ Alcohol/antiseptic wipes

_____ Soap

_____ Access to sink/running water

_____ Paper towels

_____ Disinfection solution (1 part household bleach to 10 parts water)

_____ Spray bottle (to mix water and disinfectant solution)

_____ Tissue

_____ Plastic bags that seal (e.g., Ziploc)

_____ Trash bags

_____ Household bleach

_____ Hand lotion

_____ Absorbent powder for bodily secretions

B. In addition, these infection control materials should be used when implementing procedures that could expose the professional to blood, semen, or other bodily secretions that _contain visible blood_ (e.g., oral peripheral examinations, procedures involving tracheostomy tubes, etc.)

_____ Mask

_____ Goggles

_____ Gowns

_____ Red trash bags (for disposal of materials that _could be harmful_ if handled casually)

TABLE 6.4 Infection Control Procedures

DECREASING THE POSSIBILITY OF TRANSMITTING DISEASE THROUGH TREATMENT MATERIALS.

What to Disinfect	When to Disinfect	How to Disinfect
■ Evaluation and treatment materials (e.g., toys*, games, storage boxes, therapy materials).	■ Clean tabletop and materials after each use.	■ Use soap and water or a 1 to 10 solution of household bleach to water, spray, and wipe thoroughly.
■ Work surfaces.	■ If materials, work surfaces, electronic equipment or seating surfaces contain visible blood, use Universal Precautions.	■ Use disposable materials (e.g., latex gloves, etc.) when possible.
■ Electronic equipment and accessories.		
■ Seating surfaces.		
■ Materials, supplies and instruments to examine oral mechanism.		

Note: Toys made of fabric and fur should be avoided due to the tendency to harbor microorganisms.

DECREASING THE POSSIBILITY OF TRANSMITTING DISEASE BY APPROPRIATELY DISPOSING OF MATERIALS AND BODY FLUIDS.

DECREASING THE POSSIBILITY OF TRANSMITTING DISEASE VIA SKIN CONTACT.

What to Do	When to Do It	How to Do It
■ Wash hands (effective if skin is intact).	■ Before and after seeing each client.	■ Use vigorous mechanical action whether or not a skin cleanser is used.
	■ After removing gloves.	■ Use antiseptic or ordinary soap under running water.
	■ Immediately if in contact with potentially contaminating blood or body fluids.	■ Wash for 30 seconds or longer if grossly contaminated.
		■ Dry hands thoroughly with a paper or disposable towel to help eliminate germs.
		■ Put on hand lotion so hands do not become chapped.
■ Use gloves (to give protective barrier) if your skin or client's skin is broken.	■ Before touching blood or other body fluids, mucous membranes, or non-intact skin of *all* clients.	■ Put gloves on.

110

What to Dispose of	When to Dispose of It	How to Dispose of It
■ Dressing and tissues.	■ Immediately.	■ Place used dressing and tissues (e.g., diapers, gauze, towelettes, alcohol wipes, gloves) in plastic bag and tie securely. ■ Discard bags carefully.
■ Urine, feces, sperm, vaginal secretions, menses.	■ Immediately.	■ Wear gloves. ■ Flush urine and feces down the toilet. ■ If it is necessary to use a portable urinal, potty chair, etc., empty it into the toilet and thoroughly clean and sanitize before replacing it or returning it to storage.

■ When performing an examination of the oral speech mechanism using laryngeal mirrors, middle ear testing, handling or fabricating earmolds and other prostheses.	■ If a glove is torn or other injury occurs, remove gloves, wash hands thoroughly and use new gloves.
■ When you have a cut or abrasion.	■ After removing gloves, wash hands immediately. See instructions above.
■ When client has a cut or abrasion.	■ Discard gloves. ■ Change gloves after each client.

Precautions developed by the Center for Disease Control and are applicable to the educational setting.

The intent of using such procedures is to prevent transmission of diseases, protect the health of students and professionals, and ensure individuals' rights to privacy.

DISCUSSION QUESTIONS AND PROJECTS

1. Why must school programs in speech-language be held accountable for students' learning outcomes? To whom are programs accountable?

2. Obtain a copy of a letter written about a student to another educator or health care professional. Critique it based on issues raised in this chapter. Would you make any changes? Find a report that has been written to the speech-language pathologist by another professional. Critique it based on issues raised in this chapter.

3. Start a collection of record and report forms used in the schools. How would you organize the report forms for a school system?

4. Write five outcome-based IEP goals for a student in a school program.

5. Write to ASHA to obtain the latest version of the National Outcomes Measures project and the Treatment Outcomes forms. Complete an Entrance Form on one of your students. Ask a fellow student to do the same. Compare results.

6. Check the clinic at your university or school to see if they have appropriate infection control procedures in place.

7. Discuss procedures you should follow if you learn that a child has a communicable disease. Who should you contact? What precautions should you take? Should services for the child be discontinued?

8. What would you do if a child on your caseload came in for therapy and announced that he has ringworm? What if a sibling of one of your students is reported to have hepatitis?

9. List three essential components that student's SLP records must contain.

CHAPTER SEVEN

CASE FINDING AND CASE SELECTION

Determining the composition and size of the caseload is one of the SLP's most challenging responsibilities. He or she must make difficult decisions regarding the procedures to use for case-finding and caseload selection. The ultimate task of the SLP is to identify and treat the student whose communication problem interferes with his or her educational achievement. The SLP makes decisions about how students are to be identified, how they are to be assessed, and which children should receive treatment. These processes are the cornerstones of accountability. While the SLP has the final responsibility for determining which students are eligible for speech-language pathology services, that decision cannot be made independently. The decision must be made in collaboration with other team members including the family, educators, school administrators, and others who can make significant contributions during the decision-making process.

School SLPs are expected to comply with federal and state standards in screening, diagnosis, case selection, and delivery of service. At the same time they are accountable for meeting the local education agency requirements as well as the professional code of ethics. In districts where funding is contributed by a number of sources, the clinician is also responsible for meeting the requirements established by the payers. Sometimes these requirements may seem to conflict with one another. The information in this chapter is presented to help the school SLP formulate the many decisions that must be made in these areas.

A PHILOSOPHY: THE BASIS ON WHICH TO BUILD

Knowing who and what you are and where you fit into the educational scheme will provide the basis from which to make many decisions and plans for the speech-language intervention program. Traditionally, the concept of categorical labeling, whereby children with disabilities were diagnosed, tested, and labeled according to the functional area of the impairment, has been the approach to dealing with children in a classroom. This psychological-medical orientation failed to provide information about the impact of the communication impairment on educational performance for individual children. To provide better services for children in the school it is necessary to describe the problem in terms of the educational deficits it is imposing on the child. Furthermore, it is important that the classroom teacher as well as the parents understand the connection between the communication handicap and the child's ability to profit from the instruction in the classroom. For example, it is not enough to describe a child as having a brain injury and cognitive-communication disorder and let it go at that. In the school, it is necessary to describe how the cognitive-communication disorder affects the child's ability to understand the teacher's classroom instructions; to play with other children on the playground; to monitor his or her own speech and language behaviors; to comprehend reading passages; or to recall information presented in spoken and written forms. The effect of the brain injury on the child's self-image should also be explained.

Speech, language, and hearing clinicians work in many settings. Clinicians who choose to work in an educational setting have the responsibility of removing or alleviating communication barriers that may hinder the child from receiving the instruction offered in the school. The clinician also has the responsibility of evaluating the communication problem and assessing its impact on the learning process. Another responsibility of the school clinician is to serve as a resource person for the classroom teachers and special education teachers who have children with communication disabilities in their classrooms.

Perhaps it is the term *special education* that has led our thinking astray. It is in reality education for children with special problems. The education of children with disabilities is not something distinct and set apart from education; it is a part of the total school program.

DEFINING THE PROCESS AND THE TERMS

Case finding (or case identification) refers to locating the preschool and school age students who demonstrate communication impairments or who are at risk for educational or social failure due to inadequate communication skills. Where it is not in conflict with state law and practices and court order, case finding would also include those students who are ages 18 to 21. Case finding in schools is accomplished by referrals and screening programs.

As a starting point, clinicians and educators must establish common operational definitions and terminology for communicating about youngsters with communication problems. The World Health Organization (WHO) (1980) suggests the following distinctions. Speech-language pathologists work with youngsters with communication patterns that lead to their characterization as *impaired, disabled,* or *handicapped.* Some clinicians don't make distinctions between the three terms. However, WHO provides a definition of the terms that can be useful in determining the extent of services to be provided. According to WHO, impairment is an abnormality of structure or function at the organ level. This would include speech, language, hearing, cognitive, and voice impairments. A disability is the functional consequence of impairment. People with impairments experience communication problems in the context of daily living situations and activities. A handicap is the social consequence of an impairment or disability. Depending of the nature and severity of the impairment, individuals may experience isolation, joblessness, and dependency. Their quality of life is effected (World Health Organization, 1980; Frattelli, 1998).

Case selection refers to the process of determining which students are eligible for speech and language intervention services. Neither all students referred for services nor all students who fail screening criteria are candidates. Those who exhibit communication problems are determined through the following steps:

- Obtaining appropriate background information, that is, a case history, including onset, past development, present status, and other relevant information from parents and teachers
- Appraising the problem by observing, interviewing, describing, and testing when appropriate
- Diagnosing, which includes making a tentative identification of the problem and determining probable causes

It should be pointed out that the SLP must use judgment in determining how rigorously these steps are followed. For example, the third-grader that exhibits what appears to be a serious voice problem may be suffering from a cold and sore throat at the time they are observed. That information would preclude interviewing parents or obtaining a case history.

Caseload composition refers to the size of the caseload, or the number of students comprising it, and the range of communication problems represented in it. Unfortunately, many state and local education agencies mandate the number of students that comprise the caseloads of speech-language pathologists. Thus, the numbers of students served may be higher than would be recommended if clinicians were given full control and responsibility for determining caseload size. Due to this situation, SLPs in most school districts serve inordinately high numbers of students. In addition, there is little or no agreement at this writing among state and local education agencies concerning what is an appropriate caseload size. The American Speech-Language-Hearing Association has established a team of clinicians from around the country to debate this issue and make recommendations for the most appropriate guidelines for establishing the school clinician's caseload.

Let us now look at each of these issues in greater detail. Each process will be examined in the order in which the SLP would carry it out.

CASE FINDING

Case finding is usually accomplished by utilizing two procedures, either singly or in combination—*referral* and *screening*. The purpose of both referral and screening is the identification of students with communication problems that are *educationally relevant*. In many school systems referral is becoming widely used because of its perceived efficiency and effectiveness.

Screening has two facets. One, screening groups of youngsters to determine those who need additional testing. Second, the process of obtaining a sample of the youngster's communication skills to determine if more in-depth diagnostic testing is warranted to confirm the presence of a communication disorder and to determine eligibility for intervention services.

Following referral from teachers, the SLP may elect to administer screening tests, rather than in-depth tests, to determine the next steps. In some situations, it may be more efficient to utilize group-screening methods, for example, on the preschool, kindergarten or first-grade level.

REFERRALS

Unfortunately, the efficacy research comparing screening versus referral methods for case finding is limited. Finn and Gardner (1984) recommend using teacher interviews in combination with other screening procedures. Miller's (1989) data supports teacher referral over mass screening programs for the elementary level. No longer under state regulation to conduct mass screenings, clinicians across the country have begun to initiate a teacher referral-based model versus mass screening methods of case finding. The success of any referral system is providing information to teachers about communication disorders in a simple and understandable way. In addition, so that there is a context for the referral, teachers must understand the impact of speech and language disorders on the youngster's school performance.

Let us look at the process of referral. The school clinician needs to be aware that a particular child might have a communication problem. The clinician, in the final analysis, is the one who is responsible for determining if such a problem exists; however, referrals can be made by anyone who has the child's welfare in mind and suspects a problem. This would include the child's parents, teachers, family doctor, school nurse, school counselor, principal, peer, or the child. Outside the school, the social service agencies within the community, physicians, health care specialists, and voluntary agencies such as childrens' service agencies, the Brain Injury Foundation, and others may all be considered valuable referral agencies. The school clinician will need to understand and comply with the school system's policy regarding referrals. The process for referring students for speech-language intervention services should be clearly defined and consistent throughout the school district. Referral forms should be made available to school staff and other individuals.

Referrals should not be discouraged even though the clinician may sometimes feel that the classroom teacher is referring too many children or referring children who have problems other than those in speech, language, and hearing. The door should always be kept open for referrals. Educators should be encouraged to refer any child they feel might have a problem. Teachers generally are good referral sources because they have a good sense of how children should speak at a particular age or in a particular grade. Because of staff turnover and changes in service delivery requirements and eligibility criteria, the procedures and opportunities for referral should be presented to the teachers periodically. It is especially good if the information can be presented during a staff meeting or as an in-service presentation. The school clinician will soon learn which teachers in a school are able to identify the children with communication impairments with a high degree of accuracy.

Some school districts have created school-based interdisciplinary problem-solving teams who help teachers understand and deal with students who present problems in the classroom. Oftentimes, members of this group are the first to realize that a student may have communication impairments and refer the child for further evaluation by the speech-language pathologist.

Following the initial referral from the classroom teacher or the problem-solving team, the speech-language clinician will have to make a decision about whether the student is to receive a battery of screening tests or a more complete assessment. According to state and federal laws, parental and/or guardian permission must be obtained before comprehensive testing is undertaken.

Helping Educators Make Referrals. Educators and communication disorders professionals can work together to identify children who exhibit inadequate communication skills. The key is to identify those students whose speech and language skills interfere with their learning. If others are to function effectively as referral sources, they will need to develop awareness and understanding of the following: how speech and language skills develop, types of communication impairments children present, and ways that impairments interfere with learning. They should know the behaviors and characteristics associated with language, articulation, stuttering, voice, and hearing problems. They need to learn the definitions and terminology used by professionals to discuss these disorders. It is extremely important for educators to understand that communication is the basis for learning and the negative impact speech, language, and hearing impairments can have on classroom performance. In the discussion of communication disorders, it is especially important to discuss the adverse effect the communication disorder has on the youngster's ability to participate in school and learn the general education curriculum. The quality of referrals will be improved if teachers become skilled at observing students and relating their communication problems to learning difficulties they may be experiencing.

Some colleges and universities offer introductory courses about speech, language, and hearing problems for students majoring in education. Others integrate information about communication development and disabilities into coursework on topics such as human development and learning or characteristics of children with special education needs. It would be helpful to the school clinician if all teachers were to learn about communication impairments during their preprofessional training, but this is not always the case. The school clinician may want to consider offering an in-service presentation to teachers or teaching a course lecture on communication disorders at the local university. This would give the clinician the opportunity to define and describe the various types of communication problems as well as discuss their impact on learning and procedures for making referrals.

Following is a list of topics that should be discussed during an in-service presentation to teachers and other referral sources.

- Normal speech, language, and hearing development
- Nature and causes of speech-language-hearing impairments
- Terminology used by speech-language pathologists and audiologists to describe and discuss children with communication impairments
- Impact of communication disorders on academic and social performance
- Factors communication disorders professionals consider when evaluating students' communicative performance
- Referral procedures to be followed
- The goals of the speech-language intervention program
- Ways to collaborate with speech-language pathologists and audiologists

Demonstrating typical disorders will enhance in-service presentations. As a prospective clinician, are you able to imitate or simulate various kinds of communication problems? A library of tapes about various types of problems would be helpful for demonstration. Regional resource centers and universities may have audio or videotapes available for loan to school clinicians for teacher in-service programs. Some publishers sell CD-ROMs that depict various disorders.

Referrals can be initiated in person, by telephone, or in writing. The teacher is able to observe children in a variety of communication-based learning activities. Consequently, the information he or she has to offer regarding performance is quite valuable. It is most helpful to provide a simple questionnaire or checklist to assist teachers and others in describing the communication behaviors they have observed, their concerns, and their reasons for referring. Figure 7.1 is an example of the type of checklist teachers might find helpful when observing a child's communication skills. Notice how simple the questions

FIGURE 7.1   Teacher's Referral Form

Teacher's Name: _____

Grade:_____

Read the following statements and (✓) if the child's speech, language or hearing behavior is described *CHILD'S NAME & AGE*					
1. Voice quality is noticeably different from other children (hoarse, breathy, nasal)					
2. Speech is nonfluent (hesitant, jerky, repetitive, prolonged)					
3. Child is noticeably frustrated if unable to get message across					
4. Articulation is difficult to understand					
5. Child is unable to ask and/or answer simple questions					
6. Child cannot carry on a conversation (relay events, give explanation)					
7. Child cannot formulate 5 and 7 word sentences; grammar and vocabulary are not age appropriate					
8. Generally nonverbal					
9. Has frequent colds or runny nose					
10. Attends to speakers face more than other children do					
11. Frequently responds to statements or questions with "what?" or "huh?"					
12. Does not follow simple directions					

and form are. The initial referral form should be brief so busy teachers can quickly complete it. More extensive information can be obtained through guided teacher observation as part of the evaluation process once the child has been identified as exhibiting communication impairment.

Case Finding at the Secondary-School Level.   It is more realistic to carry out case finding in middle schools and high schools by teacher referral rather than by any other screening procedure. School clinicians, while recognizing the need of improved case-finding procedures at this level, point out the difficulties of a screening program because of the inflexibility of middle and high school class schedules and the greater mobility of high school students, who are changing classes throughout the day.

Another factor that hinders both a screening program and a teacher referral program on the secondary level is that the higher the grade taught, the less aware the teachers may be of speech disorders. This is most likely the result of differences in preservice training for elementary teachers versus high school teachers. It may also be related to the demand and structure of the secondary curriculum. Secondary teachers often do not see students for as great an amount of time as elementary teachers see their students. In addition, in many classes, communicative interaction is limited because teachers use a lecture style for teaching. English and language arts teachers are good referral sources because they are sensitive to communication and they have greater opportunity to hear students communicate during classroom activities. Guidance counselors, coaches, and teachers who sponsor extracurricular activities also converse with students in informal situations with great frequency.

On the high school level, self-referrals or parental referrals are often good sources of identifying individuals with communication problems. High school students who have a speech, language, or hearing problem will have to know about the services offered if they are to refer themselves. This means that the clinician will have to find ways of letting students know the services are available, as well as make it easy for them to refer themselves.

Students can be informed of the times and days the speech-language clinician is in the school building through announcements over the public address system, through the school newspaper, or through signs posted on bulletin boards throughout the building. The message should inform students about the services offered by the speech-language pathologist. It should provide brief explanations of speech, language, and hearing behaviors which may cause concern and which they might want to check out. It should also describe how to schedule an appointment. In some districts, students may have to inform the guidance counselor of their interest. Middle school and high school students are sensitive about other people knowing they experience difficulties. Therefore, discretion is advised about the testing appointment, location, results, and recommendations. One way to encourage participation is to stress the self-improvement aspect of the speech-language program.

Paul-Brown (1991) provides a compilation of various methods, which can be used to identify communication problems in adolescents. She includes assessment tools, classroom observation procedures, and methods for obtaining teacher referrals. By providing instructions and guidelines for making referrals during an in-service program, you can develop a systematic referral program with a core group of teachers who see every student in the building. Provide teachers with instructions for observing the students' skills in the following areas of cognition and communication. Explain how these areas interfere with classroom performance:

- *Thinking*—organizing and categorizing information; identifying and solving problems; finding, selecting, and using information; and thinking about ideas and events
- *Listening*—understanding complex sentences and words; understanding main ideas and events; following complex directions; and listening effectively
- *Speaking*—planning what to say; organizing information in a logical sequence; using grammatically correct sentence structures; using language to give directions, make reports, tell stories; providing relevant and complete answers
- *Survival language*—demonstrating language skills necessary to cope with daily living situations

Differences in findings between teacher referral and screening is most likely related to the adequacy of teacher preparation for the referral process. It is suggested that you work with the principal and guidance counselors to determine the best methods for finding secondary students with communication problems in your school district.

SCREENING

Screening is a process whereby students in need of further evaluation are identified. While the referral process is the most efficient, there are still times when screening programs are considered useful. The SLP must decide when and where the screening activities will take place and which children will be screened. It is inefficient and it creates ill will to collect data through referrals and screenings in schools and classrooms where the SLP does not expect to conduct therapy.

There are some general factors to be considered before making these decisions. Answering the following questions can help determine how to implement the screening program so the screening time can be used in the best way possible:

- What are the goals of the speech-language-hearing program?
- Will different populations be served in the coming school year?
- Are speech-language pathology services new to the building, district, or community?
- Will the screening program be conducted by SLPs independently or will there be a team approach involving educators, assistants, or clinicians from other school buildings?
- Are there unique aspects related to the student population (socioeconomic status, mobility, cultural diversity, special education needs) that support the need for screening?
- Have there been significant changes in school personnel or resources?

When the answers to these questions have been obtained, the goals of the screening program can be established. It is important that these goals are not only established, but also provided in writing and made available to the school administration. When the goals are established, the procedures for carrying out the screening program can be made. The procedures should also be in writing and should be available to the superintendent, the director of special education, the elementary and secondary supervisors, the principals of each school, and the teachers in each of the schools to be screened.

Screening all children in the kindergarten and first-grade levels of schools to be serviced, however, may be the best way to identify children in need of further evaluation. This method should always be combined with teacher referrals as well as with parental input.

The purpose of screening is to determine (1) if a problem exists, (2) if further evaluation is needed, and (3) if referral to other professionals is needed. The first step in a screening process serves to identify children with communication impairments. A second screening would be made of those children identified by the first screening or by referral as having possible communication problems. The second screening would be somewhat more extensive and would help the clinician pick out those children who are candidates for intervention. The third step would be complete diagnostic evaluation for children who need therapeutic intervention and/or referral to other professionals.

Screening programs can be structured in many different ways. One procedure used successfully by many clinicians is to take three to five children at a time. While one is being tested the others can observe and will know what to do when their turn comes without the clinician having to explain. As each child is finished he or she goes back to the classroom and gets the next child in the row. This procedure creates little interruption of the teacher's schedule, and the classroom activities go on as usual. A class of 25 children can be screened in approximately 30 to 40 minutes.

The same general screening procedures may be applied to small groups of children. The clinician takes a group of six to eight children to the therapy room where the screening is carried out, returns the group, and gets the next group. If speech-language pathology assistants are available, they may take the children to and from the classroom.

In many school systems a team approach is used in the preschool screening program. The team members often include the school nurse, psychologist, speech-language pathologist, educational audiologist, and other specialists who test vision, hearing, speech and language, motor coordination, dentition, general health, and physical well being. Paraprofessionals or volunteer aides also assist in this type of screening program. If using assistants in this way, they should be trained and supervised by certified, qualified professionals.

General Considerations.   Because the purpose of the rapid screening is detection, not diagnosis, the clinician will have to resist the temptation to spend more time than is needed with a child who obviously has a problem. Also, the clinician will have to tactfully discourage a talkative child from telling a lengthy, complicated story. The results of the screening task should be recorded immediately after each individual is seen. All absentees should be noted, and arrangements should be made to screen them later.

Keeping Teachers Informed.   Teachers should be informed in advance of the referral and screening program procedures and schedule. This will help them prepare their students and plan for the interruption in their teaching schedule. Following is an example of the type of message that can be sent to teachers to announce the screening program:

■ ■ ■ ■ ■ ■

MARK YOUR CALENDARS TODAY!
SPEECH-LANGUAGE REFERRALS AND SCREENINGS

Children in your class will be screened for speech and language impairments during the **week of September 7.** Prior to that time, please observe the children in your class closely. Refer all children whose communication skills concern you.

Return the teacher referral form to my mailbox by September 3.

Children referred by their teachers plus all children in kindergarten, grade 1, and the special education classes will be screened individually. I will confirm the schedule with you after reviewing the referral forms.

If you have questions about communication behaviors that are significant or about the screening program, please let me know.

I'm looking forward to working with you this year.

Cordially,

Yvonne Smith
Speech-Language Pathologist

Screening Procedures

The major purpose of the screening process is to determine whether or not a problem exists. The screening must be done quickly and accurately; that is; it must be done with a maximum degree of professional expertise and with a minimum expenditure of time, money, and professional energy. Planning is absolutely essential. In addition to a general plan, there must also be a plan to encompass all the details and follow-up contacts after the screening.

Screening of preschoolers is generally completed in the spring preceding their entrance into school. Kindergarten screening is usually carried on during the first few weeks of school, but it may be done at any time of the year. As mentioned previously, referrals by teachers in the upper elementary grades, middle school, and high school can be obtained with the guidance of the SLP. This process can replace screening at those grade levels.

Federal regulations do not require written permission of the parents prior to a group screening program; however, some states and some school districts do require that parents be notified that screenings will take place. This can be done by a letter sent home with the children or by announcements in the school newsletter or local newspaper.

Screening programs can be carried out by one clinician, by a team of clinicians, or by a team composed of clinicians and trained assistants. If more than one person is involved in a screening program, the procedures should be clearly understood by all to ensure uniform administration and greater reliability.

Screening Instruments

Clinicians use a variety of methods for screening children ranging from observing informal conversations to using formal, standardized screening tests. Clinicians may use published or informal screening tools including checklists, questionnaires, observations, or clinician-made instruments. There are advantages and disadvantages to each. For example, through observation during informal conversation, one can observe the child's overall intelligibility and the impact of the child's communication skills on communicative interactions. However, this method reduces the quantifiable information which can be obtained, reduces accountability, and may miss children who are reluctant participants or shy (Westman & Broen, 1989). Formalized methods have the advantage of enabling the clinician to compare the child's performance to others of the same age, implementing the testing consistently across children, and facilitating documentation and accountability.

Instruments for assessing communicative abilities during a screening program differ according to the ages of the children. The instruments should be easily administered and should identify quickly those children needing further testing. In a school screening, whether one clinician or several are involved, the screening devices should be the same, and the standard for judging the results should be consistent from one tester to another. The screening procedures should also take into account differences in ethnic and in socioeconomic backgrounds of the children being tested. The examiners need to keep in mind that they are attempting to detect differences in speech, language, voice quality, fluency, or any other problems in communication that might be potentially limiting to the child's ability to learn in school or function as a useful member of society.

It will be necessary for the school SLP to become familiar with the various speech and language tests. The clinician should find out what the test purports to measure and what it actually measures. The most appropriate test or tests should be utilized for the particular situation. Check the reliability, norms, and standardization of the test, know the difference between "norm-referenced" tests and "criterion-referenced" tests, and utilize clinical judgment and expertise in synthesizing the information from the tests.

A comprehensive screening battery carried out by the speech-language specialist or as a part of a comprehensive screening program could include the following:

1. Audiological evaluation
2. Language appraisal (receptive and expressive) on the semantic level, syntactic level, phonological level, morphological level and pragmatic levels
3. Articulation/phonological process appraisal
4. Intelligibility appraisal
5. Voice appraisal
6. Fluency appraisal

Screening procedures on any age or grade level are subject to some degree of error. Some children will slip by undetected, and others may not be identified correctly. School clinicians and classroom teachers must work together to recognize any of these children.

Teacher Interview Screening

A method that combines screening and teacher referral was developed by Finn and Gardner (1984) at Heartland Area Education Agency 11, Ankeny, Iowa. Known as the Teacher Interview Screening, it is comprised of two processes: mandatory teacher in-service programs and the teacher interview. It was developed to utilize the teachers' expertise in observing communicative behaviors. To facilitate the in-service, a Communication Competency Screening Scale (Figure 7.2) which describes communication skills was developed. Teachers were interviewed and asked the following question about each student in the class: "Considering the skills outlined on the communication competency scale, do you feel this child's communication skills are adequate when compared to his/her classmates?" The teachers and clinician then had three options available to them. They could *pass* the child who had adequate skills, *fail* the child who obviously had inadequate skills, or conduct a *follow-up screening* for those children whose skills were questionable. The follow-up screening consisted of a classroom observation or a more traditional one-on-one screening depending on the concerns that were expressed.

Finn and Gardner evaluated the effectiveness of the teacher interview, comparing the results to the traditional screening method in terms of cost, reliability, and compatibility with intervention philosophies. A two-year study was conducted to make appropriate cost estimates. The results indicated the total time spent by the staff doing the new screening method was 100 hours and 42 minutes or approximately 13 working days. The traditional mass screening method took 897 hours or approximately 120 working days. Given clinicians' per diem salaries, this amounted to significant savings. Reliability was examined by selecting several of the second grade classrooms. Each child who failed either the traditional screening or Teacher Interview Screening was evaluated and the results were compared. Interpretation of the data showed 84 percent agreement between the teacher interview and traditional methods of screening. It should be noted that there were no students with disorders (those having a severity score of 4) who were missed by either group. There were no students with a score of 3 missed by the teacher group, while there were two children missed in the group screened by the traditional method. With the completion of this project it was concluded that using a well-developed teacher interview procedure for screening can be efficient, permit sampling a student's communication skills in his or her natural environment, and utilize the skills teachers have or can develop to identify students in need of our services. This is the kind of study the profession needs to continue to encourage in order to determine the most effective and cost-efficient methods of conducting our services.

Screening for Phonological Disorders in Primary Grades

According to studies, children in kindergarten, first grade, and second grade exhibit many phonological errors. Some of these children will overcome their errors through the process of getting a little older and being exposed to the school environment; however, there are children in this group who will not improve without intervention. Differentiating between these two groups creates a dilemma for the school clinician. Obviously, because of the large numbers, all these children cannot be included in the direct service program. Through

FIGURE 7.2 Communication Competency Screening

	POOR	POOR	ADEQUATE	SUPERIOR	SUPERIOR
Skill in communication	Limited awareness of listeners; speaks with little effort to evoke understanding from others; pace of words and inflection of voice not adjusted to listeners				Adjusts pace and inflection to listener; is aware of need to make self understood and can adjust content to listener's needs and responses
Organization, purpose, and control	Rambles; limited sense of order or of getting to the point; rattles on without purpose; cannot tell a story in proper sequence				Plans what is said; gets to the point; controls language, can tell a story in proper sequence; speaks fluently
Wealth of ideas/ amount of language	Seldom expresses an idea; appears dull and unimaginative; doesn't originate suggestions or plans during play periods; seldom talks; rarely initiates; needs to be prompted to talk				Expresses ideas on different topics; makes suggestions on what to do and how to carry out class plans; shows imagination and creativity in play; talks freely, frequently and easily
Vocabulary	Uses a meager vocabulary, far below that of most children this age; uses ambiguous words				Uses a rich variety of words, has an exceptionally large and growing vocabulary
Quality of listening	Demonstrates poor comprehension of spoken language; inattentive; easily distracted				Superior understanding of spoken language; attentive
Quality of sentence structure	Omissions of structural elements, including word endings; uses only simple active, declarative sentences; word order difficulties in question formations				Includes all structural elements; mature sentence patterns; maintains constant tense reference within a paragraph or story; mature use of phrases and clauses and conjunctions

(continued)

FIGURE 7.2 Continued

	POOR				SUPERIOR
		POOR	ADEQUATE	SUPERIOR	
Articulation	Child is difficult to understand due to speech sound errors; speech draws attention to itself				All speech sounds are produced appropriately
Voice	Distracts listener from meaning of the message; denasal or nasal quality; frequent loss of voice; recurrent hoarseness				Voice is pleasing to the listener; does not draw attention to itself
Fluency	Frequently repeats parts of words and whole words; demonstrates long periods of silence while attempting speech; demonstrates struggle behavior				Speaks smoothly

Adapted by: Heartland Education Agency from LOBAN'S ORAL LANGUAGE SCALE .

126

prognostic and predictive testing, school clinicians will be able to sort these children into two general groups: those who need intervention and those who would benefit from a general speech-language improvement program.

Numerous prognostic factors related to phonological errors have been explored including rate of change toward correction, number, type, and/or consistency of errors, phonemic proficiency, and evaluation of the specific sounds or phonological processes exhibited. Clinicians must conduct procedures that will enable them to discriminate between those children who will and those who will not have acquired normal mature articulation by the time they reach third grade.

Generally, SLPs take steps to assess the child's degree of stimulability (the ability to repeat sounds, nonsense syllables, words, and a sentence); the ability to move the tongue independently of the lower jaw; and the ability to detect errors in the examiner's speech. Some SLPs believe that another effective and reliable predictive variable is the total number of errors in all positions within words produced by the youngster. Westman and Broen (1989) and Peterson and Marquardt (1990) state that the persistence of specific types of error patterns are more important as predictors than the number of errors. There are several error patterns which are characteristic of children who are unintelligible or phonologically delayed (Westman and Broen, 1989; Hodson and Paden, 1981; Weiner and Wacker, 1982). These include errors involving deletion of phonemes or syllables, change in the manner of phoneme production; substitution of more anterior sounds for more posterior sounds, and change in the phonotactic structure of the word.

Another factor related to the predictability of the correction of functional phonological problems is the inconsistency of errors. It has been generally accepted that the more inconsistent the child's phonological errors, the more possibility there is that he or she will outgrow them. The rationale is that the child may be able to produce the sound correctly sometimes but has not learned the appropriate times to produce it. Children exhibiting inconsistent error patterns or phonological processes inappropriate for their age should be further tested with instruments that provide more comprehensive and systematic testing on the way sounds are produced in all possible phonologic contexts. There are several instruments available that can be used to yield helpful information. Care should be taken to learn the premise upon which the judgments will be based (number of errors, type of error patterns, stimulability, and so forth).

Some instruments provide estimates of the number of correct productions expected for children at various age levels from age three to eight. Spontaneous speech samples will yield information on the overall intelligibility of the child, but to be used effectively, the tester must have an understanding of expectations at each age milestone. To make informed clinical decisions, SLPs must be familiar with normative development. Lawrence, Katz, and Linville (1991) surveyed the literature on suppression of phonological processes. A chart summarizing their findings is presented in Table 7.1.

Screening for Phonological Disorders in Older Elementary Children

In older elementary children, speech and language screening can be accomplished by having them give their name, address, and telephone number, by counting to 25, by naming

TABLE 7.1   Ages of Suppresssion of Phonological Processes (Lawrence, Katz, Linville, 1991)

PHONOLOGICAL PROCESSES	GRUMWELL	LOWE	HAELSIG & MADISON	INGRAM	KAHN-LEWIS
Deletion final consonants	3:2		4:6	3:0	Suppressed first
Deletion initial consonants					Nondevelopmental*
Consonant deletion (includes initial, final)		4:0–4:5			
Syllable reduction	4:2	5:0–5:5	Beyond 5	4 and after	Suppressed first
Cluster reduction	3:9	6:0–6:5	4:6		Suppressed first
Cluster substitution		6:0–6:11			
Reduplication	2:5			1st 50 words	
Consonant harmony (assimilation)	2:10			3:0–4:6	Intermediate suppress
Initial voicing				4 and after	Suppressed first
Final devoicing			4:0		Suppressed last
Context-sensitive voicing	3:0	3:0			
Fronting		5:6–5:11	3:0		
Velar Fronting	3:3			Early	Intermediate suppress
Palatal fronting				Early	Suppressed first
Backing to velars		3:0–3:5			Nondevelopmental*
Stopping of fricatives, affricates		6:0–6:5	4:0		Suppressed last**
/f/	2:8				
/v/	3:6				
/θ/	2:8				
/s/	3:0				
/z/	3:7				
/ʃ/	2:9				
/tʃ, dʒ/	3:1				
Affrication		3:0–3:5	3:0		
Deaffrication		4:6–4:11			Suppressed first
Labialization		8:0–8:5			
Alveolarization		6:0–6:5			
Liquid simplification (includes gliding, vocalization)					Suppressed last
Gliding of Liquids	Beyond 5	6:6–6:11	5:0		
Vocalization of Liquids		6:6–6:11	4:6		
Glottal replacement			4:0		Nondevelopmental

*Nondevelopmental: not usually frequent in normally developing phonological systems
**Age of suppression inflated by late use of b/v and d/ð in normal phonological development

the days of the week or months of the year, or by responding to pictures of objects designed to test sounds. The best screening test is spontaneous speech because it is most likely to yield a sample of the child's habitual speech and language. If the child is asked to read words, sentences, or paragraphs, the clinician must be sure that the material is within his or her reading ability.

Screening for Language Disorders

The identification of language disorders in the preschool and school-age child is a complicated, difficult, and often frustrating task. A thorough knowledge of speech and language development is required of the examiner as well as an appreciation of the fact that both the identification and the assessment of language disorders is a continuous process shared by the persons who are best able to observe the child in many situations. These persons are the parents and the teachers as well as the speech-language pathologist.

The data and research on language development and disorders is extensive, while at the same time, much of it is inconclusive. Professional speech-language pathology journals contain many reports of studies comparing language tests and measurements, which simply means that more is being added to the body of knowledge.

In the schools, many learning behaviors are dependent on language abilities: reading, spelling, speech, writing, mathematics, problem solving, creative thinking, comprehension, and others. An intact language system is important in the learning process. The SLP plays a necessary role in the identification, assessment, and treatment of the student with a language disorder.

Keeping in mind that screening is an identification process, we therefore need to identify the student with the language disorder. The facets of language are reception (decoding) and expression (encoding). The components of language are phonology, morphology, syntax, semantics, and pragmatics. A complete language evaluation should include all of these aspects. On the screening level it is important to ascertain whether or not the language behavior is adequate and commensurate with the age of the student. The in-depth diagnosis would follow after the individual has been identified.

One of the most important steps in the identification process is to obtain information from the teacher about how the language impairment may be impacting upon academic performance. Valuable information can be gained by asking teachers to observe their students and respond to a few key questions relating language skills to classroom performance. Figure 7.3 illustrates a simple observation checklist designed to guide teacher's observations and descriptions.

Screening Secondary School Students

Most students with communication problems will have been identified by the time they reach middle school or high school. Since preparation for the world of work and post-secondary education is of primary importance to secondary teachers, some effort should be made to identify those secondary students who may experience difficulty transitioning from school to post-secondary activities due to communication problems. Teacher referral is one method of identifying students who may be at risk. A second method is to conduct an observation

FIGURE 7.3   OBSERVATION TO DETERMINE LANGUAGE FUNCTIONING IN THE CLASSROOM

STUDENT _____   DATE _____

TEACHER _____   GRADE _____

TO THE TEACHER: Read each of the following statements. Indicate those statements which are representative of the student's behavior. Refer children who cause you to be concerned to the speech-language pathologist for further testing.

1. _____   In your opinion, the student demonstrates a noticeable communication problem which may be affecting educational performance.

2. _____   The communication problem is most noticeable during:

   _____   Comprehension tasks (Written _____   Verbal _____)

   _____   Classroom discussion

   _____   Social communication

   _____   Mathematics

   _____   Language arts

   _____   Spelling

   _____   Oral reading

   _____   Other

3. _____   The student has difficulty understanding subject-related vocabulary.

4. _____   The student has difficulty understanding subject-related concepts.

5. _____   The student has difficulty following written or spoken directions.

6. _____   The student does not understand figurative language.

7. _____   The student has poor reasoning and problem solving ability, showing difficulty with cause/effect relationships.

8. _____   The student's response to questions is inappropriate.

9. _____   The student has difficulty participating in class discussions.

10. _____   The student has difficulty expressing ideas or relating stories and experiences.

11. _____   The student's sentence structure, word choice, or sentence organization interferes with his ability to clearly express the message.

12. _____   The student's speech production (articulation, voice, fluency) makes the conversation difficult to understand.

13. _____   Other students in the class seem to have difficulty understanding the student.

screening procedure. Observing students during a class where they make oral presentations offers an opportunity to screen a large number of students in a brief amount of time. The English classes are ideal because in most school systems, all students must take this subject. The screening procedure should be planned cooperatively with the teaching staff. The SLP does not necessarily have to be the individual who actually listens to each student. Rather, arrangements can be made in advance for students to read or recite a specific passage, which would enable the teacher and/or clinician to obtain a quick impression of each student's communication performance. If a sufficient amount of coordination is done in advance, the task of screening the English classes on the junior-high and high school levels could be accomplished in a short period of time. Another alternative method for reaching high numbers of students is to team with the school nurse during screening programs for hearing and vision.

Screening devices for adolescents often include reading short passages, answering questions posed by the examiner, and recounting events. Voice quality can be noted at the same time. Spontaneous speech can be elicited by asking questions, which will give the examiner some information about expressive language.

The examiner needs to be aware of the possibility of fluency disorders during the screening. Verification would have to be made by consultation with the teachers who would be most likely to have heard the student in an informal speaking situation. These teachers might include the physical education teacher, the English teacher, the guidance counselor, and other people active in extracurricular activities.

When the list of students who may be at risk is completed, the SLP can complete a screening test of those students. Few screening tests for adolescents have been developed at this writing.

CASE FINDING: SPECIAL POPULATIONS

Classrooms in schools throughout the United States are populated with students representing varying levels of learning capability and diverse cultures. Children who present developmental, physical, or mental disabilities such as learning disabilities, mental retardation, cerebral palsy, and emotional disturbances may go undetected because the other handicapping conditions are more obvious. In some instances, children may have been misdiagnosed as having a particular type of learning disability when in reality their primary problem is a hearing or speech-language impairment. Communication problems in children who do not speak English may be particularly difficult to identify if the clinician is unable to speak the child's language or an interpreter is not available.

It is important for the school clinician to be aware of these children and apply the appropriate screening and diagnostic evaluations. The school SLP needs to be sensitive to differences in children when selecting screening or evaluation instruments. Children's performance may be affected by the selection of test items and materials, performance requirements (e.g., cognitive, motor, and communicative), the verbal style used by the tester, or the testing situation itself (Peterson and Marquardt, 1990).

Children receiving special education services or being considered for placement in special education classes should receive a communication status evaluation as part of the multifactored assessment process. When facilities for further evaluation of these children are not available in the school, they should be referred for services to a university clinic, community hearing and speech center, or hospital clinic.

Many city and county school districts and regional resource centers have centralized diagnostic facilities. These programs accept referrals from education and health professionals within the district as well as from parents. The benefits of such a centralized service are that the time, which is needed to conduct a comprehensive evaluation, can be taken and recommendations for treatment can be derived from input from professionals representing a variety of disciplines.

CASE FINDING: CHILDREN WITH HEARING IMPAIRMENTS

Hearing impairment of any type and degree is problematic (Bess, 1988; Northern & Downs, 1991). Even mild hearing impairment can interfere with the language and learning process (Osberger, Moeller, Eccarius, Robbins, & Johnson, 1986). Flexer (1999) states that "any type and degree of hearing impairment can present a significant barrier to an infant's or child's ability to receive information from the environment." Hearing impairment can have harmful effects on social, emotional, cognitive, and academic development. This may limit the students vocational and emotional potential (National Institutes of Health, 1993). Screening for hearing impairment should be included in the general developmental screening of all children.

How many children are we talking about? Flexer (1999) provides an extensive discussion of the prevalence of hearing impairment. Of the 40 million school-aged children in the United States, approximately 7 million have some degree of hearing impairment (Niskar et al., 1998; Ross, Brackett, & Maxon, 1991). Adams & Marano (1995) report fewer cases, indicating that approximately 1.2 million children under the age of 18 have either a congenital or an acquired hearing loss. According to Matkin (1991), approximately 1.4 percent of the school-age population (or 14 of every 1,000 children) demonstrates a significant hearing impairment relative to verbal communication, social and emotional growth, and academic achievement. These figures can be further interpreted as follows: 1 of every 1,000 children have severe or profound bilateral sensorineural hearing impairment, 7 of every 1,000 children have mild or moderate bilateral sensorineural hearing impairment, 2 of every 1,000 school age children have permanent unilateral hearing impairment, and 4 of every 1,000 school-age children have significant speech-language delays associated with a history of recurrent otitis media and conductive hearing impairment (Matkin, 1991). These figures may actually underestimate the magnitude of the problem. Flexer (1999) believes that there may be as many as two-thirds of the children in kindergarten and first grade classes who have persistent conductive hearing losses. This would greatly interfere with the overall development of children who are in the process of learning language and acquiring knowledge.

The early identification of children with hearing impairments, regardless of the extent of the hearing loss, should be of concern to the educational community. The effects of hearing loss on speech, language, social-emotional, and academic development are well documented (Baker-Hawkins & Easterbrooks, 1994; Quigley & Kretschmer, 1982; Bess et al., 1998). Flexer (1992) uses a computer analogy to describe the potentially negative effects of any type and degree of hearing loss on academic performance. She states, "data input precedes data processing." In other words, in order to learn, children need to have information or data. In the classroom, the primary way information is entered into the brain is via hearing (Berg, 1987). If data are entered inaccurately the child will have incomplete or incorrect information to process and their performance will be affected.

Northern Downs (1991) defines a hearing loss in children as "any degree of hearing that reduces the intelligibility of a speech message to a degree inadequate for accurate interpretation or learning." The term "hearing impaired" implies a hearing loss of at least 15 dB HL. A person with a loss of 70 dB or more is considered to be deaf. Two to three million children may demonstrate some form and degree of hearing impairment (Ross & Giolas, 1978).

There are numerous causes of hearing loss in children including middle ear infections, genetic causes, bacterial infections and viruses, prenatal causes, and noise exposure (Flexer, 1999). The following factors may place infants at risk for hearing loss:

- Family history of childhood hearing impairment
- Congenital perinatal infection
- Anatomic malformations involving the face, head, or neck
- Low birthweight (less than 1,500 grams)
- Hyperbilirubinemia (jaundice) at levels exceeding indications for an exchange transfusion
- Bacterial meningitis
- Severe asphyxia

Educationally, children with even mild and intermittent losses due to middle ear infection can have difficulties in the classroom. School children with hearing losses may be affected in three ways. They may experience delay in the development of communication skills, they may demonstrate poor academic achievement, or they may become socially isolated and have a poor self-concept due to reduced ability to understand and interact with others.

There are a number of problems a child may encounter in language learning if even a mild hearing loss exists. They may have difficulty abstracting the meanings of words due to inconsistent categorization of speech sounds. The noisy classroom may interfere with reception and their ability to discriminate sounds. They may encounter difficulty with perceiving meanings resulting in confusion in word naming and multiple meanings. It may be difficult for children with hearing problems to detect grammatical rules or identify relationships between words. Recognition of intonation and stress patterns or the emotional content of conversation will be challenging.

Referrals for Hearing Problems

Teachers and parents are excellent referral sources for hearing problems. As with identifying speech and language disabilities, the quality of the referral will be increased if groundwork is laid in advance. Referral sources must have an understanding of the importance of hearing for learning, those behaviors which might be representative of hearing problems, referral procedures, and follow-up recommendations. If a hearing loss is detected, the parent should be notified immediately of the results and recommendations. If warranted, the parent will be responsible for seeking medical assistance and informing school personnel of the results of any evaluations. Information about signs and symptoms individuals should consider significant needs to be provided through in-service meetings or written materials.

In 1995 The American Speech-Language-Hearing Association established the Panel on Audiologic Assessment to review and update pertinent policies and reports on guidelines for audiologic assessment and screening. The guidelines were adopted in 1996 (American Speech-Language-Hearing Association, 1997). The panel identified the following groups of children at high risk for potential outer and middle ear disorders: children who experience an episode of acute otitis media prior to 6 months of age; infants who have been bottle fed; children with craniofacial anomalies; ethnic populations with documented increased incidence of outer and middle ear disease; a family history of chronic or recurrent otitis media; children exposed to excessive cigarette smoke; youngsters living in crowded and unclean conditions; and children diagnosed with sensorineural hearing loss. The history can be obtained by interviewing parents or requesting information in the letter sent to inform them of the screening program and schedule.

Educators and parents can be encouraged to refer children who display the following behaviors (The Ohio Department of Health, 1990):

- *Appearance*—mouth breathing, discharge from the ear canal, malformation of the ear, ear wax impaction, damaged or poorly maintained hearing equipment
- *Behaviors*—constant tilting of the head toward the sound source, inability to follow verbal directions, inattention, pulling or rubbing the ears frequently, asking for repetition of words or phrases, misunderstanding conversation of others
- *Symptoms*—poor language development, buzzing or ringing in the ears, soreness or pain in or about the ears

Screening for Hearing Problems

Because of the importance of hearing to learning, school communication disorder professionals need to establish an ongoing identification program which will enable them to screen all children periodically during their school years. In addition, they should work closely with teachers to obtain referrals based on teachers' observations of the student's performance in the classroom. It is also helpful for parents, teachers, speech-language pathologists, and others to provide descriptions of the student's listening behavior when making a referral for a hearing evaluation. Pertinent information about the child's communication characteristics is particularly useful including:

- Child's ability to understand spoken directions and ability to follow directions with spoken words or gestures
- Child's ability to express needs with gestures, sounds, words, signs, and other symbols
- Ability of listeners to understand what the child is trying to say
- Child's behavioral response to sounds (startles, blinks, searching for sound, localizing sound, turning head in direction of sounds, and so on)

The members of the ASHA Panel on Audiologic Assessment (1997) recommended guidelines for audiologic screening across the life span. The guidelines consider several aspects related to screening including: (1) the principles of screening; (2) screening test performance; (3) screening program development, management and follow-up; (4) operating definitions; and (5) organizational framework. Screening involves a pass/refer procedure to identify children at risk for significant outer and middle ear disorders that have been undetected or untreated. The process includes an optional case history, visual examination, and acoustic immitance testing (ASHA Guidelines for Audiologic Screening, 1997).

The ASHA Panel on Audiologic Assessment developed guidelines for audiologic screening of infants and children birth through 18 years. The guidelines recommend the clinical processes for screening for outer and middle ear disorders among older infants and children and for screening for hearing impairment among newborns and infants (age birth through 6 months); infants and toddlers (age 7 months through 3 years); preschool children (age 3 through 5 years); and school-age children age 5 through 18 years. It is recommended that infants and children from 7 months through 6 years of age be screened. If it is not possible to screen those children, Bluestone and Klein (1996) recommend that children be screened if they present any of the significant clinical indications. The panel addressed several aspects of the clinical screening process including personnel, expected outcome, clinical indications, the clinical process, pass/refer criteria, follow-up procedures, facilities and equipment, and documentation. They also made a statement about inappropriate procedures. Since SLPs should be aware of these recommendations, the key points are highlighted in the following sections.

The student should pass the screening if no positive results exist for test criteria in both ears. He or she should be referred for a medical examination of the ears if ear drainage is observed; if there is previously undetected structural defects; if there are abnormalities in the ear canal; if the tympanometric equivalent ear canal volume is outside the normal range. The pass/refer criteria may need to be modified to optimize performance; but this should be done only by a qualified person.

Screening programs include procedures for detecting impairments of auditory sensitivity as well as peripheral auditory disorders. The goal is to identify individuals with hearing impairments that will potentially interfere with communication and/or individuals with potentially significant ear disorders that have been undetected or untreated. Children who fail the screening should have a complete audiological evaluation and medical examination.

The screening protocol requires an otoscope or video-otoscope, and a screening or diagnostic tympanometer. You should participate in training to use the equipment. All equipment should be appropriately calibrated and maintained for electrical safety. Appropriate infection control procedures should be followed.

As with the speech-language screening program, mandates requiring that specific age or grade levels be tested vary from state to state. It is a generally accepted practice to screen preschoolers prior to school entrance, children in kindergarten, first, third, fifth, and ninth grades, all new students, transfer students, teacher and parent referrals, and students at risk for hearing loss due to noise exposure or other conditions.

Parents should be informed that the screening is being conducted. There should be an educational component designed to inform parents about the screening and the likelihood that their child might have an ear disorder. The information should be presented in a language they understand. Follow-up procedures should be recommended.

Hearing Testing Procedures for Preschoolers and Students with Severe and Profound Developmental Disabilities

When evaluating youngsters with developmental disabilities, who may not be performing at age level, the Panel on Audiologic Assessment recommends that the guidelines followed should be appropriate for the youngster's developmental abilities. A key aspect for successful screening is the instruction and preparation of children for the situation. Infants, toddlers, young preschool children, and students with multiple, severe, and/or profound developmental disabilities may not be able to respond to traditional audiometric testing procedures. Testing of these groups should be conducted by an educational audiologist familiar with methodologies for assessing children who are difficult to test. In addition to information supplied by family and teacher observers, the testing is accomplished through multiple behavioral and objective testing procedures (Flexer, 1999).

Responsibility for the Hearing Screening and Testing Program

Who carries out the program of identifying children with hearing deficits in the schools? The Public Laws require the completion of an Individualized Education Plan or Individualized Family Service Plan for all children with special needs. This, of course, includes children with hearing impairments. Screening for hearing disorders requires professional expertise. The ASHA Guidelines for Audiologic Screening (1997) recommends that screening and testing be done by certified and licensed audiologists. SLPs who are certified and licensed may also conduct the screening; however, audiologists prefer that the program and protocols be devised and supervised by a qualified audiologist. Support personnel may conduct screening under the supervision of a certified audiologist.

Because the development of an audiologic screening program requires careful planning, implementation, and follow-up, it is recommended that it be designed, implemented, and supervised by a qualified audiologist. In many school systems educational audiologists are not available, nor do the school systems have access to audiological services in the community. If an audiologist is not available in the school district or region, SLPs would be wise to seek the advice and direction of a qualified audiologist. In some states school and public health nurses are licensed to conduct screenings in the schools. In many school systems the screenings are carried out by SLPs, nurses, or the cooperative efforts of both, often augmented by volunteers and aides. The personnel who administer the screening program should be adequately trained in the screening and referral procedures to ensure that the results they obtain are accurate and reliable. Ideally, the screening program should be at least supervised by an educational audiologist. Regardless of who implements the actual testing (educational audiologists, speech-language pathologists, or volunteers and aides), it must be implemented according to accepted standards of practice for identification audiometry.

The SLPs can provide a valuable service to youngsters with hearing impairment by promoting an understanding of hearing; helping others understand the impact of hearing loss; aiding in screening programs; providing intervention for speech and language disorders; monitoring the functioning of hearing aids and assistive listening devices; and helping teachers employ educational management strategies that improve classroom performance. Where no audiological services are available, the SLP often assumes the responsibility of the hearing-conservation program, including the screening program. Other options include contracting for educational audiology services or sharing service providers with nearby school districts.

There should be a record of identifying information, screening/rescreening results, and recommendations for follow-up. Give complete information about the procedures performed, the results obtained, and the personnel who performed the procedure.

Hearing Testing Facilities

School clinicians encounter a number of problems in screening programs. One major problem is the lack of an adequate environment that is conducive to achieving reliable test results. It would be extremely unusual to find a space with an ambient noise level that meets standards. Testing in unsuitable rooms results in a large number of false failures and eventually, in an inappropriate number of referrals. This can be translated into time wasted by the clinician and both time and money wasted by parents. Middle-ear problems are often associated with slight conductive losses, so it is a possibility that many children with middle ear pathologies will not be detected if there is not strict compliance with recommended screening procedures. When good testing facilities are not available within the school buildings, some schools and communities have attempted to solve the dilemma by taking the service to the client. Mobile testing units have been used with success in many parts of the United States and Canada. These vehicles, often custom designed, are self-contained units with their own water supply systems, heating and cooling systems, electrical power generators, and other necessities needed in such laboratories. The vehicles are fitted with soundproof rooms; noise-reduction barriers in the walls; clinic areas with desks, tables, and chairs; storage space for records; testing equipment; electronic calibrating equipment; and space for therapy equipment, supplies, and other materials needed.

ASSESSMENT

According to federal and state laws, all children with disabilities must be assessed before being placed in a special education program or before receiving related services. During the assessment process, data and evidence to support the presence of a communication disorder are gathered. Assessment is different from evaluation, which means interpreting or analyzing data. During assessment, information is gathered about the student's communication skills, the demands and expectations of the environment, and the manner and style of communication of the people in the child's environment. It is important to determine how these variables interact with one another.

Assessment cannot be discriminatory based on race, cultural diversity, or disability. In 1991, ASHA's Task Force on Clinical Standards established a draft of "preferred practice patterns" for the professions of speech-language pathology and audiology (Task Force on Clinical Standards, 1992). The document specifies the "professionals qualified to perform the procedure, the expected outcome(s), clinical indications for performing the procedure, clinical processes, environmental and equipment specifications, safety and health precautions, and documentation aspects" (p. i). Several recommendations for practice, regardless of setting, are addressed.

Assessment procedures are designed to produce a description of the communication behavior and gather information that will permit conclusions to be drawn about the student's strengths and deficits. It should help define contributing factors and functional implications. The results of the assessment must permit the clinician to determine the student's communication needs and how the communication impairment impacts on the student's educational performance. In addition, it should yield information about the positive and negative factors present in the communication situations that the student encounters.

During the assessment, information is gathered from numerous sources. A history is completed through interviews and review of available records. The child is observed in the school and class setting so that the communication performance within typical contexts can be determined. Safety and health precautions such as infection control procedures should be followed. After the assessment and evaluation are completed, the clinician should be able to develop a statement of the diagnosis and clinical description of the disorder, make recommendations for intervention, and make appropriate referrals.

Assessments must be administered in the child's preferred communication or linguistic system and must consider the child's age, medical status, and sensory status. This was also mandated in the 1997 reauthorization of IDEA. If these steps are not taken, the student may not be accurately assessed and the results will not honestly reflect the child's true achievement and aptitude level. Valid testing methods, standardized and nonstandardized, should be used. The materials, equipment, and environment selected for testing should be appropriate to the student's chronological and developmental age, physical and sensory abilities, education, and cultural/ethnic and linguistic background. For example, testing for a child who does not speak English should be conducted in the child's native language. Native language is defined as the language used by the child, not necessarily by the parents. A child who uses English at school but Spanish at home could be evaluated in English. However, if it is obvious that the child is more competent in Spanish, the testing must be done in Spanish.

Clinicians have successfully used many different methods for assessing students' communication skills. Valuable information can be obtained by interviewing parents and educators. A variety of materials can provide substantial insights into the youngster's capabilities. During any assessment, it is imperative to maintain a perspective that students develop at different rates and that each student is different. Assessment materials and procedures should be individualized and developmentally appropriate. They should yield information about how the student learns and what would be the best way to teach him or her.

Materials commonly used include portfolios of student work samples, language samples, journal entries, audio or video recordings, or class assignments. Student-created materials paint a much broader picture of the skills that are present. Schools maintain educational records that contain significant information. Completion of checklists or developmental scales enables comparison with other children in the same age group. Curriculum-based assessment methods such as reading inventories, proficiency tests, or other performance based reviews permit documentation of the performance within the educational context. SLPs have begun to use dynamic assessment methods that consider how the student performs after being provided with instructions and assistance. This permits insight into how the student might be able to benefit with intervention. Of course, many norm-referenced and standardized instruments are available for assessing students' communication skills in specific communication domains. Clinicians' experience and knowledge of communication development as well as acute observational skills provide a framework for conducting all assessment activities.

The process for learning is equally as important as the content of the curriculum. Cognitive-communication impairments may interfere with the learning process. Any data the SLP can contribute to increase education team members' understanding of this concept will likely result in better program planning for the student.

Documentation of procedures, findings, recommendations, and prognoses should be prepared. If treatment is indicated, recommendations of the frequency, estimated duration, and type of service required should be included.

MULTIFACTORED EVALUATION

Federal and state laws mandate that each child with disabilities should be assessed in several domains, not just the suspected area of deficit. This is necessary for developing an educationally relevant educational and treatment plan. The evaluation should be multifactored. This means that the evaluation will be conducted by a multidisciplinary team. More than one area of the student's functioning will be evaluated so that no single procedure will be the sole criteria for determining an appropriate educational program placement. This is very important and ensures that students are not misclassified or unnecessarily labeled as being disabled.

The communicative status of all students suspected as being disabled should be at least screened by a speech-language pathologist to rule out the presence of communication impairment. If the screening results suggest a communication problem, appropriate comprehensive assessment should be initiated. A key goal is to identify the difficulties the student is having with relationship to the general education curriculum and environment.

Diagnostic-educational teams provide a comprehensive multifactored assessment for children with potentially significant problems, including children with communication problems. The child must be assessed in all developmental domains. The domains include curricular areas that represent early childhood development: the adaptive domain, the aesthetic domain, the cognitive domain, the communication domain, the sensorimotor domain, and the social-educational domain. The areas related to the suspected disability are assessed, and include, if appropriate, assessment of health, vision, hearing, social and emotional status, general intelligence, academic performance and achievement, communicative status, motor abilities, interests, preferences, employability, and adaptive behavior.

Clinicians work in collaboration with other professionals. Professionals from related disciplines will complete many portions of the evaluation. This satisfies the requirement that the evaluation be multidisciplinary. Administration of the assessment protocol should be unbiased and given in such a way that it ensures that the student is not discriminated against regardless of cultural background, race, or disability.

The composition of the team may vary from district to district. The following personnel may be represented on teams: audiologists, guidance counselors, occupational therapists, physical education teachers, physical therapists, physicians, principals, reading specialists, regular classroom teachers, regular education supervisors, school nurses, school psychologists, social workers, special education supervisors, special education teachers, speech-language pathologists, and vision specialists. Parents, of course, contribute much to the evaluation process because they possess knowledge about their child's educational, social, and medical history.

Not all children with speech, language, or hearing impairments necessarily require a comprehensive evaluation, but such an evaluation of children with concomitant psychosocial or learning problems can be important in determining their placement and intervention follow-up. Many types of assessment tools and procedures should be used to gather data during the multifactored evaluation process including:

- Assessment of physical and development factors
- Administration of norm-referenced measures, criterion-referenced measures, standardized tests, and developmentally based tasks
- Observation of performance in different situations, including the classroom and elsewhere in the school environment
- Completion of interviews with significant persons including parents and teachers
- Analysis of class work samples
- Criterion-referenced tests, standardized achievement tests, and other educationally relevant evaluation procedures
- Review of family, school, and medical history

The data gathered are used to determine eligibility for special education or related services. If standardized tests are administered but the conditions under which they are administered are not standard, then a description must be included in the evaluation report indicating the extent to which the administration differed. An example of forms used by school districts for the multifactored evaluation can be found in Appendix C.

Steps in the Multifactored Assessment Process

Several steps must be followed during the multifactored assessment process including:

1. Appointing a multidisciplinary team to conduct the assessment
2. Developing of an assessment plan that addresses obtaining a comprehensive description of the problems the student is demonstrating; specifying the information needed; and selecting appropriate evaluation instruments
3. Conducting the multifactored assessment
4. Analyzing the results
5. Preparing a report of findings and reviewing the findings with other team members and the child's parents

6. Determining recommendations for placement and intervention
7. Developing a plan for an individualized education program, individualized family service plan, or individualized transition plan

After all team members have completed their evaluation procedures and analyzed their findings, the information gathered by each member should be integrated and synthesized into one report. A sample comprehensive multifactored evaluation report form (see Appendix C) illustrating the extensive amount of information that was gathered and analyzed in order to plan an individualized education program for a student is provided for your review (Akron Public School, 2000).

SPEECH-LANGUAGE PATHOLOGIST'S RESPONSIBILITY

The speech-language pathologist in the school system has the responsibility of providing diagnostic services for children referred by the multifactored assessment team (of which the specialist may be a member). This includes all the children picked up during speech, language, and hearing screening and those referred by teachers, nurses, parents, and others.

A minimal diagnostic appraisal would include an assessment of the pupil's articulation abilities and language competencies, fluency, voice quality, and hearing acuity, and perception. Figure 7.4 provides a listing of components of communicative status that should be evaluated for children with various disabilities (Ohio Statewide Task Force on Language, 1991). There should also be an examination of the peripheral speech mechanism. It is also important to have additional information, which can be obtained through a case history. Such information would include developmental history, family status and social history, medical history, and educational history. A physical examination may be needed as well as a psychological and educational evaluation.

Parental permission is required for the evaluation procedures. Protocols should be developed to ensure confidentiality. The permission should be in writing, and usually a form is utilized for this purpose. In some cases the school system may not be able to provide some of the diagnostic procedures because of lack of specialized personnel. In this event the school system may arrange to have these procedures carried out by a qualified agency with qualified personnel in the immediate community or nearby. It is the responsibility of the school system to see that the required procedures are carried out. Such referrals are made only after written permission is obtained from parents.

It should be kept in mind that the purpose of the appraisal and diagnostic procedures is to select children who may be placed in the speech-language program in the school. The school clinician must be prepared to describe how the pupil's disability will interfere with his or her ability to profit from classroom instruction. The final decision regarding eligibility for program services rests with the school team.

IDEA describes a speech or language impairment as "a communication disorder, such as stuttering, impaired articulation, a language impairment, or a voice impairment that adversely affects a child's educational performance" [Section 300.7 (b)(11)]. States may establish definitions for clinicians and others to follow that differ from the federal definition.

FIGURE 7.4 Suggested Components of the Evaluation of Communicative Status for Disability

DEVELOPMENTALLY HANDICAPPED
- listening comprehension
- oral expression
- written expression
- articulation/phonology
- pragmatic skills survey

HEARING HANDICAPPED
- audiological/auditory tests
- articulation screening/evaluation
- listening comprehension
- oral expression
- written expression
- sign expression
- pragmatic skills survey

MULTIHANDICAPPED
- listening comprehension
- oral expression
- written expression
- articulation/phonology
- assessment of augmentative potential (if nonverbal)

ORTHOPEDICALLY AND/OR OTHER HEALTH HANDICAPPED
- oral/motor examination
- articulation screening/evaluation
- listening comprehension
- oral expression
- written expression
- assessment of augmentative potential (if nonverbal)

SEVERE BEHAVIOR HANDICAPPED
- listening comprehension
- oral expression
- written expression
- articulation/phonology
- pragmatic skills survey

SPECIFIC LEARNING DISABLED
- listening comprehension
- oral expression
- language sample
- written expression
- pragmatic skills survey
- observation of classroom language
- articulation screening/evaluation
- meta-linguistic skills assessment
- auditory segmentation skills

SPEECH HANDICAPPED
- specialized assessments in phonology, articulation, voice, fluency, pragmatics, semantics, syntax, morphology, auditory processing, and memory
- language sample
- observation of language skills in the classroom
- analysis of problem areas in curriculum and school
- teacher-student interviews
- auditory segmentation skills
- written expression

VISUALLY HANDICAPPED
- listening comprehension
- oral expression
- articulation/phonology
- pragmatic skills survey
- assessment of augmentative potential (use of Braille and other devices)

Reprinted with permission of The Ohio Department of Special Education.

SCANNING AND ANALYZING THE ENVIRONMENT AND PEOPLE IN THE ENVIRONMENT

Clinicians must be prepared to conduct comprehensive assessments of many elements in order to determine a student's problem and to confidently make recommendations for intervention. There is a planning concept that businesses and organizations use when determining their plans for the future. It is referred to as "scanning and analyzing the environment" (see Figure 7.5). Speech-language pathologists can benefit from borrowing this concept (Blosser & DePompei, 1994). In this process, the SLP obtains a clear picture of the child's communication problems by conducting assessments of the following four aspects:

- The communication problems the student presents (medical and educational history; communication skills; strengths; needs; results from evaluation)
- The environment in which he or she lives, plays, and learns (expectations; demands; capabilities; modifications required)
- The people in that environment who serve as significant communication partners (understanding of the student's problem; the partner's communication characteristics; ability to provide assistance)
- The student's opinion, desires, understanding, and impressions (understanding of the communication problem; goals; feelings; and recommendations for assistance)

This model will be further explored throughout the book.

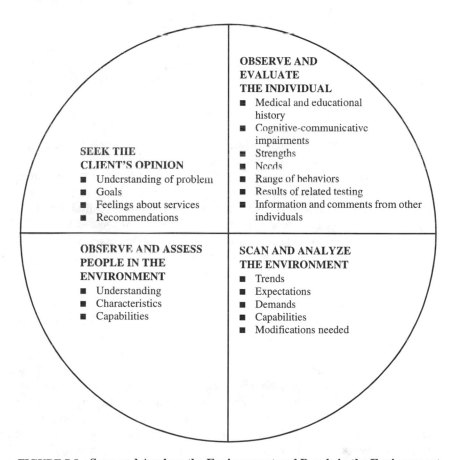

FIGURE 7.5   Scan and Analyze the Environment and People in the Environment

When assessing the student's communication skills, it is necessary to gather as much pertinent information as possible through a case history, medical history, and educational history. Information can be obtained by conducting interviews with the parents, the teachers, and if possible, the child. Records and reports can also be useful. Each informant contributes information vital to the construction of a whole picture of the child. The parents can give background information on the development of the child and the teachers may provide needed information on the present academic status of the child. The teacher should be interviewed to determine the communication requirements for success within the classroom setting and the student's present communication performance on educational and social tasks. This aspect of the assessment permits the team to determine the student's communication strengths and needs, the range of behaviors exhibited, and the results of tests that have been administered.

Observing the student in the home environment, classroom, and at play as a component of the appraisal process will yield valuable information for formulating the diagnosis and developing an intervention plan. Observations should help the team gain an understanding of the varying demands and expectations present in different situations and the student's capabilities for meeting those demands.

Holzhauser-Peters developed the observation checklist for conducting classroom evaluations presented in Figure 7.6 (Holzhauser-Peters and Husemann, 1988).

Observing those individuals who will communicate with the youngster on a daily basis will provide significant information about their understanding of the student's problem, how that problem impacts learning, and how their own communication characteristics can help or hinder the child. This will be explored further in Chapter 10. Increasing significant communication partners' awareness of the dynamics of the communication disability and explaining how they might contribute to the child's success by altering their own behavior will lead to a more effective treatment plan.

Children should be incorporated into the planning of their own treatment as often as possible. The SLP can contribute to the development of strong self-advocacy skills in the child by providing opportunities for better understanding the disability. If provided with guided questions geared toward the child's developmental age and level of understanding, the student may also be able to contribute to the development of intervention goals and activities. Youngsters can provide information that may be of great value to the clinician. Figure 7.7 illustrates a student interview form developed by Blosser and DePompei (1994). Note the questions that are asked of students that can lead to goals that meet students' needs and interests.

After the background information is obtained, the clinician needs to add to it by describing the problem. Observing the child's performance on appropriate tests that measure the degree of the problem and suggest associated aspects does this. The clinician must be an astute observer and must be able to record information objectively and without bias. In other words, the clinician must be a good "reporter." After all the information has been gathered, the clinician makes a diagnosis of the communication problem (or problems).

A diagnosis, or identification of the problem, is in reality a tentative diagnosis because as a human being grows and changes, the problem changes. A diagnosis is much more than putting a label on a person. It is convenient for professional persons to use diagnostic labels when communicating with one another if all parties concerned understand that the label is

FIGURE 7.6   Classroom Observation Checklist for Use by SLPs

Student's Name_____   Time of Observation _____

Classroom Teacher _____   Class Observed _____

School _____

1. Presentation of information

Where does teacher stand to present information?

- ☐ front of room _____
- ☐ side of room _____
- ☐ walks around _____
- ☐ Lecture _____
- ☐ Oral reading by various students in class _____
- ☐ Drill _____
- ☐ Hands-on activities _____
- ☐ other _____

_____

2. Presentation of assignments/homework

How are assignments presented?

- ☐ written on board _____
- ☐ verbally presented _____
- ☐ both _____
- ☐ other _____

_____

3. Seating arrangement

Where is student sitting?

- ☐ front _____   ☐ back _____
- ☐ center of room _____   ☐ by window _____
- ☐ other _____

_____

4. Environment—overall

- ☐ Relaxed—time to do things at an even pace
- ☐ Fast—pushed for time
- ☐ Noise level _____
  - noisy _____
  - quiet _____
  - moderate _____

(continued)

FIGURE 7.6   Continued

Comments: _____

_____

5. **Distractions**

☐ Is child distracted by other children? _____

noise _____

other _____

☐ Does child distract others? _____

Describe: _____

_____

6. **Textbooks**

Look at

☐ vocabulary _____

☐ language complexity _____

☐ concepts presented _____

☐ concepts needed to understand _____

☐ other _____

Textbook format

☐ topic headings _____

☐ summary at end of chapter _____

☐ other _____

_____

7. **How does this child indicate what he or she knows? How does teacher determine competency level?**

Worksheets

☐ Are worksheets used a great deal?

☐ What skills must student possess to complete the worksheets? _____

☐ Are worksheets   black _____

blue _____

clear _____

Written Essays/Papers _____

Tests

Types of tests given

☐ worksheets _____

☐ multiple choice _____

☐ fill in blank _____

☐ other _____

_____

8. Does student have option of taking test?

☐ orally _____

☐ written _____

☐ both _____

9. Does child participate in class?

☐ Raises hand appropriately _____

☐ Shouts out _____

☐ Does child have time to respond when called upon? _____

Does child respond

☐ immediately _____

☐ need more time to respond _____

Comments: _____

_____

10. Transition

When class moves from one subject or task to another, how does teacher cue children into transition?

☐ physically (with body movements) _____

☐ verbally _____

☐ bell _____

☐ other _____

☐ Does student pick up on this cue? _____

11. Child's organizational skills

Does child remember?

☐ homework assignments _____

☐ books needed to take home _____

☐ what books and materials to take to next class _____

☐ schedule of classes and daily events _____

Comments: _____

_____

12. Study skills

Does child know how to study?

☐ to remember only important information _____

☐ scan chapter first to review headings _____

☐ read chapter summary first _____

(continued)

FIGURE 7.6   Continued

☐ get clues by looking at worksheet first to determine how to do and then read directions

_____

☐ how to take notes _____

☐ how to outline _____

Comments: _____

_____

13. Verbal organizational skills

Student:

☐ answers simple questions requiring a one word or 1–2 sentence response

☐ relates information in an understandable cohesive manner

☐ during conversations with adults

☐ during conversations with friends

☐ during class discussions through

written assignments _____

oral presentations _____

☐ communicates wants and needs

☐ relates the sequence of events in the proper order

☐ communicates something that has happened recently _____

in the distant past

will happen in the future

☐ relates feelings

☐ relates thoughts

☐ relates opinions

Comments: _____

_____

14. Requests for assistance

When the student has difficulty with a task he

☐ requests assistance   ☐ gives up   ☐ other (Describe) _____

_____

15. General

Does child seem to exhibit skills comparable to other children in the class or does the student stand out? Describe how the student "stands out" from the group. Give examples of specific situations when the student "stands out" and also when he "fits in."

_____

_____

_____

FIGURE 7.7   Student Interview Questions

LET US KNOW HOW TO HELP YOU

You are the best judge of how other people can cause problems for you or help you do better. Answer these 10 questions and let's work together to think of some helpful solutions.

1. What problems are you experiencing in class (at home, at work)? Briefly describe the problems you are having since you returned to school (your home, work, and so on).

2. How do you usually act when you are experiencing problems or frustrations in class (at home, at work)? **List some of the ways you behave when you are having problems.**

3. What classroom (home or work) situation causes you the most problems?
   - noise
   - temperature
   - pictures and wall decorations
   - other people in the room
   - other things

4. List several ways your teachers (family, classmates, coworkers) help you when you experience trouble in class (at home or work).

5. What do you think people should do to help you?

6. List several things your teachers (classmates, coworkers) do to frustrate you or cause you more problems.

7. What do you think people should stop doing when they are around you?

8. At what time of day do you do your best? Why do you feel this is your best time of day?
   - early morning
   - mid-morning
   - around noon
   - mid-afternoon
   - early evening
   - late evening

9. If you could choose three skills to improve, what would they be?

10. Tell five things that are great about you that you wish other people knew.

---

not the diagnosis. A diagnosis involves weighing all the evidence, discarding some of it as not being pertinent, and keeping the information that merits further investigation.

On the basis of the gathered information, the testing, and the tentative diagnosis, the clinician then determines the prognosis and sets up a long-range plan for the intervention procedures. The long-range plan includes therapy appropriate to the communication problem as well as other strategies and treatment. The school clinician is involved in a collaborative team approach with others who are interested in the child's welfare, and these individuals work as a team in establishing an individualized education program (IEP), individualized family service plan (IFSP), or individualized transition plan (ITP). The school clinician is responsible for the appraisal and diagnosis of the communication problem, but the clinician is a team member in the overall appraisal, diagnosis, and treatment of the child. Final decisions about the student's educational placement rests with the team, including the parents.

CASE SELECTION

After students with communication impairments have been identified and the assessment data gathered, the clinician evaluates the data and comes to a conclusion about the nature and severity of the disorder. It is at this point that the SLP and fellow team members face three difficult tasks. First, the team must determine if the student meets the *eligibility criteria* for treatment and services. Second, children selected need to be *prioritized on the caseload.* Third, the *service delivery model* most appropriate to meet the student's needs must be determined. The type of services to be provide as well as the service providers and the frequency and intensity of treatment are critical aspects of the caseload selection process.

Educational colleagues and school administrators responsible for determining policy for special education programs in the district should be aware of the decision-making criteria that is being followed to determine eligibility, severity, and priority case selection. The case selection system should be in written form and made available to administrators and educators within the district in order to improve accountability and understanding of the functioning of the program. The understanding of the case selection system and the cooperation of other school personnel would have to be enlisted for the system to function satisfactorily. The principal is a key figure in the success of such a program. Teachers also have to be familiar with case selection procedures in order for them to work well with clinicians and youngsters in their classroom. Having a documented system for selecting cases can also be useful in helping parents understand the rationale for recommendations regarding their child's program. It can also be used to provide information about why youngsters are not eligible for services should questions arise.

ELIGIBILITY CRITERIA

Clinicians develop eligibility criteria to enable a more definitive means of identifying the population to be served and to provide a more consistent means of applying criteria across the school district (Work, 1989). The eligibility criteria established should be standardized within the school district and appropriate to the population served with respect to age, culture and/or linguistic diversity, cognitive factors, and health status. Some state departments of education have established eligibility criteria for speech-language intervention programs as well as for other special education programs. Where statewide criteria are not available, clinicians often establish criteria for their local districts. ASHA has provided some guidance on determining eligibility criteria over the past several years. Task forces and committees continue to work on interpretations that are helpful to practitioners. Two documents that are available are *Issues in Determining Eligibility for Language Intervention* (1989) and *Admission/Discharge Criteria in Speech-Language Pathology* (1994).

Clinicians within a district should work together to determine how they will interpret specific aspects of the eligibility criteria including terminology and application to certain populations such as adolescents or students who are mentally retarded. Eligibility criteria provide a mechanism to ensure consistency of case selection among clinicians in a district. It also serves as a framework for evaluation of the demographics of the caseload (numbers, types of disorders, and severity of students served). A fully certified speech-language pathologist must base eligibility for speech and language services on a comprehensive evaluation. The clinician and team must then consider the relationship between the student's speech and language disabilities and the adverse effect they may have on the student's ability to learn the general school curriculum including academic, social-emotional, or vocational aspects. Thus, the team must consider the need for services as well as the eligibility for services on the basis of federal and state mandates and local policies and procedures (ASHA, 1999).

THE DEFINITION OF TERMS

A good place to start any process is to come to an agreement on the definition of terms. Clinicians who work together in a particular school district, region, or state will find it useful to mutually agree on definitions to be used to describe and discuss children with communication disabilities.

Over the years many ASHA committees have reviewed terminology and submitted definitions to the membership of ASHA for agreement. Definitions for communication disorders and treatment have been accepted by the association and disseminated for use by federal, state, and local agencies and others concerned with programs for those with communication impairments. The school pathologist must be able to define and interpret the terminology to parents, teachers, medical personnel, and legislators. The definitions of communication disorders and variations are presented on pages 152–153.

CLASSIFICATION OF PROCEDURES AND COMMUNICATION DISORDERS

In 1987, the ASHA Executive Board approved The American Speech-Language-Hearing Association Classification of Speech-Language Pathology and Audiology Procedures and Communication Disorders, commonly referred to as the ASHA Classification System (ASHACS). This provides a standardized system for coding and indexing procedures and diagnoses commonly used by speech-language pathologists and audiologists. The school speech-language pathologist or audiologist can use the nomenclature and classification system to uniformly describe communication disorders and the procedures being used. The system is especially valuable for clinicians who are interested in analyzing their service programs, generating research data about their caseloads, or developing a computerized information management system. While the actual code numbers used in the system do not correspond to those used by third party reimbursement sources, the terminology used in the ASHACS is widely accepted by payers. The Classification System is presented in Appendix A.

A communicative disorder is an impairment in the ability to (1) receive and/or process a symbol system, (2) represent concepts or symbol systems, and/or (3) transmit and use symbol systems. The impairment is observed in disorders of hearing, language, and/or speech processes. A communicative disorder may range in severity from mild to profound. It may be developmental or acquired, and individuals may demonstrate one or any combination of the three aspects of communicative disorders. The communicative disorder may result in a primary handicapping condition or it may be secondary to other handicapping conditions.

I.   A speech disorder is an impairment of voice, articulation of speech sounds, and/or fluency. These impairments are observed in the transmission and use of the oral symbol system.
   A. A voice disorder is defined as the absence or abnormal production of vocal quality, pitch, loudness, resonance, and/or duration.
   B. An articulation disorder is defined as the abnormal production of speech sound.
   C. Fluency disorder is defined as the abnormal flow of verbal expression, characterized by impaired rate and rhythm which may be accompanied by struggle behavior.

II.   A language disorder is the impairment or deviant development of comprehension and/or use of a spoken, written, and/or other symbol system. The disorder may involve (a) the form of language (phonologic, morphologic, and syntactic systems), (b) the content of language (semantic system), and/or (c) the function of language in communication (pragmatic system) in any combination.
   A. Form of language
      1. Phonology is the sound system of a language and the linguist rules that govern the sound combinations.
      2. Morphology is the linguistic rule system that governs the structure of words and the construction of word forms from the basic elements of meaning.
      3. Syntax is the linguistic rule governing the order and combination of words to form sentences, and the relationships among the elements within a sentence.
   B. Content of language
      1. Semantics is the psycholinguistic system that patterns the content of an utterance, intent, and meanings of words and sentences.
   C. Function of language
      1. Pragmatics is the sociolinguistic system that patterns the use of language communication which may be expressed motorically, vocally, or verbally.

III. A hearing disorder is altered auditory sensitivity, acuity, function, processing, and/or damage to the integrity of the physiological auditory system. A hearing disorder may impede the development, comprehension, production, or maintenance of language, speech, and/or interpersonal exchange. Hearing disorders are classified according to difficulties in detection, perception, and/or processing of auditory information. Hearing impaired individuals frequently are described as deaf or hard of hearing.
   A. Deaf is defined as a hearing disorder that impedes an individual's communicative performance to the extent that the primary sensory avenue for communication may be other than the auditory channel.
   B. Hard of hearing is defined as a hearing disorder whether fluctuating or permanent, which adversely affects an individual's communication performance. The hard of hearing individual relies on the auditory channel as the primary sensory avenue for speech and language.

IV. Communicative Variations
   A. Communicative difference/dialect is a variation of a symbol system used by a group of individuals which reflects and is determined by shared regional, social, or cultural/ethnic factors. Variations or alterations in the use of a symbol system may be indicative of primary language interferences. A regional, social, or cultural/ethnic variation of a symbol system should not be considered a disorder of speech or language.
   B. Augmentative communication is a system used to supplement the communicative skills of individuals for whom speech is temporarily or permanently inadequate to meet communicative needs. Both prosthetic devices and/or nonprosthetic techniques may be designed for individual use as an augmentative communication system.

Prepared by: The Committee on Language, Speech, and Hearing Services in the Schools (1982). Various definitions and eligibility criteria may exist for determining degree of handicap and disability compensation. The definitions in this document are not intended to address issues of eligibility and compensation.

PRIORITY SYSTEM OF CASELOAD SELECTION

Clinicians often have difficulty determining which youngsters to serve, how frequently to see them, and what type of service delivery model to provide. These decisions are especially difficult when there are numerous children who present communication disorders. Priority ranking enables the clinician to systematically determine those students most in need. Eligibility and priority ranking systems developed by clinicians range from very simple to very complex. It is most important to create a system that makes sense and all are willing to implement.

The development of an eligibility and priority rating system should be directed by several guiding principles. In this way, the process of case selection will ensure continuity and consistency among all clinicians within the school district. Consequently, it can then be used to organize the service delivery program according to pupils' needs. A rationale can be determined for the allocation of treatment time. There will be accountability for decisions. If a method is appropriately designed, it will incorporate observation of consistent variables by SLPs, teachers, parents, and other professionals without compromising clinical judgment. It will assist the clinician in case selection and suggest the intensity of service, the treatment providers, and the delivery model for the least restrictive alternative in a continuum of service delivery options.

Some priority and severity rating scales provide a numerical index to facilitate the rating process. Categories can be made for (1) standardized (norm-referenced) test results; (2) nonstandardized (descriptive) assessment results; (3) educational relevance and potential impact on educational performance; (4) specific types of disorder; and, (5) prognostic indicators that indicate low potential for success. Following is an explanation of each category.

Standardized Test Results.   Students are provided with a complete multifactored, multidisciplinary test battery. A basic numerical factor is obtained from the results of the evaluation. Some protocols assign numeric value to test scores.

Nonstandardized (Descriptive) Assessment Results.   Clinicians use a variety of methods to collect data about a student's functional communication skills and needs. Common procedures include checklists, interviews, developmental scales, review of student's work, curriculum-based assessment, samples of speech and language performance, and observations in different settings. Again, support for eligibility will increase or decrease based on the findings.

Educational Relevance and Potential Impact on Educational Performance.   Upon evaluation of the assessment data and determination of the type of disabilities that are present, the SLP and team should determine how the communication impairment may interfere with the student's learning. Three key educational areas that may be affected are academic, social-emotional, and vocational performance. If the SLP, teachers, and family all agree there is an adverse effect upon educational performance, the eligibility for treatment would increase.

Specific Type and Severity of Communication Disorder.   Some types of disorders the student exhibits may interfere more with successful educational performance than do others. Likewise, the severity of the disorder will cause differing levels of performance. When SLPs complete their evaluation of specific speech and language areas, they are able to discuss the likely impact of the presenting disorder on the youngster's performance on specific aspects of the curriculum such as reading, writing, oral speaking, mathematics, and so on.

Prognostic Indicators.   Some aspects of the student's performance may, in fact, indicate that treatment is not warranted. By considering those prognostic factors that do not support treatment, the clinician can provide documentation and rationale for not providing services or for reducing and limiting services to students. This includes consideration of factors such as comparison of communication skills to mental age or communication characteristics of peers; potential change due to maturation; lack of stimulability; reaching a plateau in performance or maximum potential; and poor attitude or prior attendance.

   The diagnostic and eligibility factors determine the type of service that should be provided and lead to recommendations regarding who will provide the services and the frequency and amount of treatment time. A student whose communication is within normal limits is ineligible for services. The child with a mild communicative problem may be served effectively through indirect or alternative service delivery models. The student with severe disabilities generally needs more direct and frequent services. In all cases, it will be important for the SLP and education staff to plan collaboratively to determine how the student's needs can be best met.

   While a system that is developed for one school system may not be applicable to all school districts, it is important to adhere to a conceptual framework when thinking about how to make caseload selection and service delivery model decisions. Using systematized methods will enable the clinician to be accountable for the decisions. Ultimately, this type of information is necessary in order to document the importance and effectiveness of the speech-language intervention program. Data generated will help the clinician support discussion of changes in program design and implementation of new service delivery models.

DESCRIBING THE FUNCTIONAL STATUS OF THE COMMUNICATION

Over the last several years, ASHA has supported the development of a project to obtain data about treatment outcomes. This project, called the National Outcome Measurement System (NOMS) project, is the first step in a national effort to develop a common language for describing and rating students' communication skills. The NOMS, while still being investigated to determine reliability and validity, offers a framework and mechanism that clinicians can use to generate data about treatment outcomes. It provides a systematic method for measuring different aspects of a student's functional communication or related disorders. The Functional Communication Measures (FCMs) can be used by school-based clinicians to report descriptive data about their caseloads and service delivery models. They can also be used to measure the effectiveness of treatment over time (Blosser, Ehren, Subich, & Ribbler, 1999).

The NOMS includes a seven point rating scales ranging from least functional to most functional or independent. Functional communication is defined as the ability to convey or receive a message regardless of the mode of communication. The mode should not affect the communication performance rating score unless the child requires assistance or prompting to use the mode of communication. For the instrument, the following definitions were developed for evaluating the functional status measures using a scale of independence as a benchmark:

No Basis for Testing—Circumstances in which a behavior cannot be observed, directly tested, and/or the information is not available from other sources.

Cannot Do—The child cannot perform the communication behavior, even with maximal assistance and/or prompting.

Can Do with Maximal Assistance—The child performs the communication behavior only with constant assistance and/or prompting.

Can Do with Moderate to Maximal Assistance—The child performs the communication behavior but very frequently needs assistance and/or prompting.

Can Do with Minimal to Moderate Assistance—The child performs the communication behavior, often needing assistance and prompting.

Can Do with Minimal Assistance—The child performs the communication behavior, rarely needing assistance and/or prompting.

Can Do—The child performs the communication behavior, needing no assistance and/or prompting.

As the NOMS project continues and the results are verified through additional research, there will be opportunities for determining how these instruments can be used to describe students' communication behaviors and to help make clinical decisions.

RATING THE SEVERITY OF THE COMMUNICATION IMPAIRMENT

The severity of the impairment is an important factor in determining the need for treatment, the appropriate program placement and/or service delivery model, the intensity and frequency of services, and intervention strategies for children with communication disabilities.

Unfortunately, there are no uniform procedures or guidelines for rating severity which are common to the profession. Clinicians have developed different methods for rating severity. Generally the models developed are based on a continuum of performance model. Descriptive statements are provided to assist the user in deciding the rating number or category to assign. For example, a rating scale for articulation may consider intelligibility, phonological processes, error types, and development. The language category may considers results of informal assessment measures, impact on educational performance, pragmatic skills, results of formal measures, and other factors. A voice scale might rate symptoms, reactions of casual listeners, reactions of significant others, pupil awareness, and the overall effect on communication. The fluency category would most likely consider the interference with communication interaction, the number of stuttered words per minute and percentage of words stuttered, speech rate, duration, awareness, and secondary characteristics. Some considerations should be made for children with disabilities in addition to communication impairments such as mental and developmental disabilities.

These aspects of communication should never be considered in isolation. They should be made in relation to the student's age, the demands and expectations of the communication situation, and the impact on learning and performance in the educational setting.

CLINICAL JUDGMENT

Regardless of the rating procedure or scale used, we cannot dismiss the importance of clinical judgment. In conjunction with assessment methods, the speech-language clinician needs to consider the following factors:

- The consistency of the inappropriate communication patterns
- The pupil's ability to interact verbally with others
- The effect of the communication problem on school performance
- The possible impact of the communication problem on the listener
- The ability of the pupil to communicate well enough to satisfy his or her needs
- The status of speech and language stimulation in the home
- The student's response to stimulation of the deficit in speech and language structures
- The student's chronological age in comparison with the expected age for developing the communication skills which are in deficit or missing

PROGNOSTIC INDICATORS

Speech-language pathologists also exercise their clinical judgement when determining which youngsters to serve and which service delivery models to provide. They consider the prognostic indicators, or variables which are likely to contribute to a students' success or lack of success in the speech and language program. Some prognostic indicators that are considered include:

- Chronological and mental age of the child
- Overall intelligibility

- Type of communication problem detected
- Response to intervention methods
- Intelligence
- Responsiveness to correction
- Cultural variables
- Gross and fine motor skills
- Auditory memory span
- Orofacial functioning and structure
- Discrimination skills
- Personality and adjustment
- Length of time in therapy
- General health
- Support and cooperation provided by family and teachers
- Academic performance
- Self motivation

CRITERIA FOR DISMISSAL FROM THERAPY

In the process of selecting students for therapy, diagnosing, providing therapeutic intervention, and maintaining students in therapy, sometimes too little attention is paid to dismissal. The question of when a pupil should be dismissed from treatment may be predicated on when the pupil reaches maximum anticipated performance or when the pupil's communication problem has been completely improved.

After the pupil has been placed in a therapy program the short- and long-term performance objectives are identified and written in the intervention plan. The objectives are based on what is identified through testing, observation, comments from parents and teachers, and discussion with the pupil. In this way it is determined what the student needs to learn.

The long-term objectives are what are hoped the student is able to do at the termination of the treatment program. They are the desired outcomes of treatment. The short-term objectives are the steps through which the student must progress successfully to reach the long-term objectives. This, in effect, means that long-term (or terminal) objectives constitute the exit criteria, or the point at which the student is dismissed from therapy. This is part of the intervention plan (IEP, IFSP, or ITP). Example of an Individualized Education Plan form and steps in the planning process are presented in Appendix C.

Obviously, the nature of the disorder will have a direct bearing on the expected outcome of treatment. For example, a student with cerebral palsy and apraxia of the speech musculature may not be expected to attain "normal" speech patterns, depending on the extent of the involvement. This dismissal point for this pupil may be "adequate" speech or understandable communication using an augmentative device. A student with a phonological problem may be potentially able to attain a more complete mastery of the distorted sounds, and the dismissal point for this pupil would be when the student could use the sounds correctly.

The SLP must develop dismissal criteria that is unique for each student and terminate therapy when these criteria are met. This means that dismissal from therapy may occur at any time during the school year. This is a change in practice for some clinicians who are used to carrying students on their caseloads throughout an entire academic year. Students who have not reached optimum improvement at the end of the school term are often continued into the following term. Students who transfer to another school are referred to the SLP in that school system. Parents should be urged to inform the new school that their child has been in therapy and that they wish it to continue. In this situation, the referring clinician secures the proper release forms to transfer the student's therapy records to the new school.

Dismissals need not be absolute. No clinician is wise enough to be able to dismiss a child from therapy with the absolute certainty that the child will never again need it. When a dismissal is made, the child should be scheduled for periodic rechecks to find out if the therapy has held. In a school it is important to have the classroom teacher check this also. It will be necessary to be very specific with the teacher on what to check. The same holds true for parents. A dismissal, then, could be called a temporary dismissal.

What we are doing as clinicians is trying to make each client his or her own clinician. In other words, we try to bring students to the point where they are able to monitor their own speech, language, or auditory problem to such an extent that they no longer need us. This is sometimes painful for clinicians to do, and at times the student is reluctant to be dismissed from therapy. Both these factors must be objectively viewed by the clinician. When the student has reached the optimum levels of performance, it is time for dismissal. The criteria for dismissal are unique to each child and must be carefully established, evaluated, and reevaluated during the course of treatment. If necessary, they must be adjusted or modified in the light of more knowledge about the student. In addition to providing rating scales for determining selection for the caseload (entrance criteria), it is also important to provide clear guidelines for determining readiness for program completion (exit criteria). Some examples of exit criteria are listed below:

- Speech and language goals and objectives have been met.
- Speech and language skills are developmentally appropriate or are no longer academically, socially, personally, or emotionally affecting the student. Documentation must be presented by one or more of the following: pupil, teachers, parents, speech and language clinician.
- The pupil has made minimal or no measurable progress after one academic school year of consecutive management strategies. During that time, program modifications and varied approaches have been attempted and a second opinion has been obtained.
- Maximum compensatory skills have been achieved or progress has reached a plateau due to cognitive ability level, structural deviations (e.g. severe malocclusion, repaired cleft lip or palate, physical condition of the vocal mechanism, or other physical deviations or conditions); or neuromotor functioning (e.g. apraxia or dysarthria).
- Limited carryover has been documented due to the pupil's lack of physical, mental, or emotional ability to self-monitor or generalize the behavior in one or more environments.
- Lack of progress or inability to retain learned skills due to poor attendance and participation, although program IEP goals and objectives have not been met. Poor attendance and participation records should not stand alone, rather it is the lack of progress or retention which is of primary concern when utilizing this criteria.

In addition to providing rating scales that can be used for determining selection for the caseload (entrance criteria), it is also important to provide clear guidelines for determining readiness for program completion (exit criteria). Examples of reasons for dismissal from the NOMS project include:

- Goals met and no further intervention needed
- Summer recess and discontinued intervention planned for the coming year
- Family moved
- Illness or medical complications
- Student withdrew from the school
- Educational team has moved the student from the school
- Other

WHO DETERMINES ELIGIBILITY FOR SPEECH-LANGUAGE PROGRAM SERVICES?

A placement team comprised of those individuals with the greatest knowledge of the child must always make the decision regarding eligibility for services and appropriate placement of the child with disabilities. This includes the child's parents or guardians. The federal law also specifies that the team should include a representative of the local educational agency, the teacher, and if appropriate, the child. Although the law does not state that other individuals are required to be present, good educational practice would suggest that other team members also attend. This list would include those persons who by virtue of their professional backgrounds and the child's unique needs would reasonably be expected to be involved. It might include the principal, psychologist, reading teacher, occupational therapist, physical therapist, vision consultant, and speech-language pathologist and audiologist. The results of the multifactored evaluation and the possible placement options should be available when the placement team meets.

Coordinator of the Placement Team. The representative of the local educational agency usually is the team captain and coordinator, and as such arranges for the meeting, presides over the meeting, determines that all necessary persons are present, and acts as spokesperson for the school system. The chairperson presents the necessary information and data or calls on the person responsible for presenting it. The chairperson also has the responsibility of informing the parents of their rights. Setting the tone of the meeting and seeing that all the basic ingredients of the individualized education program are present, and that the procedures are carried out according to state and local guidelines, are also within the responsibilities of the chairperson.

The Teacher as a Team Member. The teacher is the person most responsible for implementing the child's educational program. The teacher in the case of the child with communication handicaps may be the speech-language and hearing clinician or the classroom teacher. The teacher's responsibilities as a team member at the meeting include explaining to the parents the learning objectives, curriculum, and various techniques that are used to meet the annual goals. The teacher will also explain to parents why one particular strategy was used instead of another. In addition, the teacher will answer questions parents might have about events that occur within the classroom. In effect, the teacher is the main emissary between the school and the parents.

Speech-Language Pathologist's Role on the Team.   The role of the speech-language clinician on the placement team may vary according to the guidelines and practices of the local education agency. If the child in question has a communication problem, the person providing the language and speech services in the school needs to participate in the placement process. While the full placement team has the responsibility of developing an educational program for each pupil, the school clinician should be prepared to provide input into the process of establishing goals, objectives, prognosis, and intervention strategies. The school clinician will also be responsible for reporting to the placement team the results of any diagnostic and assessment testing and may recommend further testing.

Family as Team Members.   Family members can provide insights about the home situation, the impact of the disability on interactions and home activities, and factors that may be contributing to the child's problems. Making family members team members gives them and speech-language pathologists, as well as other members of the team, an opportunity to observe each other's interaction with the student, The family may be team members in the actual diagnosis, treatment, and carrying out of the IEP, IFSP, or ITP. Furthermore, the more the caregivers are included in these processes, the smoother and the more consistent is the delivery of instruction to the child. Both family and SLPs gain from the insights of the other, and both will be able to use each other as a source for added ideas. Also, family and SLPs will be able to keep each other informed about the progress of the child.

Reports to caregivers, both oral and written, should be in clear, understandable language and not in professional terminology, sometimes referred to as jargon. Clear explanations of the diagnosis and treatment strategies should be made to caregivers. The SLP should make it plain to caregivers that diagnosis is an ongoing process and that, as the child changes and progresses, the assessment of his or her condition will likely change.

Speech-language pathologists should avoid labels as much as possible when talking with family. If labels have to be used, it should be made clear to family that the terms are merely words for explaining the communication disorder.

The Placement Team's Purpose.   The ultimate result of the placement meeting is to develop an IEP, IFSP, or ITP for the child and to achieve agreement to that plan by the parents and professionals. The plan must be a written document, prepared and distributed according to the policies of the state and local education agencies. Policies also regulate who shall have access to the report and how copies shall be made available. A copy of the report is made available to the parents. All placement team members sign the report.

In most cases the speech-language pathologist is a member of the team if the child displays communication difficulties. If the clinician is not on the team (an unlikely but not impossible situation), a copy of the document should be made available to the clinician.

ETHICS AND RESPONSIBILITIES

Our selection of testing procedures and, ultimately, of those students who will or will not receive services in our programs, should be guided by our professional ethics and standards of practice. For example, if during the testing session with a child you learn of a need in another area, it is your responsibility to refer that child for services by the appropriate professional. This may mean a medical referral for a physical condition you might observe, the school psychologist for a learning disability you detect, or the guidance counselor for an emotional or social problem. This necessitates looking at the "whole child" not just the speech and language behaviors displayed. Children are complex creatures. We cannot diagnose or treat them in isolation. We must report the total picture we observe when we create our description of the child's behaviors and needs (Peterson and Marquardt, 1990).

DISCUSSION QUESTIONS AND PROJECTS

1. How would you introduce yourself to a kindergarten class you were about to screen for speech-language problems? How would you explain to them what you were going to do? Role play this situation in your class.

2. The third-grade teacher sends not only the students who have articulation problems but also all the "problem" readers as well, when you ask for referrals. How would you handle this situation?

3. How would you generate self-referrals on the high school level?

4. Compose a memorandum to the teachers of Gibbs Elementary School in which you explain the procedures of the speech-language referral system you will be conducting there.

5. Interview a school-based SLP to find out what procedures are used to identify and select students for the speech-language caseload.

6. Survey several SLPs in the schools to find out how they identify students who may have a hearing loss.

7. Find out how preschool children with communication disorders are identified in your area.

8. Explain those modifications which can be made in your assessment procedures to appropriately test children with the following characteristics or impairments: inability to speak; severe sensory impairment (blind or hearing impaired); unable to move or use hands; or unable to be understood.

9. Develop a library of examples of speech and language disorders.

10. Develop a listing of materials that can be used to present an in-service meeting.

CHAPTER EIGHT

MODELS OF SERVICE DELIVERY AND SCHEDULING

The roles and responsibilities of the speech-language pathologist working in the educational setting have changed greatly in the past few decades. The roles will continue to change as understanding of the needs of children and youth with communication disabilities expands, as the impact of communication impairments on learning becomes more clearly defined, and as methods for delivering services improve. Clinicians still function as specialists who work with children with communication disabilities. However, they are no longer implementing their programs in isolation from the rest of the educational system. Speech-language pathology services are an integral part of the total educational program for children with disabilities. Clinicians now have increased responsibilities for demonstrating how communication disabilities impact the learning process. There is a demand to design programs that will increase youngsters' potential for benefiting from the educational process.

Public Law 94-142, a legislative landmark, had the greatest impact on the role of the speech-language pathologist in education. The law specified requirements for identifying children with impairments, providing appropriate services based on individual needs, and making available a broad range of service options. Legislation that followed in subsequent years continued to mandate changes in practices. Schools are required to align all programming, including speech-language pathology services, with the curriculum and state standards. Schools are being challenged to adhere to state standards and comply with federal legislation.

In this chapter, we will explore service delivery options for children and youth with communication disabilities. Emphasis will be placed on explanation of alternative models of service delivery. We will also show how services can be provided in different contexts and discuss curriculum-based treatment and outcome-based goals. The definitions of communication disorders and an understanding of the range of service delivery options are basic tools for the school speech-language pathologist. They may be considered the building blocks of good program development and management. We will explore the complex issue of determining which children will be placed on the caseload. We will also consider scheduling alternatives and variables of importance when scheduling different age or disability groups.

Speech-language pathologists and special educators have vigorously debated many of the issues raised in this chapter. There is not always agreement on what is the right way or the wrong way to approach and solve these problems. But fortunately, the discussions continue, often generating more research, and eventually common ground is reached.

CLASSIFICATION OF PROCEDURES AND COMMUNICATION DISORDERS

In 1987, the ASHA Executive Board approved The American Speech-Language-Hearing Association Classification of Speech-Language Pathology and Audiology Procedures and Communication Disorders, commonly referred to as the ASHA Classification System. This provides a standardized system for coding and indexing procedures and diagnoses commonly used by speech-language pathologists and audiologists. The school speech-language pathologist can use the nomenclature and classification system to uniformly describe communication disorders and the procedures being used. The system is especially valuable for clinicians interested in analyzing their service programs, generating research data about their caseloads, or developing a computerized information management system. The Classification System is presented in Appendix A.

ASHA has also developed a resource describing practice approaches that are essential to good service delivery. Referred to as the Preferred Practice Patterns for the Profession of Speech-Language Pathology, these statements define universally applicable activities that are directed toward providing service to clients/patients (The American Speech-Language-Hearing Association, 1997). This includes the requisites of the practice, the processes to be carried out, and expected outcomes. The idea behind the Preferred Practice Patterns is to provide an informational base to promote the delivery of quality care. They are flexible and yet definitive enough to enable decision making for appropriate clinical outcomes. They reflect the generally accepted professional response to a particular set of client characteristics or circumstances. School-based clinicians can use the Preferred Practice Patterns as a tool for discussing common practices that can be utilized throughout the school district or for discussing service delivery needs. In addition, they can be given to administrators to promote better understanding.

ALTERNATIVE SERVICE DELIVERY OPTIONS

Before a comprehensive speech and language intervention program is organized by the school clinician, some basis must be established for its implementation. We will call this basis a model.

A model is an approximation of the real world. In the process of trying to determine the most appropriate practices, clinicians manipulate, change, add to, and expand models until they find the one that meets the needs of their program. The speech-language pathologist in any school district is the decision maker who must take into account all the information available. Using the model as a guide, he or she must construct the program in speech-language intervention for that particular community.

Numerous models for delivering speech-language pathology services are being practiced across the country. They were designed based on the requirements of the federal and state laws, the needs of the school district, the unique demographics of the community, and the insights of professionals. There are variations in service delivery models from school district to school district. Differences may be due to the populations served, funding capabilities, administrative support (or nonsupport), and professional expertise and energy. One of the primary factors in the numbers and types of options available is the availability and expertise of staff. Many models have historical roots, with patterns of service delivery being passed from clinician to clinician through the ages.

The laws regulating special education are very clear on one major point. Regardless of the model implemented, the school district should make available alternative service delivery options for providing services. The real intent of this mandate is that the service delivery model selected should be matched to the student's unique characteristics and needs. Over the past several years, there have been many discussions of alternative service delivery models in the literature (ASHA, 1999; Blosser & Kratcoski, 1997; Crais, 1995; Creaghead, Estomin, 1992); Holzhauser-Peters and Husemann, 1988; Montgomery, 2000; Simon, 1987).

Traditionally, service delivery options are presented as though they are discreet programs with unique characteristics. In fact, they are often presented in a hierarchical structure based on factors such as frequency of services, location of services, and amount of direct contact between the speech-language pathologist and the student. Discussions of the range of service delivery options for speech-language pathology are generally assigned labels such as direct therapy, pullout services, home-based intervention, residential services, parent training programs, diagnostic intervention, center-based, classroom-based, community-based, consultation/collaboration model, resource rooms, self-contained classrooms, in-service education programs, and many more. Notice that these descriptors are focused on the roles performed by the clinician (collaboration), the location of the service (resource room), the context for delivery of the service (classroom-based or community-based), or the scheduling pattern (pullout).

Unfortunately, there is limited consensus concerning the definitions of many of the service delivery models used by SLPs in the schools. It is even more unfortunate that there are no commonly shared definitions of service delivery models among professionals and educators. This presents a problem for educators, parents, administrators, and third party payers. There is often confusion and misperception about the type of service to be provided, the reason that model was selected, and the appropriateness for the particular student.

In lieu of definitions that are uniformly accepted by all professionals, following are examples of definitions that have appeared in the literature (ASHA, 1996; Homer, 1997). These are provided only as a frame of reference for the discussion of the concept of alternative service delivery options. There is no intent to suggest that one model is better than another or that there is a prescribed movement from one model to the next.

Monitoring Speech-Language Behavior.   Not all students must be seen on a routine (daily or weekly) basis. For example, children who demonstrate developmental delays but do not warrant direct intervention can be monitored for a period of time until the clinician and education team determines that intervention would be beneficial. When monitoring students, the SLP observes the student's communication behaviors over a period of time. The child may be monitored to see if immature speech and language patterns show change over time (thus decreasing the need for therapy). Or, the SLP may be watching to see if the student's behavior changes when stimulated or motivated by a certain situation or person. In addition, children who have been enrolled in therapy temporarily are also monitored to determine if generalization has occurred and new patterns are stabilized.

Pullout Intervention. This mode of delivery has historically been referred to as the primary model used by the speech-language pathologist to deliver service in a school setting. Speech and language services are provided as a supplementary service to regular or special education programs. The student leaves the classroom to receive direct intervention from the speech-language pathologist. Pullout intervention may be aimed at an individual student or a group of students. Criteria for grouping students into a particular session may include age, grade level, type and degree of communication disorder, and functional level. Traditionally sessions are scheduled for an average of once or twice per week for an individual student or group of students. Group size may average from two to four students but may include as many as ten students. The number of sessions per week, length of time per session, and number of students per session are influenced by the nature and degree of the students' problems and the speech-language pathologist's caseload demands. Creative use of learning centers, technology, and volunteers are sometimes used by clinicians to maximize the benefits of pullout intervention.

Unfortunately, in many school districts the pullout scheduling pattern has become the norm. Clinicians are stuck in a routine that does not enable them to evaluate each child from a creative, flexible, unique point of view. It is this pattern that has restricted many clinicians from implementing a more individualized, variable service delivery approach. Clinicians must ask themselves: How can it be that the majority of students served need to receive direct services twice per week (Monday and Wednesday; Tuesday and Thursday) for one half hour? This scheduling pattern defies the notion that the intervention model selected should match the student's needs. Doesn't it make more sense to consider alternative approaches that are suited to each child's needs?

Collaboration/Consultation. In recent years, leaders in the professions of speech-language pathology and special education have recommended increased use of collaboration and/or consultation as models for service delivery. In such approaches, the SLP (or educator) works closely with others to facilitate a student's communication and learning. They jointly determine goals and objectives for intervention. This is considered an indirect service delivery model.

For example, to make collaboration work, the speech-language pathologist observes a class and assembles information about the various levels of speech and language competence among the students. Following analysis of the information, the speech-language pathologist meets with the teacher to share observations and recommendations to enhance the students' language skills and incorporate language development into the curricula. The speech-language pathologist demonstrates or suggests specific teaching strategies and techniques and may provide supplementary materials to the teacher.

When an IEP is developed for a student, goals and objectives are indicated linking the student's language performance with the educational curriculum. The speech-language pathologist may provide specific suggestions to the teacher so he or she can help the student reach the goals and objectives specified in the IEP. Following are some examples of successful collaboration. The SLP explains or demonstrates specific techniques that the teacher, tutor, peer, or parent can use to assist the student in carrying over appropriate language skills into everyday life. The SLP provides informal analysis and suggestions for modification of the classroom environment, the teacher's communication style and delivery, or student-learning strategies. Language materials that may include pictures and word lists are provided on a routine basis for others to use with preschool, kindergarten, or high-risk students. The SLP demonstrates language and speech enrichment sessions in the classroom as needed.

Classroom-Based Delivery.   Some practitioners refer to this model as integrated services, curriculum-based, transdisciplinary, or inclusive programming. Of all of the definitions for service delivery, this one causes the most confusion. For example, one clinician may interpret "classroom-based model" to mean that the SLP incorporates classroom-based materials in therapy. A second clinician may define classroom-based as working with the teacher. In a third interpretation, the clinician may be working with a small group of children within the classroom structure, whereas a fourth SLP might present a language or listening-based lesson to an entire class. A fifth interpretation describes classroom-based as team teaching. This type of confusion becomes especially troublesome when a team of educators is trying to develop an IEP for a student with communication disorders.

Community-Based Intervention.   Programs for children with low-incidence disabilities are beginning to emphasize community-based instruction. In this model, the speech-language pathologist collaborates with the special education teacher and other staff members to assist the student with functional speech and language in community sites. As part of their school program, severely involved students learn how to function in their own communities. The speech-language pathologist provides direct or indirect services to students on-site in such community settings as restaurants, stores, libraries, banks, post offices, etc. The speech-language pathologist helps students with communication skills, monitors their progress, and assists in planning instruction. As a collaborator in a community-based intervention program, the speech-language pathologist assists the teacher, occupational therapist, physical therapist, or other staff members in developing plans and strategies to encourage the growth of the students' functional communication areas.

Because the school is a community site, emphasis can be placed on development of the student's functional communication skills and carryover of those skills into everyday life. The speech-language pathologist can enlist the support of many resources in the school to aid in development of a student's communication skills. In community-based sites, the speech-language pathologist analyzes the experience and site to identify relevant vocabulary to be learned. He or she develops language concepts relevant to assigned tasks, and guides staff in using instructional language most likely to clearly convey instructional messages to students.

INCLUSIVE MODELS OF SERVICE DELIVERY

At present, speech-language pathologists in school settings are seeking ways to incorporate inclusive models of service delivery that merge speech and language services with educational programming. Inclusive practices are based on the unique and specific needs of the individual and are provided in a setting that is least restrictive (ASHA, 1999b). Clinicians across the country are striving to develop services and acceptable service delivery environments for all children with special needs. Personnel working in educational settings must demonstrate that their services will support the student so that he or she can participate to the maximum extent possible in social and learning contexts (Hales & Carlson, 1992). These directions would indicate that the general education classroom should be considered the first step in the options for service delivery for students with communication disabilities (Huffman, 1995).

Clinical effectiveness is defined in terms of helping students reach measurable, functional outcomes so they can participate in school, community, family, work, and play activities. Service delivery has been expanded to encompass all settings. These issues are causing practitioners to seek different options for serving their caseloads.

One major challenge that poses a barrier to accomplishing goals for inclusion continues to be the relationship between the classroom teacher and the speech-language pathologist. Teachers may lack the understanding and preparation they need to provide assistance to students who are in their classes. In addition, SLPs are not always aware of the curriculum or other aspects of educational programming that make a difference to student learning. The amount and type of intervention that is needed to change a student's communication behavior is yet an unknown. Unfortunately, there are not common guidelines for decision making. As McKinley explains, "the least restrictive environment is mandated by law, but is the classroom really the most restrictive environment for all children?" Maybe the law is being overinterpreted by educators. The legislation really mandates that children are supposed to be served by the best intervention model for them. For some children, this will be through inclusionary approaches within the classroom setting; for others, it will mean pullout programming or some other model. SLPs are charged with using their skills and clinical judgement to determine the most appropriate model for each child. That is really the intent of the law.

MATCHING SERVICE DELIVERY MODELS TO INDIVIDUAL STUDENT'S NEEDS

If alternative service delivery approaches are to be effective, the options will not be mutually exclusive and the clinician will be able to use them individually or in combination to best serve the needs of a particular student. The service delivery option selected should be the most appropriate to meet the child's needs and should be the least restrictive in terms of enabling the child to participate in the activities of the school as much as possible.

Consideration should be given to the student's level of functioning and should serve children and youth with communication disabilities ranging from severe disorders to developmental problems. The model needs to be applicable to children of all ages in regular education as well as special education programs. It should also make provisions for providing preventive services to the overall school population.

The caseload size and service delivery options selected should be based on several variables relating to the student and personnel available. This includes the type and severity of the student's communication impairment; the effect of the communication disorder on academic performance; the relationship of the communication disorder to other learning conditions; the stage of development of the communication disorder; the student's history in the speech-language intervention program; amount and type of contact needed to implement intervention strategies; and scheduling constraints. (ASHA, 1984; Eger et al., 1990). Because students' needs are constantly changing, these factors should be reevaluated and the program adjusted periodically. Consideration needs to be given to the number of children who can be adequately served using particular service delivery options or combination of options. Federal, state, and local requirements for serving students with communication disorders must also be considered.

Decisions regarding a group versus individualized or combined group/individualized program should be based on student need rather than factors such as administrative direction and time or budget constraints. Service delivery models selected should allow adequate frequency and intensity of help for optimum progress. As with group size, decisions regarding the length and frequency of intervention should be based on the student's needs and clinical factors rather than budgetary and administrative issues. The option selected should provide students with the best chance for functioning successfully within the school setting and in their future lives.

THE PAC FRAMEWORK FOR ALTERNATIVE MODELS OF SERVICE DELIVERY

When devising a comprehensive service delivery model, there are four major concepts of service delivery that should be considered. First, the model should recognize that communication impairments affect learning success. Second, the model should create an optimal environment for providing speech-language services. Third, the model should incorporate collaboration and sharing expertise to develop effective program goals, objectives, and intervention strategies for children. Fourth, the model should integrate speech-language goals, objectives, and techniques into the student's learning experiences.

Blosser and Kratcoski (1997) developed a conceptual framework for guiding decisions about selection of appropriate services to meet particular clients' needs. They define alternative service delivery as determining the unique combinations of *providers, service activities,* and *contexts* (PACs) necessary to meet the specific needs of the individual with communication disorders.

The conceptual framework is based on three premises. First, there are essential characteristics that define good service delivery. Second, service delivery must be creative and flexible. Third, the provider, activity, and context must be clearly specified in the Individualized Education Plan (treatment plan), the Individualized Family Service Plan (IFSP), or the Individualized Transition Plan (ITP).

Premise One—Characteristics of Good Service Delivery Models

According to Flower (1984), the essential characteristics of good service-delivery models fall under five headings: efficacy, coordination, continuity, participation, and economy.

1. *Does the service make a difference to the child?* The first obvious criterion, efficacy, is whether the service makes any difference to the consumer. Screening services can usually be judged in fairly objective terms; however, other services are often more difficult to assess. Evaluation by the clinician and the insights of families, clients, and other professionals all provide information of a subjective nature, but it is frequently difficult to determine whether achievements have, in fact, occurred.

2. *When multiple professional services are provided to the same individual, are all services coordinated and working toward the same end?* Several different types of professionals serve clients with communicative disorders. Some of these may provide services that are directly related to the communicative disorder, for example, the learning disabilities specialist working with a child with problems in language acquisition. Other professionals provide services with only peripheral relevance to the communicative disorder, for example, the teacher of a classroom in which a young stutterer is enrolled. Whenever multiple professional services are provided to the same client, the effectiveness of any of those services will often depend on the coordination of all the services.

3. *Is there an uninterrupted sequence of services, and is each phase staged and integrated?* Good care depends on the continuity of sequential services over a period of several months or sometimes several years. This often requires multiple professional services, that is, a total plan for services, with each phase staged and integrated into an uninterrupted sequence toward the ultimate goal.

4. *Are the individual's wishes, motivations, and interests considered by incorporating the individual and family members in the decision-making process?* Professional services carried out with little regard for the clients' wishes or little concern for their understanding of what was occurring seriously impair the effectiveness of those services. Participation by the client and the family in all decision-making processes ensures the opportunity for excellent services.

5. *Are the time, energy, funding, and other resources used most efficiently to accomplish the goals?* Economy does not only mean spending as little money as possible. It refers also to the conservation of time and energy. The conservation of financial resources, as well as the orderly management of services to avoid waste, and the achievement of efficiency through careful planning constitute the broader definition of economy.

Flower's five criteria are helpful in assessing service delivery models. Each school system is unique. The school clinician needs to implement the service delivery options that best fit the organization of the school system, needs of the students, and professionals on staff. A number of factors may influence the number and types of options a school district is able to make available to its students including:

1. The geographic location of the schools, the clinician's "home" office, and the distance and travel time between these locations
2. The availability of working space in each of the schools
3. The type and severity of the communication problems within the schools
4. The number and population of the schools (would some schools warrant a full-time clinician?)

5. Time allotted for coordination activities, including in-service training; supervision of paraprofessionals or aides; preparation of records; parent conferences; placement team conferences; and collaborating with classroom teachers, special education personnel, and administrators; administration of diagnostic tests; and so on
6. School policies affecting the transporting of students from school to school to place them in locations where they may receive the appropriate services
7. The level of the school (it is entirely probable that the junior high schools and the senior high schools may have smaller population of students with communication impairments than elementary schools)
8. The support of the school administration and teaching staff

Premise Two—Service Delivery Must Be Creative and Flexible

The service delivery option selected must fit the needs and lifestyle of the student. In addition, it must be integrated into the school context. This means that various key aspects of service delivery must be manipulated to meet the student's unique needs. The aspects that can be tailored include:

- The type of services provided
- The amount of contact time the speech-language pathologist actually spends with the student
- The location for providing services (resource room, therapy room, classroom, lunch room)
- The provider who delivers the services (SLP, teacher, parent, peer, aide)
- The mode of service delivery (technology-assisted, written format, verbal interaction)
- The materials and techniques used for assessment and intervention (curricular, clinician made, commercial process oriented, product oriented)

Premise Three—The Provider, Activity, and Context Must Be Clearly Specified

In most discussions of service delivery, collaboration is treated as a distinct and unique service delivery model. In the PAC model, collaboration is a necessary component for providing services for all students. In other words, unless others are integrated into the intervention process, treatment will not be effective.

Providers (P).   In the PAC Model, communication partners who can foster meaningful change in a student's communication performance are referred to as "providers." They make changes by knowing how to implement appropriate procedures such as eliciting, modifying, and/or reinforcing communication responses. Traditionally, the SLP is viewed as the only person who can make changes and who has the ultimate responsibility for this role. However, in the PAC model the SLP is not assumed to be the only or even the best provider. To improve efficacy, both assessment and intervention require shared responsibility among all of the student's significant communication partners. Numerous providers should be involved in the assessment and intervention process. Several factors are used to select the providers. They are determined by the student's needs at a given point in time, the activity to be completed, and the context in which the activity is to be conducted. Providers may change over time as the child's communication skills improve and intervention needs or goals change. Clearly this model assumes that there should be several providers for each student.

When implementing alternative models of service delivery, the SLP's role includes guiding the team as they weigh the following question: "Who are the most appropriate persons to conduct or provide specific communication-related activities with this student and in what context?" Several factors must be weighed when making the decision regarding who can be an effective provider. The person should have a meaningful relationship with the student (teacher, parent, sibling, or friend). The severity of the disability also makes a difference. Sometimes the problems are so severe that providers need to be introduced more slowly and over an extended period of time. The partner's general knowledge and understanding of the communication disability will also impact the decision. Sometimes they will need to be educated about the disability before being brought into a more active role. The individual's willingness to participate in the program, and situations and contexts of interactions, also will help determine the involvement and the success of the involvement. In determining providers, the SLP and fellow team members should consider the following questions:

1. Who are the key communication partners in this youngster's life (parents, other caregivers, teachers, coworkers, tutors, peers)?
2. Are there barriers that would prevent the person from delivering specific assessment and/or treatment procedures (time constraints, location, motivation, conflicting philosophies, fear, lack of information, inadequate skills)?
3. Can these barriers be resolved through training and/or counseling (in-servicing, support groups, workshops, written materials, audio and video materials, observation, demonstration)?
4. What is the most appropriate provider role for each communication partner considering the outcomes/goals for the client at the specific point in time (observe and report behaviors, model, question, prompt, correct, reinforcing)?

Examples of potential providers in addition to the SLP are parents, siblings, regular educators, special educators, tutors, intervention specialists, psychologists, friends, administrators, occupational therapists, and physical therapists. Key roles played by individuals such as these will enable services to be carried out throughout the student's daily routine.

Activities (A). Those tasks that comprise the total case management for clients with communication disorders are referred to as "activities" (A) in the PAC model. The primary tasks can be grouped into four major categories:

1. Planning to determine courses of action in all aspects of case management
2. Assessing to determine strengths and needs
3. Implementing treatment procedures
4. Evaluating services to determine the efficacy and outcomes to identify if modifications are necessary

Clearly, the SLP is not the only person qualified to perform these activities. Through shared responsibility, the team can gain more valuable information and make more efficient use of shrinking resources. Each of the activities can be explained to team members in the following way.

Planning.   A significant portion of the SLP's service delivery time involves planning. Teams must spend adequate time and effort to determine the appropriate course of action needed to meet each student's needs. Planning involves tasks such as discussing assessment findings, reviewing pertinent data, determining goals and objectives, selecting appropriate intervention procedures, and modifying intervention plans. This planning often takes the form of meetings where several participants from various disciplines come together to present their perspectives. Within the PAC model, the emphasis during planning efforts is on who the providers will be and what activities they will conduct and in what context.

Assessing.   The purpose of assessment is to identify the communication strengths and needs of the client as well as the extent of services necessary. Unless information is also gathered regarding the priorities and concerns of the client, his or her family, and other important individuals, an appropriate service plan cannot be developed. Within the assessment process, all individuals who can contribute information are considered providers. In the PAC Model, the goal of the identification and assessment aspects of service delivery is not to identify what is wrong. Instead, the goal is to *identify what works for a particular client in a particular setting when assisted by particular people.* Thus, the SLP's role is to provide a framework for obtaining, organizing, and synthesizing the information.

Implementing Interventions.   Perhaps the most primary activity in service delivery is providing intervention. As the intervention plan for a student is developed, different providers will inevitably assume different roles for implementing intervention. For example, one provider (such as the SLP) may introduce a new skill to the client, while a second provider (the parent) reinforces the targeted behavior and a third provider (the teacher) observes the child's performance to determine additional communication skill areas to be targeted in the future. Clinicians working within the school setting often express confusion about how to work collaboratively with teachers. Following the PAC model provides a useful way of understanding how to make collaboration work so that it is beneficial to all concerned.

In the PAC model, the SLP assumes the responsibility of preparing providers for the activities they will conduct. For example, to involve key communication partners in implementing intervention, the SLP must prepare them for the role by teaching them to:

1. Identify when a communication breakdown has occurred
2. Recognize that it is related to the individual's communication disability
3. Know the appropriate procedures to implement to bring about change at that time

One way to help others understand the key roles they can play is to provide guidance and training. Consider this a service delivery option that is appropriate to the needs of the majority of youngsters on the caseload. Providing in-service training, both formal and informal, is a functional way to reach teachers, parents, and others. It can impact a great number of students without the SLP providing direct service. In addition, it would be helpful for the SLP to also participate in in-service training to learn more about the school curriculum and expectations for students.

There are many ways to provide training including providing information via five-minute "quick-hits" at faculty meetings, distributing written handouts, and providing materials: Share ideas with teachers during informal conversations or in-service presentations; show others how to elicit correct responses or correct incorrect responses by demonstrating speech and language techniques; loan useful materials to teachers and encourage them to try them out in the classroom; volunteer to participate on curriculum selection committees; provide routine updates about students' progress and suggest activities teachers might want to try.

Evaluating Efficacy and Outcomes.   Intervention is effective when the student's communication performance is appropriate for the contexts in which he or she participates. In the school setting, this means the student can perform the required tasks in the classroom. This can be determined only by reports provided by the astute providers in the client's various communication environments. The SLP's role is to solicit information, analyze it, and work with other providers to make appropriate modifications.

In deciding those activities that are necessary to address the child's needs, teams should contemplate these "activity related" questions:

1. What tasks do the providers need to complete for this student at this particular point in time (identify needs, design interventions, teach others to implement interventions, evaluate progress)?
2. What providers would be most appropriate for performing each task? (Consider such factors such as the person's relationship to the student; the frequency of contact the provider and student have with one another; the provider's level of understanding, experience, and training relative to the disorder and the necessary intervention; and so on.)
3. What steps should be taken to prepare the providers to perform these activities and who should take the steps? (Providing in-service opportunities, demonstrations, written materials, audio or videotapes are some examples.)
4. What materials do the providers need to conduct the activity? (Observation and data collection forms, assessment checklists and materials, surveys and questionnaires, resource lists stimulus materials, augmentative or assistive devices are some possibilities.)

Contexts (C).   The situations, conditions, environments, or interactions where communication is required are referred to as the "contexts." During planning opportunities, providers should jointly determine the most appropriate contexts for conducting specific activities necessary for case management. The range of contexts and conditions for each student is extensive. In determining contexts, the SLP should consider demands and expectations for communication required in the context. Specifically, the team must consider:

1. What are the primary contexts in which the student communicates or must transfer newly learned behaviors (home, school, learning activities, curriculum, community, work)?

2. What contexts provide natural opportunities for communication or for practicing the targeted behaviors (instruction, play, large group activities, recreation and leisure, routines, vocational settings)?
3. What contexts provide opportunities for observing and evaluating communication performance and progress?
4. Does the environment restrict or promote communication skills for this individual?

Appropriate contexts include the regular education classroom, resource room, curriculum, cafeteria, recess, home, community, vocational settings, and so on. Services can be delivered in numerous locations using a wide variety of treatment approaches. During planning, emphasis should be placed on determining the best context for implementing recommended interventions. Unfortunately, too often clinicians place students into a particular context and do not consider if it is the most appropriate match for the youngsters' needs.

The Board of Cooperative Education Services (BOCES) in Nassau County, New York has developed several different contexts for delivering services to youngsters in their service area. A quick review of their programs demonstrates the integration of creativity and flexibility of design (Cappadonna, 2000). The Collaborative Teaching Classroom (CTC) provides continuous collaboration between a special educator and speech-language pathologist. The two educators share space in the learning environment. The teacher addresses the curriculum and the SLP provides assistance with skills that are at the foundation of learning. The Child Aided Language and Literacy Model (CALL) focuses on students with physical disabilities. The SLPs and special educators collaborated to design a school environment that fosters interactive communication. Many children use alternative-augmentative communication systems. The Visual Strategies Model provides assistance to students by combining assistive technology, AAC, and visual language to enhance students' functional communication skills. The teachers design adaptations for the classroom curriculum and create visual aids. In the district's Mealtime Management Program, SLPs and other professionals work together to provide services to children with moderate to severe oral-motor dysfunctions. The Nassau BOCES also has implemented a Speech/Psychology Collaborative Project, focusing on the social pragmatic communication skills for adolescents with emotional and behavioral problems. Project speech-language pathologists and psychologists work with classroom teachers and families to enhance their understanding of the students' needs and strategies for helping. The BOCES also provides services for young children in preschool programs as well as specific disorders including hearing impairments, vision impairments, autism, and developmental disabilities. The wide range of options illustrates the type of ingenuity that clinicians across the country are demonstrating to comply with the legislation and to provide the best possible services to children in their region. Most likely the SLPs in that BOCES are excited and invigorated by the diversity of their job.

Following is a description of contexts in addition to the classroom or therapy room that some clinicians establish for the provision of various types of services.

Diagnostic Therapy.   Some school districts and regional resource centers offer comprehensive diagnostic services at diagnostic centers. Students are enrolled in these programs for only a short period of time. After evaluations are completed, results and recommendations are shared with the parents and school personnel. Individualized educational plans are formulated and implemented in different contexts.

Hospital or Home-Based Intervention. In the home and/or hospital-based context, educators and clinicians travel to serve students who are unable to attend school because of confinement to their homes or to a hospital setting. This context is employed when providing services to school-age children who have physical or mental disabilities that prohibit them from participating in the school environment. For example, children with brain injuries may receive educational services in the medical setting and then at home prior to returning to school full time.

Parent Training. Instruction is often provided to parents with children who have communication disorders, developmental disabilities, or who are at risk for either. The clinician provides guidance and instruction in techniques for assisting infants and preschoolers in developing appropriate communicative behaviors and skills. The services may be provided in the school, a center, the child's home, or other approved facility.

Residential Placement. The residential context is usually reserved for pupils with severe and profound impairments who have medical or education needs beyond that which can be provided at school or in the home. Education and specialized services are provided in addition to daily care.

Self-Contained Classroom. Some speech-language clinicians serve as classroom teachers. They are responsible for providing academic as well as curriculum instruction and speech-language intervention. The class generally serves groups of students with multiple disabilities. Naturally, the SLP must gain knowledge and certification in education as well as in speech-language pathology.

SERVICE COORDINATION

Children with disabilities and their families frequently require a broad range of intervention services. Physical and mental health care may be necessary as well as financial assistance and therapy services. Therapies might include speech-language pathology, aural habilitation, physical therapy, occupational therapy, visual training, counseling, and the like. Numerous professionals representing multiple agencies are charged with delivering the services. As a result, goals, treatment programs, and services are often fragmented and/or duplicated. In addition, complications arise for reimbursement for services because the agencies may each have different funding streams.

To improve the quality of services offered to children and their families, Public Law 99-457 mandated the coordination of services for children. The central question asked is "What help does the family of a child with disabilities need to function well?" Emphasis is placed on collaborative planning and efficient, effective service delivery. To achieve this service coordination, professionals from a variety of disciplines and agencies must strive to understand one another's disciplines. Through this model, the family is involved meaningfully in all aspects of planning, implementing, and monitoring their child's programs.

One of the agencies involved in service delivery for children is the educational system. School clinicians have opportunities to coordinate their services with professionals both inside and outside of the school system. The clinician can contribute much to the service coordination process. For example, he or she can share information about the services available in the schools. Because many healthcare professionals are unaware of services that are available and how they can be accessed, the clinician can help in this area also. In addition, he or she can explain the child's communication impairments and their impact on the child's ability to function. The speech-language program and educational program planned for the child can be explained in terms that are understandable. Elimination of redundancy and assistance with facilitating multiple goals can be accomplished through collaboration with other professionals.

SCHEDULING SERVICES

In Chapter 7, systems for case identification and selection were discussed. One aspect dealt with the identification and further diagnosis of individual children who were possible candidates for intervention. Let us now turn our attention to the scheduling of children for services. In implementing a program based on the alternative service delivery concept, the SLP would allocate his or her direct intervention time so that the children in the highest priority categories would receive the most attention. Children with lower priority ratings might be served by options that require less of the SLP's direct time and attention. Nevertheless, all children needing services would receive them but the decisions for how they would be served would depend on need versus scheduling routines.

This system is based on the needs of the child and meets the requirements and the spirit of federal legislation. Rather than servicing schools the SLP is servicing children. Too often administrators expect the SLP's time to be divided equally among schools without regard to the needs of the children. This puts at risk the reputation of the program and may result in lack of support and fewer referrals from teachers, principals, and eventually parents.

Guidelines for case selection should be flexible and adaptable for large, small, or medium-sized school systems. They can also be applied to pupils from preschool through high school. The most basic consideration in planning the therapy program is to make the best use of the time allotted. This is not much help to the beginning clinician, however, who must decide whether to schedule children for 30-minute sessions or longer; to work in the classroom or use pullout; to group or not to group. Perhaps the best approach is to take a careful look at the schedule of classes in the school and then determine a schedule that coincides with the class schedule. This does not necessarily mean that therapy sessions should be the same length as classes, but it would be helpful to both teachers and students if there were some coordination between the two. Nor does it mean that all the sessions should be planned for the same amount of time. Some sessions may be 20 minutes in length, and some may be 45 minutes. The decision about the amount of time should be made by the clinician on the basis of the child's needs. More time may be needed for group sessions. The child in the generalization stages of therapy may require 10 or 15 minutes several times a week. High school students who may be able to assume more responsibility for themselves may need only one one-hour session per week. The amount of time needed for each child may change as the child progresses. Classroom teachers should be informed of the fact that change will occur during the year and that their input would be valuable in considering any changes in the time. The key word in planning the amount of time per therapy session is flexibility and the criterion is what is in the best interests of the child. The responsibility for making good use of the time is the clinician's.

Itinerant Scheduling. Traditionally, speech and language services have been provided on an itinerant basis and have been based on state regulations that define caseload, number of child-contact hours per week, and ratio of clinicians to school populations. By providing more options for delivery of services instead of relying solely on the itinerant model, more children who need help can be reached. This does not imply that the itinerant model is not a good model when it is used in the appropriate circumstances. However, it does mean the speech-language pathology professions must break the habit of thinking of it as the only option.

Many of the children with severe communication disorders, as well as those with mild to moderate deviations, will be in regular classrooms with speech-language intervention services provided by the school clinician on an itinerant basis. The itinerant model has been used from the time it was suggested in 1910 by Ella Flagg Young, who felt that it protected the young teacher from "depression of spirit and low physical conditions resulting from confinement in one room for several successive hours while working with abnormal conditions." Not until recent years have other systems of scheduling been developed. These have come about as a result of mandatory legislation, more sophisticated tools, larger numbers of children needing services, and the recognized need for an interdisciplinary approach.

The itinerant model may be effective in situations where schools are within a few miles of each other or where school populations and caseloads are low. It may also provide continuous therapy for children who need more frequent intervention over a longer period of time, such as children with fluency problems, hearing problems, and problems resulting from such conditions as cleft palate and cerebral palsy. The itinerant (or traditional) model may take several forms. The school clinician may serve one, two, or three schools, working with a small group of children (two to five) or individual children on an intermittent basis of twice a week.

Intensive Scheduling. Another model of scheduling services is the intensive cycle, sometimes called the block system. In this model the child is seen four or five times a week for a concentrated block of time, usually four to six weeks.

Specialization Scheduling. Another possible option in a school system with two or more SLPs would be to assign the clinicians on the basis of their areas of specialization. In a variation of this model in a large school system, part of the staff might be on an itinerant schedule while several clinicians would serve as "specialists," matching their strengths to the students' needs.

Combining Scheduling Models.   Another option for scheduling services would be a combination of models. For example, the clinician may decide to combine the itinerant model with the intensive cycle scheduling system. Obviously, this would be easier to arrange if there were more than one SLP on the staff, if communication aides were available, if the program were carefully coordinated, and if the clinicians and the school administrators all agreed on the program.

Scheduling Groups of Children.   Although some therapy in the public schools is carried on in individual sessions, a great deal of it is also done in group sessions. Initially, the clinician is faced with the task of deciding which children should be placed in a group. The answer would depend on the needs of the child at any given stage of therapy. Some children may need an intensive approach to master some skills, and this may best be accomplished by working alone with the clinician. Later that same child may be ready to use these skills in a social context, and a group experience would best fit this need. The makeup of the group is an important factor in planning for optimal therapy results. Some clinicians find it more productive to work with a group of children who have similar problems, whereas for other clinicians the homogeneity of problems is not as important as grouping children of the same age level.

In deciding when children should be put in a group and the composition of the group, the SLP must consider several factors. First, there are no right or wrong ways of grouping children. Groups must be flexible and must meet the needs of each child enrolled. Second, grouping is done to control the factors that enhance learning. Third, groups should not become static. As children learn and as needs change the composition of the group should change. Fourth, groups should be structured but not rigid. A structure assists learning, and if learning is not taking place there is no purpose for the existence of the group. Fifth, the size of the group should depend on its major purposes; however, a group of more than five or six students to one instructor tends to lose its tutorial effect.

Often, several children from a single classroom are recommended for therapy. Depending on their disabilities and needs, they may or may not be able to be accommodated in the same group and scheduled for the same therapy time. The teacher's input in scheduling is essential so consideration can be given to subjects the children will miss and disruptions that will occur as they enter and leave the classroom.

Students with speech, language, or hearing disorders should not be put in therapy groups simply to accommodate more students in the SLP's caseload. The rationale for placing a student in a group should depend on the needs of the student and the purpose of the group.

WORKING WITH TEACHERS AND ADMINISTRATORS TO PLAN SCHEDULES

SLPs may encounter difficulty with scheduling because everyone is competing for the student's learning time. Required or fun learning activities that are planned for the time when therapy groups meet may result in problems if the student must routinely miss them. The wise clinician will discuss scheduling with the teachers and school principal before the beginning of the school year. Perhaps a rotational system can be developed so students do not miss the same class each week.

FLEXIBILITY IN SCHEDULING

The therapy program has many facets, many ramifications, and requires much from the school SLP. Decisions must be made, and they will not always be the right decisions. Speech-language pathologists are conscientious and intelligent people, but they are not infallible. They usually learn from their mistakes and often from the mistakes of others. The beginning clinician might be wise to avoid getting locked into a course of action that later, because of circumstances, might not be the best one. This can occur on the intervention level and on the organizational and management level. For example, if the clinician determines that the student is not responding to a particular approach in therapy, the clinician changes the procedures. On the organizational level if the SLP has sold the school administration on the idea that the itinerant service delivery model is the only feasible one, the SLP may have difficulty if it becomes apparent in the future that other service delivery models should be utilized. Allowing for some flexibility will enable the school clinician to maintain a viable program.

SCHEDULING JUNIOR AND SENIOR HIGH SCHOOL STUDENTS

Receiving grades and academic credit for participating in the speech-language intervention program often motivates junior high and high school students. The credit is usually one-quarter or one-half as much as a regular course and enrollment may be repeated. Clinicians wishing to use this model must work with administrators, teachers, and counselors to determine where the course best fits in the school curriculum. Some districts offer a course of this nature as an elective in the language arts area; others consider it a personal enhancement class. Students who might qualify for the program can be identified by reviewing caseloads from elementary programs in the district or through referral and screening programs. In this type of program, one class period of the student's schedule is devoted to work on language skills. The course might be titled "Communication Skills." During the class period, the speech/language pathologist services several students whose language learning and remedial needs would benefit from this type of scheduling. Course content may include vocabulary development, problem-solving techniques, listening skills, social and conversational speech, question-asking and answering strategies, nonverbal communication skills, study skills related to language, and survival pragmatic language. Service is provided in a more natural environment than is possible in a separate speech therapy room. Examples of language interactions, language modeling, and cuing may enhance the teacher's interaction with students. Language skills are incorporated into the academic curriculum, thus enhancing opportunities for generalization and carryover of language skills into everyday life.

In order to be considered a legitimate course, there must be a defined course content, objectives, learning activities, and grading criteria commensurate with other courses on the schedule. For example, students can be objectively evaluated on factors such as attendance, level of involvement and participation in class activities, completion of assignments, and efforts made toward reaching identified targets and goals. The course can be listed as an elective course option in the student's school handbook and scheduling can be done through the school computer along with all other academic scheduling. If the scheduling system is refined, groups of students with similar communication disabilities can be formed.

Organizing the program in this manner makes it more acceptable to students who may be sensitive about their speech or language difficulties. It also promotes interaction of students with similar concerns. This enables practice of functional speech and language skills. Another advantage to this scheduling plan is that students begin the year with the speech-language therapy program as a part of their schedule rather than an addition to it.

SUMMER PROGRAMS

One way in which many school clinicians have extended their services is to offer a summer program. There may be several reasons for carrying out a summer program: to provide more intensive therapy for children who need it, to provide services of an intensive nature to children with such problems as stuttering or communication problems associated with physical disabilities, and to offer a preventive program of therapy along with a parental guidance program.

School clinicians have provided summer programs for a number of years. Some of the programs have been financed by the local education system. Some have been underwritten by foundations, grants, or local service clubs. Many times the program is offered as a joint effort of both the school system and a voluntary organization. In this sort of program, usually the building, facilities, supplies, and so on have been furnished by the school, whereas the clinician's salary has been paid by the community group. The clinician in charge of the program will need to establish criteria for accepting children and will need to carry out the necessary diagnostic procedures. Often only a limited number of children can be accepted, depending on the number of staff members available. Summer programs are usually well received in a community, and once started are often repeated during subsequent summers.

DISCUSSION QUESTIONS AND PROJECTS

1. Why is it important to have definitions of service delivery models that are uniform and agreed on by professionals in the field?

2. You are the school SLP. How would you utilize the service delivery options model in explaining your program to a meeting of elementary teachers in a specific school?

3. Can you give examples of the various service delivery options in your community?

3. Interview some SLPs presently working in programs where the various service delivery options are employed. What questions will you ask them?

4. Using Flower's list of essential characteristics of good service-delivery models, devise a list of questions under each of the five headings. The purpose of the questions would be to evaluate the service delivery models found in a typical school.

5. Think of one therapy session you have observed or conducted. What really made that session stand out in your mind as being excellent or not so excellent? Use Flower's list of essential characteristics of good service delivery models to summarize your observations.

6. Familiarize yourself with numerous contexts within the educational system where services can be provided and identify ways to conduct services in those contexts.

7. Meet with a local speech-language pathologist. Ask that person to describe the various programs and contexts he or she utilizes for delivering services.

8. Obtain an hour by hour description of a local SLP's schedule. Find out the ages, grades, and disorders served; the service delivery models employed; and the intervention providers, activities, and contexts for each child on any one given day of the week.

9. Would you schedule children for intervention during recess? Art class? Physical education? Reading? Social studies? Explain your rationale for the answers you give.

10. Does the severity of the problem have any influence on the time of day you would provide service to a youngster?

CHAPTER NINE

DEVELOPING A RELEVANT INTERVENTION PROGRAM

The school clinician spends most of the working day involved in offering services to students. Development of the intervention plan is guided by clinical decisions made by the clinician with input from parents, teachers, and others. The plan must be relevant to the student's communication disability, the educational needs, and appropriate to the age of the child. It is not necessary at this time, nor would there be space in this chapter, to discuss the various philosophies and treatment approaches for each disorder. Suffice it to say that the school clinician should be well versed in the current treatment practices as well as the school curriculum. There are a number of approaches available to the clinician, and the choice will depend on what best serves the child. Beginning school clinicians will reflect on what they learned in academic courses as well as in clinical courses and experiences. Learning doesn't stop after college. It is your responsibility to keep up with current trends and practices in the field. In this chapter we will discuss planning, implementing, and evaluating intervention services.

PLANNING INDIVIDUALIZED PROGRAMS

Effective intervention begins with the planning process. The planning process actually starts with the referral and determination of steps to take for conducting assessments. Following the evaluation, one or more planning conferences are held. At that time, the clinician works with the student's parents, a representative of the school district, the student's teachers, and other appropriate professionals to plan the intervention program. During the conference, decisions made are based on data gathered during the multifactored assessment and evaluation. The nature and degree of special education programming and intervention is determined. The mode for service delivery is selected, and the goals, objectives, and procedures for intervention are identified. The SLP and other team members should come to the meeting prepared to discuss the nature of the student's communication impairment, its impact on educational performance, recommendations for treatment, ideas for integrating treatment into educational activities, and the roles and responsibilities of each team member. In cases where only speech and language problems are the primary concern, fewer individuals may be involved in the planning.

An Individualized Education Program (IEP) is developed for school-age children. The Individualized Family Service Plan (IFSP) is used for preschoolers. In addition to the IEP, an Individualized Transition Plan (ITP) is prepared for older students.

As an SLP you will be one of the most valuable members on the planning team. The following assessment strategies are recommended prior to planning a treatment program for students. Conduct an environmental assessment to determine communicative situations that might pose difficulty for the student. Determine the communication needs required for accomplishing classroom objectives and daily classroom requirements. Analyze the communication behaviors of key persons with whom the student will be interacting. Based on the information gathered, work with the student's family and teachers to restructure the environment and modify communicative interactions in order to strengthen communications skills.

AN APPROACH TO THE PLANNING PROCESS

Sound planning and program management are necessary for any educational or treatment program to be successful, regardless of the disability. Planning treatment programs poses education teams with substantial challenges. Careful thought, organized approach, imaginative planning, coordinated actions, and skillful management are required to achieve desired outcomes. Treatment plans must meet expectations and requirements imposed by many different entities including parents, teachers, funding agencies, and federal legislation. While these challenges seem to be insurmountable, they also offer planners opportunities for developing excellent programs if they take the time and care necessary to do so.

The education plan is supposed to be tailored to meet the unique needs presented by the child in accordance with recommendations from all significant educators and family members. Unfortunately, plans sometimes focus on correction of specific behaviors and completion of tasks. They often fail to take a comprehensive, integrated view of the student. Taking this approach limits the effectiveness of all educational efforts.

A more meaningful approach is to design a program that is more student-centered by modifying and strengthening the environment in which the student learns, lives, works, and plays.

Blosser and DePompei (1994) recommend implementing an ongoing planning process. A useful framework for understanding the planning process is to approach it as though you were planning a trip. Figure 9.1 presents the questions the planning team needs to ask as it begins to formulate a treatment plan for the student.

There are four phases to the ongoing planning process (see Figure 9.2). Phase I is the preplanning phase where groundwork is layed and the design for treatment is developed. The team is formed and each team member begins to gather pertinent data including: the student's history and current status; the environments in which learning will take place; the skills and needs of the potential contributions people in the learning environment can make on the student's success. A wide variety of assessment procedures take place during the preplanning phase. This enables planners to gain good perspective about the student's strengths and needs. Also importantly, we can begin to gain understanding of what the school and people in the school have to offer to support the student as well as the modifications needed

FIGURE 9.1   Questions for the Planning Team for Developing the Intervention Plan

1. *"Where is the individual now?"* What is the nature and extent of the student's communication impairment? From a number of perspectives, what are the resulting impairments, strengths, and needs? How do the communication problems impact on the student's overall performance in a variety of situations?
2. *"Where do we want him or her to go?"* The long-term outcomes we want the student to achieve should be determined. Consider this question especially in relation to the general education curriculum and participation in school-related activities. We want students to achieve their maximum potential. Treatment planners need to decide if the services and programs they are offering for the student will help him or her participate maximally in educational and social activities.
3. *"When do we want the person to get there?"* What is the timeline for implementing the program and achieving the desired outcomes? Treatment for communication impairments generally occurs over several months and in some cases, over several years. Evaluation of the student's performance must be continuous with ongoing review of the modifications and strategies that are implemented and how they are working.
4. *"Who do we want and need to take with us?"* In order to plan and implement the program effectively, who needs to be involved? The individuals that have the most stake in the student's success should be at the table when plans are made. Their understanding of the student's strengths and needs, the policies that will have an effect on school, the challenges that are likely to be faced, and the resources that will be available for support should be identified.
5. *"How do we want to go?"* What approaches to intervention are most effective for meeting the needs of the student? Any mode of treatment that will bring about the desired outcomes should be tried. Clinicians and educators should be willing to try creative approaches to meet the students needs. There is not a "one size fits all" to therapy. Team members need to be a part of the learning process: gaining a better understanding of the communication impairment, learning to work together as a team, identifying opportunities to promote the student's successes, and striving to continually improve the quality of the student's performance.
6. *"How much will the trip cost? What resources will be necessary to implement the plan?"* The team must decide what resources it will commit to achieve the desired outcomes they decide upon. It takes a lot to provide assistance to children. Resources include finances as well as personnel, time, and service options.
7. *"How will we know when we have arrived?"* What are the benchmarks against which the team will measure the student's success? We must know if the modifications we make and the strategies we implement are making a difference. The intervention program and student's progress should be evaluated in an ongoing manner to determine the appropriateness and suitability for meeting the student's needs.

to enable success. At the end of Phase I, we want to be able to identify the obstacles that will interfere with the student's success.

In Phase II, the planning phase, the team begins to work collaboratively to analyze information gleaned during the preplanning phase. Then together, the team determines the youngster's needs, goals, objectives, and workable strategies for preparing the youngster to function effectively in school and other environments. Meeting time is devoted to deciding the who, what, where, when, why, and how aspects of the plan. Team members collate information from family, teachers, specialists, health care providers, and others. The anticipated demands and expectations the student will confront in the classroom are identified.

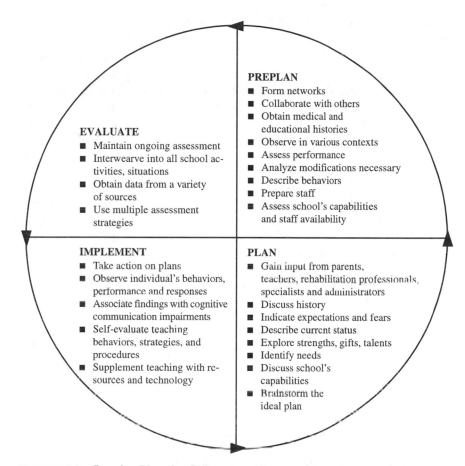

FIGURE 9.2   Ongoing Planning Process

From *Pediatric Traumatic Brain Injury Proactive Intervention,* by Blosser/DePompei. Copyright © 1995. Reprinted with permission of Delmar, a division of Thomson Learning. Fax 800 730-2215.

Thus, the student's strengths and needs are explored in the context of changes that might occur if modifications are made. The roles and responsibilities of team members (providers) are identified and clarified.

In Phase III, the implementation phase, action is taken on the plan. The climate for effective intervention and teaching is established and opportunities for learning are provided. This includes learning by the student as well as learning by educators, through in-service and other forms of training. Modification strategies are tried, with careful observation to see if the child responds positively.

During Phase IV, the evaluation and improvement phase, the plan is reviewed to determine how well it is or is not working. The degree of success at achieving desired outcomes is determined. The team determines if further modifications are necessary and discusses next steps. Thus, the planning process, including information gathering and observation, begin again.

DEVELOPING THE INDIVIDUALIZED EDUCATION PROGRAM

When IDEA was reauthorized in 1997, the law included requirements or standards for Individualized Education Programs (IEPs). The IEP is the vehicle that directs and guides the development of meaningful learning experiences, helping each child achieve the goal of becoming contributing and valued members of the community. The standards indicated that IEPs must include parent involvement, a focus on the general education curriculum, verification that team members are qualified and prepared to serve the student, accommodations, statewide and districtwide assessments, and progress reports. The IEP meeting must be held within 30 days after it has been determined that the student needs special education or related services. Services (if recommended) must begin within 60 days of the request for an initial evaluation.

Speech-language pathologists and the educators with whom they work must consider all of these elements when they develop the IEP. The school district is responsible for training staff on the components of IEPs. While these standards are intended to improve the education of children with special needs, it is anticipated that school districts will struggle with how to implement some of the requirements, especially enabling students with disabilities greater access to the general curriculum and ensuring that educators are prepared for the teaching challenges.

Table 9.1 presents the specific steps that should be followed to identify the student's needs and to recommend modifications. Figure 9.3 provides a format for conducting an interview with the teacher to determine the impact of communication disability on the student's performance.

THE INDIVIDUALIZED EDUCATION PROGRAM

Identification and Development Information

An individualized program must be developed for each school-age student identified as having a disability and needing special education placement or support services. The plan should include a description of the student including demographic information, the disability, and the educational level. The IEP also presents a plan of future goals. The IEP (or IFSP and ITP) should provide a cohesive picture of who the child is, where the child has been, where the child is currently, and where the child is going. Federal regulations specify the following content in the IEP:

- Demographic information and a description of the student's communication impairment
- A statement of the child's present levels of educational performance
- A statement of annual goals, including short-term and related services to be provided to the child and long-term instructional objectives
- A statement of the specific special education services to be provided and the extent to which the child will be able to participate in regular educational programs

TABLE 9.1   Steps to Assessing and Planning Modifications

	DATE COMPLETED

1. *Determine TASKS/ACTIVITIES TO BE ACCOMPLISHED*
   Identify the student's communication characteristics and needs
   ■ Meet with the planning team
   ■ Profile the student's performance	

Adhere to established policies and procedures for evaluating, exchanging the student, obtaining information, and communicating with potential providers.	
Obtain a concise statement of the youngster's communication problem as it appears in school-related situations from teachers and parents.	
Identify the providers who will consider the student's strengths, problems, characteristics, learning styles, and needs. Make recommendations based on findings. The student's parents must be included at this time. *In the PAC system, family members are considered to be equal providers and the home is an equal context.*	
Select a mutually agreeable meeting time that is sufficient in length to avoid having to rush discussions.	
Compile descriptive information about the students' communication skills and performance in academic and social situations. Include samples of work. Compile a portfolio and profile of performance. **(TOOLS: Formal tests; observations; teacher/parent interviews; educationally relevant assessment procedures (portfolio, work samples, etc.)** Include a student interview to determine the student's perspective of problems he/she is experiencing and ways he/she thinks other people can help or hinder. **(TOOLS: Student interview)**	
Construct a performance history and generate a report characterizing the student's skills, capabilities, and needs.	
Conduct the meeting and exchange information, taking care to relate findings to academic and social performance.	

Ask yourself and team members: "Do we have all the information necessary to develop a data-based description of this student's current level of performance that can be used to drive the formulation of intervention outcomes and strategies?"
 	
You will know the answer to this question if you can answer these two questions.
   Where is the student now?
   Where does the student need to go?	

(continued)

TABLE 9.1   Continued

If you can answer these two questions, you are ready to begin seeking the answer to this question: **How will we get him or her there?**	

2. *Determine TASKS/ACTIVITIES TO BE ACCOMPLISHED*
   ■ Identify environmental/situational characteristics and needs
   ■ Meet with the planning team
   ■ Design appropriate interventions
	DATE DONE—COMMENTS

Analyze the communication manner and style of important communication partners (Teachers, family, peers). **(TOOLS: Communication Style Identification Chart)** Help the student's important communication partners analyze their own communication behaviors (manner; style etc.) to determine if specific characteristics help or hinder the student's communicative performance. Discuss the match and/or mismatch between the partner's communicator's manner and style and the student's problems and needs. Jointly select the communicative intervention strategies that will reduce the mismatch between the partner's manner and style and the student's communication needs. **(TOOLS: Recommended strategies for modifying communication styles to accommodate the needs of students with communication disabilities)**	
Analyze the classroom instruction style and format. **(TOOLS: Classroom Observation Guide)** Help analyze the style and format of the classroom instruction to determine if specific modes of instruction help or hinder the student's communicative performance. Discuss the match and/or mismatch between the classroom instruction style and format and the student's problems and needs. Consider key aspects of teaching instruction such as planning instruction, managing instruction, and delivering instruction. Jointly select the teaching instruction strategies that will reduce the mismatch between the teaching instruction style and format and the student's communication needs. **(TOOLS: Teacher-to-student instruction strategies; classroom adaptations and modifications; student-to-student instructions strategies; student learning strategies)**	

(continued)

TABLE 9.1   Continued

Analyze the environmental factors that might influence performance.
(TOOLS: Classroom observation)
Help analyze key physical, social and psychological aspects of the learning environment to determine if specific components help or hinder the student's learning and communicative performance.
Consider components such as noise level, visual stimuli, seating arrangements, student's location in relation to typical instructional position, location of learning and work material, attitudes of teachers and peers, teacher expectations, opportunities for social-communicative interactions, etc.
Jointly select the environmental components that can be manipulated to reduce the mismatch between the environmental factors and student's learning and communication needs.
(TOOLS: Teacher-to-student instruction strategies; classroom adaptations and modifications; student-to-student instruction strategies student learning strategies)

- The projected dates for initiation of services and the anticipated frequency and duration of the services
- Appropriate objective criteria and evaluation procedures for determining, on at least an annual basis, whether the short-term instructional objectives are being achieved

The IEP must be specific for each child who receives either special education or related services or both. A single IEP is written for a child enrolled in regular or special education and receiving both special education and related services. The related service may be in speech-language intervention services, physical therapy, occupational therapy, adaptive behavior, counseling or other services that would support the student's success in school. Many students receive more than one related service in addition to their classroom placement.

The IEP Team

The IEP Team determines the impact of the disability on the student's progress in general education. Education is broadly interpreted to include academic achievement as well as social, emotional, and vocational components.

Presumably, the team will consist of people who know the student very well and who can provide information based on their knowledge of the child or the situation. The participants should be decided on a case-by-case basis based on the child's needs and best interests.

FIGURE 9.3   **Format for Conducting the Teacher Interview**

TEACHER INTERVIEW
OBSERVATION OF COMMUNICATION AND PERFORMANCE IN THE CLASSROOM

Date _____   Interviewer _____

Student _____   Teacher _____

School _____   Grade _____

INSTRUCTIONS: Through conversations with teachers, develop a profile of the student's communication skills and performance within the classroom setting. Highlight strengths as well as problem areas. Use the questions listed below to guide the discussion. Analyze the information gathered and use it to formulate recommendations and strategies for services.

TEACHER INTERVIEW QUESTIONS	
INTERACTIVE COMMUNICATION SKILLS/PERFORMANCE	**TARGET FOR SERVICE?**
How would you describe the student's overall performance in your class at this time? *Recommendations:*	
What are three successes the student has experienced recently in your classroom? *Recommendations:*	
Now describe three problems and talk about how you handle them. *Recommendations:*	
Tell me about the student's ability to tell stories, relate events, or convey information. *Recommendations:*	
Describe the way the student begins, ends, and maintains conversations. Is it appropriate for the situation? *Recommendations:*	

FIGURE 9.3   Continued

Explain how the student responds to humor, sarcasm, and figures of speech. *Recommendations:*	
Do you feel the student recognizes and uses appropriate vocabulary considering the age and situation? *Recommendations:*	
Is the student's voice and intonation level appropriately suited to the situation, place, and intent? *Recommendations:*	
Can the student locate details and facts to answer questions and draw conclusions? How does he or she go about trying to do so? *Recommendations:*	
Is the youngster able to comprehend written material from a variety of sources (newspaper, magazine, content area texts, reference materials)? Is this skill demonstrated through summarizing and recalling main ideas? *Recommendations:*	
Describe the student's performance when following written directions to complete a task (worksheet, recipes, problems, directions for building models). *Recommendations:*	
Characterize the student's written work (grammar, word choice, sentence structure, organization, appearance). *Recommendations:*	
Does the student's response time permit him or her to respond to questions when asked, participate in classroom discussions, complete assigned tasks? *Recommendations:*	

(continued)

FIGURE 9.3 Continued

What motivates the student to change or improve performance efforts? *Recommendations:*	
Identify behaviors that might be helping this student do well. *Recommendations:*	
Now, identify behaviors that might be interfering with the student's success. *Recommendations:*	
Based on your knowledge of children and your experience in teaching, what steps do you think are necessary for helping this student at this time? *Recommendations:*	
What are three specific strategies you have tried to use to help this student? Why did they work or not work? *Recommendations:*	
PROFILE OF STUDENT'S INTERACTIVE COMMUNICATION AND ACADEMIC PERFORMANCE: RECOMMENDED TARGETS FOR SERVICE AND SUMMARY OF RECOMMENDATIONS:	RESPONSIBLE PROVIDERS

The team composition would most likely include some combination of the following individuals: the child's parents, at least one regular education teacher, at least one special education teacher or special education provider, a local education representative, and an individual who can interpret the instructional implications of the evaluation results. When appropriate, the child should also be present, especially if he or she is 14 years of age or older.

Team members may perform more than one of the above roles. The local education agency (LEA) representative should be qualified to supervise specially designed instruction, know the general curriculum, and be aware of the availability of resources. The SLP would be considered a special education provider if a communication disorder were the primary disability. The parents are expected to be treated as equal participants and to play an active role in the planning and intervention process. They can provide critical information about the child's strengths and needs. They should be given opportunities to express their concerns and thoughts about the impact of the disability on the child's ability to progress in the general curriculum and participate in assessments. They should be included in decisions about the services that the student is provided. The child will be best served if the parents' expertise is sought and valued and if they are incorporated into the intervention plan. Chapter 10 provides information about how to mentor parents and teachers to be effective participants in that role.

All participants should contribute to developing, reviewing, and revising the plan. This includes proposing behavioral interventions and strategies. Dependent on the student's needs, it may also include supplementary aids and services, program modifications, or support for school personnel so that they will be able to deliver the required services. Many must be involved in implementing the plan if it is to succeed.

Some school districts have begun to "outsource" services (including speech-language intervention) in order to obtain the diverse services they need or to be more cost efficient. When out-of-school services are contracted by the local board of education for a specific child, the IEP is written by the school personnel involved and contains the information regarding the nature of the service provided. The out-of-school professional should be included in the preparation of the IEP.

Components of the IEP

Each of the major components necessary for the IEP is described in the following section. The components conform to the IEP requirements contained in the public law. Many alternatives exist for developing the IEP and complying with the law. Creativity and flexibility should be used so that the student can be properly addressed. The suggested components are designed to provide speech-language pathologists, educators, administrators, and family with information about the child and the educational demands, needs, and environment. As a secondary benefit, the information can lead to improvements in the program and case management procedures. The complexity of the IEP content will vary from student to student. The following figure and explanation indicate the required components of the IEP (Table 9.2). Examples of forms used in planning the IEP are included in Appendix C.

TABLE 9.2   Components of the Individualized Education Program (IEP)

Vision	Explore, the hopes and dreams that are held for the student for the future. Solicit the family's and student's preferences and interests.
Present level of educational performance	Review and document relevant data on the student including progress on current IEP, evaluation team report, family and student input, interventions, assessments, observations, and special factors. Provide a picture of how the student's disability affects involvement and performance on the general curriculum. Include information about strengths and needs.
Annual goals and short term objectives	Develop annual measurable goals and objectives or benchmarks/milestones which enable the student, to the extent that is appropriate, to be involved with the general curriculum. Determine the services necessary to meet the student's needs.
Amount of special education or related services	Indicate the projected beginning date, frequency, and duration of services to be provided.
Supplementary aids and services	Determine the accommodations, modifications, or assistive devices and program modifications or supports for school personnel that will be needed for the student to progress in the general curriculum and to participate in extracurricular and other nonacademic activities.
Participation with students without disabilities	Decide the extent of participation that is possible with students who do not present disabilities in regular classes or in extracurricular activities.
Test modifications	Indicate the modifications that should be provided in the administration of state or district assessments of student achievement in order for the student to participate in the assessment process.
Transition service	Focus on the student's courses of study by age 14. Focus on interagency responsibilities or needed community supports by age 16.
Notification of transfer of rights	Document that the student has been informed of the rights that will transfer to the student upon reaching the age of majority.
Evaluation procedures and methods of measurement	Specify how the student's progress will be evaluated (e.g. criterion-referenced test, standardized test, student product, teacher observation, or peer evaluation). Indicate how often the evaluation will take place (e.g. daily, weekly, monthly, each grading period/semester, or annually). Report progress as often as progress is reported for general education students.
IEP team members	Record signatures of all members of the IFP team that developed the IEP.

Assessment Information.   As discussed previously, informal and formal assessment procedures used to determine the child's needs and eligibility for special education should be included. No child can be placed in special education based on a single assessment procedure. The goal of assessment is to determine the student's ability to function and perform required learning tasks. Standardized and nonstandardized assessment methods should be used. Teacher interviews and classroom observations are especially important tools for determining how the student performs in the learning environment.

The team is responsible for reviewing the results of the multifactored evaluation or current IEP that is in place for the student. Team members must explain the student's present levels of performance including progress, strengths, capabilities, interests, and needs displayed at home, school, or in the community. The results of the assessments should be described and interpreted in a manner that facilitates understanding by other persons viewing the IEP.

The evaluation report should include complete names of all assessment instruments that were used. The date of assessment and the name and title of the examiner also should be included. It is very important to administer and score the assessment according to prescribed instructions and protocols. Assessment results are not valid or useful unless scored and interpreted according to the recommended procedures. Sometimes it is necessary to modify the administration procedures to accommodate the needs of the child. The evaluator should make notations of adaptations or modifications made during the administration of the test. It would be unethical to enroll a student in an intervention program based on a test that is incorrectly administered or scored. Based on the evaluation information presented, the team determines the student's areas of need.

Current Levels of Development, Function, and Performance. From the assessment information collected, data-based statements of performance must be developed. These statements indicate the performance level for specific tasks or behaviors. Preferably, each statement will include a quantitative (numerical) and qualitative (descriptive) reference to the child's performance level. Performance levels can be indicated for such communication areas as language, speech, reading, hearing, or any other breakdown appropriate for the child or the informational needs of the school. The description of the student's performance provides a profile from which to launch discussion about the student including strengths, capabilities, interests, and needs displayed in school, in the community, or at home.

Need Statements. Need statements show the direction of change that is to occur as the present level of performance is modified. Need statements indicate that a behavior is going to increase or decrease.

Annual Goals. Goals indicate the projected level of performance for the child as a result of receiving the special education and related services indicated in the IEP. Goals should describe and explain the behavior that should occur, when the behavior should occur, and the criterion for determining if the behavior is correct. The goals are measurable targets for achievement. Goals should allow the student to participate in the general curriculum as well as in social, emotional, and vocational areas.

Short-Term Instructional Objectives. The specific performance areas to which the instructional objective relates, for example, language or articulation, must be delineated. "Instructional Objectives" indicate the intermediate steps leading to the goal. In the legislation they are also referred to as benchmarks. They include specific behaviors that will be acquired as the child moves toward accomplishment of the annual goal. Each annual goal may have a number of instructional objectives depending on the intermediate steps needed to accomplish the goal. A significant component to the IEP is the determination of how and when each objective (and goal) will be evaluated to determine the student's progress and success. Each objective should include the components such as the procedures to be used to measure the objective, the criteria, the schedule for review, the person responsible for that objective, a review of progress, the special education services to be delivered, the length and duration of the service, and the context (or setting) in which the behavior is to occur.

The objectives should be written using terminology that links the goal to the curriculum. This will ensure that all the educators are addressing the objective and that the effect of the disability on the student's performance is the focus of the special education services.

Extent of Participation in the Regular Educational Environment.   Incorporating services into the educational setting implies that the treatment will occur within educational environments such as the classroom. In order for that to happen effectively, there are a number of modifications or supports that schools usually consider. The accommodations and special services that are necessary to ensure that the student can access the general curriculum are included. Some examples include reducing the amount of work, adapting the work in some way, assessing learning in different ways, assigning preferential seating, and other similar modifications. Educators should be creative as they explore modifications that might help the student perform better to meet learning outcomes. Materials, presentation format, task requirements, grading practices, delivery of instructions, content, and physical or environmental modifications are all examples of those aspects of the instructional process that can be modified.

Assistive technology based on the child's identified needs must be discussed by the IEP team. This includes monitoring hearing aids and ensuring that devices are made available if required. Assistive devices are equipment that is used to support a student's functional capabilities.

Primary or unique methods and materials that are needed to complete the instructional objectives are included under the recommendations section of the IEP. Recommendations should include the following components: what, how many, and how often.

The explanation of modifications also includes indicating who will provide the service. Options include individual educators or teams of educators. Parents are also given responsibilities for implementing specific aspects of the plan.

Amount and Duration of Services.   The IEP must include a statement of the amount of services, date the services will convene, and how long they are likely to be provided. This demonstrates the school's commitment of resources. The amount of time to be committed must be appropriate to the specific service and stated clearly in the IEP. When changes are to be made, parents must be notified in another IEP meeting.

Progress and Status Reports.   There is a requirement for reporting progress and a method for maintaining ongoing contact with the parents and others about the student's achievements. Federal legislation mandates that schools implement a process for evaluating and reporting progress to parents on a nine-week basis. Many methods can be used for accomplishing this task including face-to-face meetings, written notes, phone calls, or report cards.

On the date the instructional objective is to be accomplished, or on any other regularly scheduled review date, the evaluation component in the instructional objective can be executed. Using a status code or descriptive statement can indicate progress the child has made in completing the objective. By describing the student's mastery of a particular skill, staff will be able to indicate the amount of progress made by the child in those instances when 100 percent of the indicated criterion has not been met. Revisions and comments that provide insights about the student's performance should be included to provide information that can be used in developing future IEPs.

Verification and Documentation.   Schools are bound by law to inform and include parents in the planning and intervention process. The IEP form contains space for documenting the parents' address and signatures indicating their understanding of the proceedings.

Special Education and Related Services Needed.   The special education and related or support services the child needs in order to receive an appropriate education and participate in the general curriculum should be described. Statements should include information on the specific educational alternatives, the types of services to be provided, and frequency with which the service will be provided. The percentage of time the child will spend in each special education and related service program and regular education program must be indicated. The percentage can be computed by determining the total number of educational hours available during the year and dividing that number into the number of hours spent in the various special and regular education programs.

The parents' signatures must be secured to indicate they approve of the services that will be provided to their child. A summary statement indicating the recommendations and the rationale for the decisions must also be included. The IEP team meeting may be convened and the plan developed without parental attendance if the school district makes reasonable attempts to get them to attend and they refuse. The school district must maintain complete records of attempts to arrange meetings at mutually agreeable times and places. This includes the SLP program. If the SLP is having difficulty connecting with the parents, the school administration should be notified so that correct procedures are followed.

Creating IEPs for a large caseload can be a very time-consuming task. Some clinicians have made the job more efficient by using computers and word processors. They select intervention goals from a data bank of goals and objectives. Many publishers of speech-language pathology resource materials have created comprehensive resources containing functional, relevant IEP goals and objectives that are educationally appropriate for school-age children. Check the publishers' catalogues and request to review these materials. Energetic SLP staffs often create their own data banks. While this is a time-consuming approach, the result will be well worth the effort and suited to the curriculum and needs of the specific school district.

An example of an IEP form developed in a large public school district can be found in Appendix C.

INDIVIDUALIZED FAMILY SERVICE PLAN

Public Law 99-457 specified guidelines for serving the needs of infants and toddlers presenting developmental delays. Public Law 99-457 assigns responsibility to the states to establish criteria for eligibility. Consequently, criteria may vary from state to state. The law requires that the services be multidisciplinary and that service delivery plans reflect coordination of services among local agencies. Provision of services to the child's family is an integral component of the law. Federal regulations mandate that a systematic service plan be developed. This is referred to as the Individualized Family Service Plan (IFSP). The plan must span one year with a six-month review, specify outcomes for the child and family, and name a service coordinator from the profession most relevant to the child's or family's needs. Collaboration is reinforced as a service delivery model for this population.

With the exception of services provided to the family and the emphasis on the child's health-related needs, several components in the IFSP are similar to those of the IEP. A meeting is held with the family and professionals who can provide services to the child. The goal of the meeting is to establish a plan for achieving the desired outcomes. Gillette and Robinson (1992) describe a process for developing an Individualized Family Service Plan (IFSP). They include a sample meeting agenda, schedule for discussing pertinent topics, and sample planning forms. Prior to the meeting, the coordinator should gather pertinent background information about the child and family to facilitate greater understanding of the needs and possible ways to meet those needs.

The IFSP format can be used to focus the attention of meeting attendees and guide the discussion. A sample format is included in Figure 9.4. The components of the IFSP are similar to the IEP. The topics listed below should be addressed in writing and face to face during discussions:

- Introductions and background information including identifying information about the child, family, and disciplines/agencies represented
- An overview of current medical, health, and rehabilitation services being provided to the child
- A summary of the child's current health, development, and family functioning including the child's strengths and needs and the family's strengths and needs in relation to the child
- The child's health outcome, providers, and methods of service delivery including identifying the providers, the location, duration, frequency, and intensity of each service
- The child's development outcome, providers, and methods; again determining professional providers, service schedules (numbers of contacts, length of contacts, and location of service), family involvement and measures of child development to be used
- The family's life outcome, providers, and methods; determining services that may be needed in the following areas: support, child care, education, family life planning, financial resources, and community resources
- As the meeting draws to a close, a service coordinator should be identified

INDIVIDUALIZED TRANSITION PLAN

When IDEA was reauthorized in 1990 and again in 1997, it included a mandate that schools should plan for students' transitions from school to work and/or postsecondary

FIGURE 9.4   Sample Individualized Family Service Plan

Date: mm/dd/yy

Name: John

Birthdate: mm/dd/yy	Birthdate: mm/dd/yy
Age:	Age: 12 Months
Parents/Guardian:	Relationship to Child (please circle)
Address:	biological parent, foster parent, residential facility
City:	Referred by: Children's Hospital
Phone:	Referral Date: mm/dd/yy
State:	Next review date: mm/dd/yy

County:

School district/residence: Home City

I. CHILD'S CURRENT SERVICES

Primary Physician: Dr. Mosnott

Nursing: Sharon Short, R.N., County Services

Early Intervention: Nancy Hill, Teacher; Annette Manning, Speech; (County) Trevor Blosser, Physical Therapy; Cheryl Pelland, Occupational Therapy

Human Services: Respite Services; Family Resources; Nutritional Funds

Other: Denise Wray, Summer Occupational Therapy; Dr. DePompei, Neonatology Follow-up Clinic; Dr. Jackson, Surgery; Dr. McCarthy, Ophthalmology; Dr. Butler, Cardiology; Dr. Ryan, Genetics; Dr. Renick, Neurosurgery

Case Manager: Nancy Hill, Teacher

II. SUMMARY OF CHILD/FAMILY CURRENT STATUS

Child Health (Past History, Current Status):

Differences from last plan: (1) shunt revision: mm/dd/yy; (2) hernia repair: scheduled for mm/dd/yy; (3) chailasia scan mm/dd/yy—mild reflux

Immunizations: DPT: 4/91; OPV: 4/91, 7/91; MMR: HIB:

Flu shot: mm/dd/yy

Nutrition: mm/dd/yy, videofluoroscopy—swallowing mechanism intact

Hearing: mm/dd/yy, hearing evaluation—behavioral—intact hearing

Vision: follow-up scheduled for mm/dd/yy

Technology Dependence: None

Child Development (Assessment, Date, Findings):

(Battelle 1/26/92 Age Equivalents)

Movement: 5 months

Communication: Receptive—5 months; Expressive—2 months

(continued)

FIGURE 9.4 Continued

Understanding: 5 months

Social: 6 months

Living Skills: 2 months

Other: INFANIB. Abnormal muscle tone—low

Family Functioning:

Financial Resources: Provider (Name, Address, Phone)

Insurance: HMO; 1212 Trail Rd., Home City, OH 10101

Public Assistance: (Medicaid, SSI): SSI for 2 older children

Other: (MCMH, Model 50, Family Resources): for nutritional supplement allowance

Transportation: added additional family car

Child Care: none

Respite Care: grandmother and county respite

Support Systems (family, church, counseling, etc.): extended family, many friends

Child's Strengths: enjoys moving and touching people and objects; smiles

Child's Needs: needs to improve eating habits and make weight gains; development in all areas delayed

III. OUTCOMES—CHILD HEALTH, CHILD DEVELOPMENT, FAMILY FUNCTIONING

A. Outcome: John will continue toward best possible health in terms of:
1. *Eating, and Growth (Methods and Providers):*
   a. Measure and chart weight, length, head circumference weekly. (Provider—county nurse)
   b. Review measurements above monthly. (Provider—pediatrician)
   c. Continue to feed John with nutritionally supplemented formula. (Provider—mother)
   d. Regularly follow and revise oral motor skills program. (Provider—mother and county)
2. *Breathing and Hearing Patterns*
   a. Review vital signs monthly. (Provider—family and pediatrician)
   b. Attend scheduled cardiology appointments. (Provider—family and pediatrician)
3. *Neurological Status*
   a. Monitor fontanelle and shunt site
   b. Observe for signs of shunt malfunction
   c. Attend hearing, vision, and neurosurgery appointments. (Provider for a, b, and c—family and neurosurgeon)
4. *Routine Health Care*
   a. Schedule and attend appointments for follow-up of health status and immunizations. (Provider—family and pediatrician)

B. Outcome: John will continue toward his best possible development integrating the following skill areas: movement, understanding, communication, socialization, self help.

FIGURE 9.4 Continued

1. Attend classes 2 times a week for 2 ½ hours to address the four skill areas above and to plan home interventions and teach family skills.
2. Work toward self-help in feeding following plan under health.
3. Attend evaluation at orthopedic clinic to determine best intervention and appropriate equipment for low tone.

(Provider for 1, 2, and 3—county, parent-infant program, teacher, speech, occupational and physical therapists, and family)

C. **Outcome:** The family will continue to meet John's needs with their choice of health, developmental and social services.
1. Continue to provide allowance for nutritional supplement. (Provider— county)
2. Continue to take advantage of county and family for respite. (Provider— family)
3. Explore financing through county's family resources for any equipment recommended. (Provider—family)

activities. Transitions are considered "the life changes, adjustments, and cumulative experiences that occur in the lives of young adults as they move from school environments to more independent living and work environments" (Wehman, 1992). Transition can also include changes in self-awareness, body image, sexuality, work, financial needs, and mobility.

Blosser and DePompei (1994) believe that this is a rather limited interpretation of transition because it focuses only on transition from school to work. It does not take into account transition into school from healthcare settings by students with healthcare needs. Nor does it consider transition into the school setting for preschoolers with disabilities. More importantly for youngsters with communication disabilities, it does not account for the many transitions youngsters experience as they progress through school from grade to grade, subject to subject, or teacher to teacher. This expanded definition gives perspective to the problems students often experience in school throughout the day or from year to year. This explanation of transition illustrates the daily stress that is placed on students' communication performance. Transition into each situation carries with it unique and different demands and expectation for communication performance.

The law stated that a statement of needed transition services be included as part of the IEP for students with disabilities beginning no later than age 16, and when appropriate age 14 or younger, and annually thereafter. The intent was to assure that students with disabilities have the opportunity to lead rewarding and productive lives after leaving school. The goal is to provide opportunities for work or study, independent living, and community participation.

There are four essential components of transition planning as defined by IDEA: planning and services should be based on student needs and preferences; transition planning should be oriented to postsecondary outcomes; transition planning should include a coordinated set of activities; and services should promote movement from school to postschool settings.

Speech-language pathologists can be significant members on the transition planning team in school districts by helping other team members understand the difficulty students encounter as they transition from one situation to another. The success of the student's transition from one situation to another (including high school to the world of work) is influenced by the following factors: (1) the nature and extent of the student's communication impairment; (2) the demands and expectations of the specific situation; (3) the level of understanding of the people in the student's environment; (4) the quality of treatment and services the student receives; (5) opportunities for success; and (6) the student's readiness and preparation for the situation he or she is about to enter.

Transition planning differs from the IEP because it focuses on the types of services needed to achieve long-term postsecondary goals such as postsecondary education, vocational training, supported employment, continuing education, adult services, independent living, community participation, and the like. The composition of the transition team is important to the development of an effective transition plan. At a minimum, the student, parents, teacher, and other relevant staff members should be present when the Individualized Transition Plan (ITP) is developed. Speech-language pathologists can be significant members on the transition planning team in school districts.

A review of the professional literature on planning transitions for students (deFur & Patton, 1999; Clark et al., 1991; and Wehman, 1992) indicated the following guiding principles to make the transition proceed smoothly:

Transition efforts should start early. The 1997 reauthorization the Individuals with Disabilities Education Act (IDEA) recommends that educators and parents begin the transition planning process at as early an age as possible. Schools should establish a systematic K–12 transition education program where elementary students gain a strong foundation that will help them as they transition through school and after they leave school (Clark et al., 1991). Transition activities should be initiated early to ensure a seamless transition to postschool settings. Most school districts initiate transition planning when the child reaches age 14. At that time, vocational assessment is added as part of the multifactored evaluation process. The information obtained can be used to develop an ITP.

Planning must be comprehensive. Students must be looked at from a comprehensive point of view to determine their needs as they progress through school. Comprehensive transition planning includes periodic review of where the student is with regard to the following aspects: employment, further education and training, leisure activities, community participation, health (physical, emotional, and spiritual), self-determination/self-advocacy, communication, interpersonal relationships/social skills, and transportation/mobility. The speech-language pathologist has much to contribute about the dynamics of communication related to each of these areas. In some cases, the SLP will help prepare the student for the next step; in other cases, the SLP will make recommendations for the transition plan. Prerequisite skills that will be necessary for success should be the focus of treatment and intervention.

The planning process must balance what is ideal with what is possible. Special educators are often troubled and frustrated because they cannot do everything that it takes to help their students. We must learn to be satisfied with our contribution when we do what we consider to be our absolute best effort. Given that students will experience many different transitions, the individualized transition plan should be reviewed and updated on an ongoing basis.

Student empowerment is essential. Students must be at the table when plans for their future are being discussed. This may be uncomfortable for the student as well as for the professional but plans will be much more effective if the student's interests and motivation are considered. Enabling the student to participate will also foster greater independence and self-advocacy. The earlier we begin inviting students to participate in the discussions of their educational program, the more likely they will gain skills that will help them as they progress throughout life. Recommendations for students' participation in various activities are made in NEXT S.T.E.P.: Student Transition and Educational Planning (Halpern et al., 1997). Students will flourish if they are provided with options and opportunities to participate in many different experiences.

Family involvement is critical. It is valuable to have families involved in all aspects of the student's education. This is even more crucial for families of youngsters with severe disabilities. They will be the ones who must ensure ongoing services for their child, especially after the student leaves school. Seek their input and value their contributions, whatever they may be. Some families are not capable and others are not interested in participating, while others want to be a part of every decision that is made about the student's education. Professionals must learn to deal with each type of parent, providing the information that is needed when it is needed. It will be useful to gain good understanding of the family dynamics and involve them in crucial transition planning activities as much as possible.

Transition planning must be sensitive to diversity. Transition planners must demonstrate sensitivity to diversity issues including dimensions such as cultural diversity, race, ethnicity, religious beliefs, gender, and sexual orientation. It is especially important to make recommendations to the student and family with these aspects in mind.

Transition planning should help students and families access supports and services. Youth with special needs and their families should be informed of the extensive variety of supports and services available in the community. This will help them understand that they are not alone when they encounter difficult situations. There are numerous people in every community and work situation with knowledge that can be helpful to the success of individuals with disabilities.

Transition planning should include preparing the environment where the student will be going and preparing the people in that environment to support the youngster and help facilitate success. Each situation the student enters poses a different set of demands and expectations for the student's communication skills. SLPs can help identify and modify those features of the environment that might pose challenges or obstacles for the student. Family members, friends, teachers, and others can play very active roles in ensuring smooth and successful transitions. The Individualized Transition Plan should specify the persons who will be involved in the transition including describing their role, ways they can help, and skills they need to develop in order to provide assistance.

Community-based activities are important. Assessment and training should be carried out in real-life situations. That way, the student can be prepared for situations that are likely to be encountered. It will also help the student generalize practiced skills to everyday occurrences.

Interagency commitment, cooperation, and coordination are critical to successful transition. It is likely that students with disabilities will need to access many different types of services. This can be made easier if personnel in various agencies form positive relationships with one another and coordinate their services. In this way, movement from one service provider to another will be smooth and will not create undue stress or duplication of services for the students and their families.

School administrators should be involved in planning transitions. In order to implement successful transitions for students, administrative support is often necessary. Therefore, it is helpful to have administrators present when ITPs are being formulated and written.

Transition plans should be evaluated periodically to be sure they are current and relevant. Writing the transition plan is only the beginning. Similar to IEPs, the transition plan should be revisited periodically to be sure that the priorities, goals, objectives, and decisions that have been made are still suited to the student's needs and capabilities.

EDUCATIONAL STANDARDS

Education reformers suggest that there is a belief that schools should prepare students to meet specific standards. The belief is based on the premise that by raising the standards, school achievement will also increase and students will be better prepared to the world of work, postsecondary education, and citizenship in a democratic and global society. Standards explicitly state the knowledge and skills that all students are expected to master. What are those standards and where does speech-language intervention fit?

Each state is organizing its standards in different ways. However, there are many similarities from state to state. The goal is to clearly define and articulate learning expectations for all students, teachers, and schools. Efforts are under way across the nation to define "exit expectations" for high school seniors in English language arts including reading, writing, listening, and speaking. Most states are also defining learning "benchmarks" for key points along the learning path from kindergarten through twelfth grade. The intent is for the curriculum and formal instruction to consistently line up with the expectations for learning indicated by the standards. This national agenda will most likely impact the way speech-language services are delivered in the future and the interpretation which students are eligible for services. The SLP should be familiar with the standards, expectations, and curricula for each of the content areas but especially for the language arts, literacy, math, and science areas.

The standards for English/language arts generally recommend that the teaching of reading and writing should be integrated. Students should learn to read a variety of texts: fiction, nonfiction, informational, historical, political, and social/cultural. Students should learn to read visual texts such as film, television, photographs, graphics (charts and illustrations), and technological texts via the Internet. Students are expected to learn to write for a variety of purposes and audiences. They should know the various purposes of writing as well as the technical and mechanical aspects. Thus, students are expected to be able to speak, listen, view, and visually represent language to self-reflect, communicate with others, and learn. Of all of the areas of the curriculum, the greatest link between the standards and the services we offer are within the English/language arts standards. A compelling argument can be made for the need for speech-language intervention for a student who is unable to perform to the highest expectations of the standards due to communication impairment.

Regarding the mathematics standards, students are expected to value mathematics, become problem solvers, and learn to reason mathematically. They should be able to communicate about mathematics and use math-related terminology. Students are supposed to learn math so they will be able to function in society, being able to compute, estimate, and use technology. Many students with communication disabilities have difficulty learning mathematics because of the abstract nature of the concepts presented. Teachers should be advised of the impact of communication problems on understanding and communicating about mathematics.

Science, like math, has become the focus of much discussion regarding the needs for educational reform. Critics do not believe that students are being adequately prepared in the area of science in order to perform effectively in society after leaving school. Scientific literacy is considered necessary for everyone. Students must be able to make informed decisions, discuss scientific and technical issues, and understand the natural world. There is an expectation that they will be able to understand science as inquiry, physical science, life science, earth and space science, technology, and other concepts and processes. Similar to learning math, learning science implies that the student will understand abstract concepts. In addition, students must learn difficult vocabulary and be able to manipulate complex information and sequences. Again, the SLP can contribute much to teachers' understanding of why students experience difficulty with the math curriculum by explaining the link between language and learning.

The social sciences include history, geography, civics, government, and economics. The social science standards state an expectation that the student will become a responsible citizen, understanding the responsibility that is entailed. Through these content areas, students learn to respect the institutions and laws of government. In addition, they are to learn about diversity and other cultures. Students who have difficulty comprehending language in the written form and recalling facts will likely have difficulty meeting the expectations of the standards.

School clinicians must have a good understanding of the structure, scope, and sequence of the general education curriculum followed for each grade and subject area in their school district. All school districts have manuals available describing these components and the competencies students are expected to gain as they progress through school. The manuals may be referred to by a number of names including "scope and sequence," "course of study," "school curricula," or "competency guidelines."

The wise clinician will obtain a copy of the school curriculum and state standards from the curriculum director in the school district and coordinate the speech-language program with the curriculum. An example of the scope and sequence for a language arts curriculum is provided in Appendix B to show you how valuable these materials can be for program planning.

It is the SLP's responsibility to provide teachers with specific suggestions for creating a "communication positive" climate in their classroom. This can be done by jointly arranging classroom materials, space, and activities so that communication exchanges will occur. With instruction from the SLP, teachers can learn to use several interactive communication strategies to elicit correct speech-language production, reinforce children's attempts to practice what they are learning in the therapy program, and facilitate correct productions when communication errors are observed. Strategies and modifications must be incorporated into the IEP as shown in Figure 9.5. Several specific communication strategies teachers can implement are presented in Chapter 10.

FIGURE 9.5   Teaching Accommodations and Modifications

X	TEACHER-TO-STUDENT INSTRUCTION STRATEGIES
	Determine your expectations for successful communicative performance in your classroom (work) environment.
	State and clarify expectations for communicative performance to the student.
	Analyze the communicative demands made of the student by classroom activities and assigned tasks.
	Help student prioritize learning goals and tasks.
	Guide student to recognize reasons why communication attempts are inaccurate or inappropriate.
	Introduce important information at a level that is commensurate with the youngster's developmental, mental, and communicative capabilities.
	Individualize assignments and tests to accommodate special communicative needs (reduce the number of questions; alternative modes of response).
	Avoid abrupt changes in topic during class discussions (use transitions from topic to topic).
	Provide listening guides and outlines for lectures.
	Connect "who," "what," and "where" questions to information desired from student when asking questions.
	Cue the student with words such as: "first," "second," and "next."
	Introduce stories and curricular units with visual cues such as pictures, outlines, etc.
	Permit alternate response modes such as drawing, pantomime, selecting answers from choices.
	Ask probing questions to see if student comprehends important information.
	Use sentence completion strategies when you don't understand the student.
	Arrange opportunities for practice.
	Provide feedback and guidance to increase understanding of successful and unsuccessful attempts.
	Observe and evaluate performance routinely and systematically. Modify teaching strategies based on information gained.

FIGURE 9.5 Continued

X	TEACHER-TO-STUDENT INSTRUCTION STRATEGIES *(Continued)*
	Provide incentives to stimulate communicative interaction.
	Teach the student to recognize and measure components of successful performance.
	Encourage the discussion and sharing of problems the child may be experiencing. Help the child understand the relationship between the communication problems and the difficulties being experienced.
	Implement teaching approaches that actively involve the student in learning activities.
	Be observant of stressors placed on the child by others (teachers, peers, family, administrators). Reduce stressors as much as possible.
	Use additional ideas based on your knowledge of effective instructional strategies.
	STUDENT-TO-STUDENT INSTRUCTION STRATEGIES
	Use cooperative learning strategies.
	Pair the student with a buddy to use reciprocal teaching strategies.
	Provide small group activities to facilitate peer tutoring and modeling.
	Select a fellow student to act as a "buddy" to help the youngster participate meaningfully in class and school related activities.
	Select a "fellow student coach" to help the child stay aware of instructions, transitions from activity to activity, assignments, and so on.
	Directly teach peers to implement specific interactive communication strategies so they are prepared to provide models and facilitate positive responses when the student has difficulty communicating or learning.
	Encourage friendships and sharing through social and extracurricular activities based on the child's capabilities and interests.
	CLASSROOM ADAPTATIONS AND MODIFICATION TECHNIQUES TO PROMOTE EFFECTIVE COMMUNICATION
	Permit and encourage the use of assistive devices including calculators, computers, tape recorders, assistive listening devices, and more.

(continued)

FIGURE 9.5   **Continued**

X	**CLASSROOM ADAPTATIONS AND MODIFICATION TECHNIQUES TO PROMOTE EFFECTIVE COMMUNICATION** *(Continued)*
	Formulate a system to help the child maintain organization (such as schedule books, assignment notebooks, "to do" lists).
	Accompany textbooks and work pages with supportive materials (pictures, written cues, graphic illustrations).
X	**STUDENT LEARNING STRATEGIES**
	Encourage the student to reread instructions more than one time, exercising care to underline, highlight, and note important elements.
	Ask the student to repeat instructions verbatim before initiating a learning task.
	Verify the student's comprehension of directions by requesting that the instructions be restated using different terminology.
	Have the student review work after completing it. Encourage proofreading of assignments before submitting them, looking for completeness and accuracy.
	Provide the student with opportunities to repeat assignments at another time to see if performance can be improved.
	Invite the student to ask questions and to clarify information not understood.
	Have the student write instructions on a separate sheet of paper.
	Have the student self-evaluate work to see if it is appropriate, verbalizing correct and incorrect aspects of the work.
	Teach the student to use specific graphic organizers such as: flow charts, comparison/contrast charts, story map, sequence maps.

From *Pediatric Traumatic Brain Injury Proactive Intervention,* by Blosser/DePompei. Copyright © 1995. Reprinted with permission of Delmar, a division of Thomson Learning. Fax 800 730-2215.

MAKING SPEECH-LANGUAGE INTERVENTION RELEVANT TO THE STUDENTS' EDUCATIONANEEDS

School is a communication-based environment. Therefore, students who exhibit communication impairments are at risk for academic failure. This means they will not be able to progress in the general education curriculum without assistance. Success in the school setting depends on the ability to communicate effectively in classroom and social situations where functional communication skills are necessary. For example, children must respond appropriately when asked questions. They must understand the meaning of vocabulary words and concepts unique to numerous subject areas. They are expected to interact socially with adults and peers. In order to gain information, they must be able to formulate questions and use appropriate phonology, syntax, semantics, and pragmatics so others can understand them. They have to understand relationships between sounds and symbols. It is essential for them to follow written and verbal instructions, organize thoughts in verbal and written expression, and comprehend large amounts of information presented by the teacher.

The school speech-language clinician can increase students' potential for success by making the intervention program relevant to students' academic needs. There are two ways this can be accomplished. One, the clinician can incorporate objectives and materials from the classroom into the therapy program. Two, the teacher can reinforce communication skills during classroom activities. Both of these methods require collaboration between the classroom teacher and speech-language clinician.

The creative clinician needs only to look to the classroom to obtain materials and resources for the intervention program. Textbooks, workbooks, and teaching kits provide materials and activities that are age appropriate, interesting, and motivating to children. By developing speech-language therapy goals around the curriculum, the clinician can increase the student's chances of using appropriate communication skills while responding in the classroom. Following are examples of functional treatment goals based on curricular objectives and communication needs:

- To appropriately respond to questions *from the end of the social studies chapter*
- To correctly produce target phonemes taken *from the student's weekly spelling list*
- To generate and combine sentences *about life's events to create an autobiography*
- To verbally recall details *from a story assigned in reading group*
- To verbally describe (in sequence) four steps *in a science experiment*
- To correctly explain *the rules of a sport being taught in gym class*
- To comprehend mathematical concepts *stressed in math class*
- To produce syntactically correct sentences *using the weekly vocabulary list from language arts class*
- To use appropriate pragmatic skills *during a small group craft activity*
- To use fluent speech to practice an *oral book report for English class*

PLANNING AND EVALUATING THE TREATMENT SESSION

There are considerations the school SLP needs to make when planning instructional objectives for individual lesson plans. First to be considered are the goals for that particular lesson. What does the clinician hope to have the student accomplish? Are the clinician's aims reasonable? Is the student aware of the goals for that lesson? Has he or she helped formulate them? Do the clinician and student agree on the goals? Will these goals bring them closer to the final goal? Along with the specific goals for each treatment session, the clinician and student must be in agreement on the general, or long-range, goals. In other words, what is to be finally accomplished in the way of improvement of communication?

The next thing needed in the lesson plan is the list of materials. If the list contains classroom and curricular materials, the subject, text, page numbers, and worksheets should be listed. The list should be so complete that a person unfamiliar with the session would be able to assemble the materials from the list. A complete listing of materials will provide a ready future source of reference not only for the beginning clinician but for the SLP as well.

Following the list of materials, the lesson plan would then go on to the steps or the procedures in the lesson. These can be listed in order of use and include the estimated time for each. This would be particularly helpful to the beginning clinician, who has not yet been able to judge accurately the amount of time needed for each step. It is a common occurrence for the novice to complete all the activities of the lesson in half the time allotted or else to complete only the first few steps in the entire amount of time. It should be a comfort to the beginning clinician to know that more accurate judgment skills will be developed with continued experience.

The steps in the lesson should be based on the child's needs, the general and specific goals of therapy, and the evaluated results of the previous lesson. The clinician may wish to consult with the parents concerning home assignments or with the classroom teacher on generalization.

The clinician must have justification for listing the steps in a particular order; otherwise the therapy session becomes a hodgepodge of activities unrelated to the goals. On the other hand, the order of activities must not become so sacred that it cannot be changed. I recall one professor's lecture to a class in which she said, "I expect each student teacher to teach from a lesson plan, complete with goals, materials, estimated time for each activity, and the activities listed in order of presentation. But if I come into the room and find the student teacher teaching the right activity at the right time according to the clock and the lesson plan, I'll know there's something wrong with the lesson."

Her point, of course, is that any lesson plan, no matter how carefully thought out, should be abandoned or rearranged to suit the needs of the student. Unexpected teaching moments should be seized. For example when Jimmy comes to speech therapy and proudly announces that he has a new baby sister, or if Susie wants to show off her new shoes, or if the first snow of the season has fallen during the night, use these instances to develop interactive language skills.

By using meaningful activities, curricular materials, and real-life situations, generalization becomes much less of a problem. The clinician doesn't fall into the trap of playing endless, meaningless games with the student. In most schools, classroom teachers are required to submit lesson plans each week to the principal or curriculum supervisor. This is done for two reasons. One, if the teacher becomes ill, a substitute teacher can take over the class. Two, the teacher's plans can be monitored to make sure that curricular objectives are being met. Speech-language pathologists also need to keep their lesson plans current and available for review if asked.

Developing individualized lesson plans for large numbers of children can be a time-consuming and complex task for school clinicians. Experienced SLPs often evolve unique systems for preparing their lesson plans using abbreviations, numbers, and codes to record therapy objectives and procedures for each child on the caseload.

MOTIVATION

Much has been written about motivating students. Everyone seems to be in agreement that motivation is necessary to produce good and lasting results. It is not uncommon to hear clinicians express the wish that they could motivate their clients. This would imply that motivating is something one does to another person. However, motivation is something that is within the person, driving him or her to achieve. It is not realistic to think that clinicians are able to motivate clients. Rather, the recipients of our services will make a change in communication behavior only if personal values and attitudes compel them to do so.

The use of games—negative reinforcement, positive reinforcement, rewards, punishment, shaping behavior—provides incentives and inducements that may bring about changes in behavior. If the inner drive, or the motivation, is absent, however, there may be regression or lack of what is commonly referred to as carryover or generalization; or there may be no change in behavior.

Although the clinician is highly anxious to change the child's speech behavior, it does not necessarily follow that the child will share that feeling. In some cases the child may be highly motivated to hang onto an immature speech and language pattern because it may be a way of controlling, satisfying, or coping with other members of the family. Or a child may enjoy the attention that immature speech brings.

What are the implications for the clinician in regard to motivation in students? Much can be accomplished by shifting from a teacher-centered orientation of motivation to an understanding of the attitudes and values present in the child's motivation for learning. A child-centered approach is suggested. In this approach, the SLP focuses on the child's interests and needs when designing the session. Developing a sense of the child's emotional state of being and the meaning of his or her nonverbal responses helps the astute clinician shape the tone of treatment. It is desirable for the clinician to have some background in developmental psychology, a sensitivity to the nuances of the therapeutic relationship, and a willingness to learn as much as possible about an individual child's emotional functioning. Understanding the feelings of the child may be as important as any diagnostic information that is gathered.

EVALUATING THE EFFECTIVENESS OF THE SESSION

Following each session, the clinician should evaluate the effectiveness of the lesson. What should the evaluation include? In order to decide, let us look at the goals. Did this lesson accomplish the specific goals set forth in the lesson plan? Did the techniques employed bring about the desired results, or could the same results be accomplished by simpler, more direct methods? Did the student understand why he or she was doing certain things? In other words, did this lesson make sense to the student? Did it include an opportunity for generalization? For practice? For review?

Did this lesson have any relationship to the student's specific needs? Were the techniques and materials adapted to the appropriate age level, gender, interests, level of understanding? Paradoxically, it is possible for a lesson to be well taught and interesting to the student yet still not have any bearing on the communication problem and its eventual solution!

Was the clinician able to establish good rapport with the student? Was the clinician genuinely interested in both the student and the lesson? Did the clinician talk too much or too little? Did both clinician and student seem to feel at ease? Was the clinician in charge of the lesson or did the student take over?

All of these questions need to be answered concerning every lesson. Too often the criteria for a treatment session are based on whether or not the student enjoyed it and whether or not good rapport existed between the student and the clinician. Although both are important, there is much more to a successful lesson. Careful preparation and careful evaluation of therapy sessions, both group and individual, are essential ingredients of good therapy.

The most effective clinicians we have observed have kept a running log of therapy, usually written immediately after each session. This is in addition to the lesson plan.

Lesson plans may serve still another purpose. When progress reports, case closure summaries, periodic evaluation reports, and letters are required, the lesson plan may serve as a source of referral and an evaluation of progress of therapy, and it could facilitate the writing of letters and reports.

Considerations for Special Populations.   Since the early 1970s the role of the SLP in the schools has moved into new areas. Much of the terminology has changed, research has added new dimensions, and service delivery methods are becoming more flexible and diverse. In the early days programs known as "speech improvement" were designed to help preschool and early primary children improve speaking and listening "habits."

Interestingly enough, programs for special populations today have their roots in the concerns of the early practitioners. Today's clinician must be interested in an ever-expanding list in communication disorders and issues related to treating special populations. Attention must be directed toward prevention of speech, language, and hearing problems in infants and preschool children. School districts are wrestling with ways to handle the communication difficulties of bilingual and nonstandard speakers of English. Language disorders in children and adolescents constitute the major focus of the SLP's time and interest.

There are many options for the delivery of educational services. The individual needs of the children determine the amount and type of supplemental services required. The speech-language clinician may be working with teachers of children who are developmentally delayed, emotionally disturbed, hearing impaired, or learning disabled. The children in these modules may also require the help of the reading teacher, physical therapist, occupational therapist, academic tutor, psychologist, and others. This means that the school clinician will be working closely with the child's classroom teacher as well as with other specialists and the parents of the child. All personnel must keep in mind that instruction should be student centered and child oriented. The specialists involved work as a team, and each team member has specific responsibilities that are known to themselves and other team members.

The literature in the field of communication disorders provides professionals with extensive discussion of approaches for treating children with communication impairments. It is not the intent or purpose of this book to suggest specific methodologies. There are many books and resources available that discuss specific communication impairments. However, there are considerations that need to be made for developing an intervention program that meets the needs of special populations.

As mentioned earlier, SLPs must be prepared to continually review the literature about new intervention approaches that might have promise. Then, they need to be discriminating in their use with students while determining if the approach has promise for their population or not.

LITERACY (READING AND WRITTEN LANGUAGE) DISORDERS

The National Education Goals (U.S. Department of Education, America Reads Challenge, 1997) state that all children in the United States will start school ready to learn and that every adult American will be literate. The National Literacy Act of 1991 (U.S. Congress, 1991) defines literacy as "an individual's ability to read, write, and speak and compute and solve problems at levels of proficiency necessary to function on the job and in society, to achieve one's goals and to develop one's knowledge and potential." These issues are important for all educators including speech-language pathologists. Since language is the foundation for learning and there is a relationship between spoken and written language, speech-language pathologists have an important role to play in developing children's literacy skills. In 1999, ASHA established an Ad Hoc Committee on Reading and Written Language Disorders to develop a technical paper and position statement describing the roles and responsibilities of speech-language pathologists related to reading and writing in children and youth (ASHA Ad Hoc Committee on Reading and Written Language Disorders, 2000). The position statement provides an understanding of why speech-language pathologists should plan an active role in this initiative. The technical paper clarifies how this can be done. Speech-language pathologists who are striving to link their programs with the educational curriculum should refer to these valuable resources.

Many of the same children who exhibit communication impairments also demonstrate reading and writing difficulties (Blachman, 1997; Catts & Kamhi, 1999). It is important, therefore, for SLPs and other educators to understand the relationship between spoken and written language. The ASHA position includes the following statements: Language is the foundation for the development of listening, speaking, reading and writing skills. Spoken and written language build upon one another, thus there is a reciprocal relationship. Youngsters who present spoken language impairments frequently have difficulty learning to read and write. Instruction in spoken language can result in gains in written language. The committee recommended that SLPs can and should contribute to the reading component of the language arts curricula through the following actions (ASHA Ad Hoc Committee on Reading and Written Language Disorders, 2000):

- Implementing prevention programs designed to foster language acquisition and emergent literacy
- Identifying language behaviors that place children at risk for later reading problems
- Assessing children's literacy abilities
- Providing intervention that builds on and encourages the relationships between spoken and written language
- Collaborating with other educators to shape or modify the curriculum to strengthen understanding of the link between language and learning
- Documenting and monitoring outcomes of language intervention
- Advocating for effective literacy practices in schools

The speech-language pathologist may be the first to recognize that a youngster is at risk for reading and written language problems. If the following characteristics are present, the SLP should begin to alert other educators and the family of potential problems: difficulties in phonological processing, including phonological awareness; multiple articulation problems; word retrieval difficulties; language comprehension problems; delayed discourse abilities; verbal memory difficulties; limited megalinguistic or metacognitive awareness (ASHA Ad Hoc Committee on Reading and Written Language Disorders, 2000).

Current research supports using language based approaches to develop spoken as well as written language skills. This recommendation is based on the philosophy that language learning should be an integrated process involving interactive and naturalistic intervention practices. Emphasis is placed on teaching language and reading skills using real conversational contexts and situations. The components of language and reading are not fragmented into separate components (such as phonology, morphology, syntax, semantics, and pragmatics). Rather, communication is presented as a whole process to be used to understand and transmit meaning. Clinicians who are involved in working with students' literacy suggest that the SLP work closely with the classroom teacher to plan meaningful learning activities, provide realistic and functional opportunities for facilitating communication, and encourage the student to actively participate during the learning activities.

One of the most valuable roles SLPs can play is to work with classroom teachers to improve reading proficiency in the classroom. SLPs have much to contribute to educators' overall understanding of how language skills relate to the learning process, especially reading, writing, and language arts. The SLP should share information on the "language-reading connection" with the teacher, and together they plan ways of structuring and achieving goals for the language-delayed child at risk for reading problems.

To avoid fragmented learning experiences, the child's language program in areas such as writing, spelling, reading, speech, and auditory training should be coordinated and based on concepts of language acquisition. Following are several language procedures that can be recommended to improve students' reading skills:

- Teach the correspondence between graphemes and phonemes
- Establish phonemic awareness of speech sounds
- Help children learn to identify how speech sounds relate to the written alphabetic symbol
- Teach students to discriminate various stress patterns across words
- Help students learn to recognize when one word stops and another begins
- Develop semantic awareness of word labels and functions
- Deemphasize reading accuracy and encourage rhythm and melody during oral reading
- Acknowledge and permit the student to read in his or her native dialect
- Write stories composed by the children using their language patterns
- Recommend that adults read various types of materials to children
- Involve children as active participants in meaningful language and reading activities
- Explain how stories are typically organized
- Demonstrate how to ask questions to obtain additional information
- Stress comprehension skills
- Incorporate vocabulary and reading material from the child's classroom reader into therapy activities
- Present the reading words in the context of a phrase using a modifier or verb, not in isolation

Reading is one of the most important skills taught in the school. Classroom teachers in the primary and early elementary grades are responsible for teaching reading, and the reading specialist in the school system is responsible for helping the child with a reading problem. Sometimes this is done directly with the child and sometimes it is accomplished indirectly through the teacher. Children having reading difficulties are referred for a thorough reading analysis, which may be done by the reading specialist. The speech-language clinician and the reading specialist should strive to learn one another's professional terminology. Often they are talking about the same things but using different terms. The reading specialist and the SLP have much in common and much to offer one another. A close working relationship between them is an important aspect of the speech, language, and hearing program.

CULTURALLY AND LINGUISTICALLY DIVERSE POPULATIONS

The issue of providing speech and language intervention services to children whose native language is not English or who speak different dialects has been a topic of intense discussion among professionals. Public Laws do not permit federal funds to be designated for services that are elective or for children who are not handicapped. The United States is a multicultural population. There is an increase in the percentage of the school-age population from ethnically diverse backgrounds.

School districts vary greatly in the type of services they offer to youngsters who are from diverse cultures. Some districts employ a cadre of specialists who provide English-as-a-second-language (ESL) services. Some SLPs perform that role. Unfortunately, in some areas of the country, no one particular discipline has claimed this population group. Therefore, students may be served inadequately or not at all.

Much of the intervention process is dependent upon the relationship established between the individual with a communication difference or impairment and the clinician. Therefore, the relationship is affected when the client and clinician speak different languages or come from different cultural backgrounds. Clinicians need to have an understanding of the various cultures they will encounter in their communities. Acceptance of speech-language services may be affected by cultural variables such as traditions, customs, values, beliefs, and practices. It is important to know about the speech, language, and behavioral characteristics associated with specific cultures. It is essential to have knowledge of the unique aspects of a language in order to assess or remediate the phonemic, syntactic, morphological, semantic, lexical, or pragmatic characteristics. The clinician should become aware of specific assessment materials and treatment strategies known to be effective for particular ethnic populations. Caution must be taken to avoid making generalizations and formulating erroneous expectations. It is necessary for clinicians to modify intervention paradigms to incorporate alternate strategies and culturally distinct styles of learning.

With so much blending occurring in the world, it is hoped that future professionals demonstrate a high degree of cultural sensitivity. Clinicians can increase their awareness of the cultures they serve by gathering the following information about the ethnic groups in their communities:

- The countries of origin, languages spoken, and numbers of individuals from the ethnic group living in the community
- The social organization of the ethnic group and resources available within the community
- The prevailing belief system within the community including the values, ceremonies, and symbols important to that culture
- The history of the ethnic group and current events directly and indirectly affecting the culture
- The methods used by the members of the community to gain access to social services
- The attitudes of the group toward seeking assistance

Various degrees of English proficiency may be observed in speakers from diverse populations including those who are bilingual English proficient, limited English proficient, and limited in both English and their native language. Assessment and intervention should be conducted in the student's primary language for those who are limited in English.

Dialectal differences cannot be construed as speech or language disorders; however, we must make sure that the student does not present a disorder in the native language. Experts in second language suggest that dialectal differences are differences from Standard American English which are based on the rules of the dialect, not on the speaker's ability to understand or speak. They reflect the internalization of the language rules of a primary culture or subculture.

In discussing the bilingual population in the schools, Work (1989) stated, "To consider these children speech-language disordered would be improper. Their difficulty with English is not due to a language disorder but to a language difference. Differences may be found in the linguistic structure, the phonological system, and the inflectional use of voice. Differences also exist in the cultural background at verbal and nonverbal levels."

There is little doubt that speech, language, and hearing deviations and disorders do exist among minority populations, including Hispanics, Blacks, Asians (including Pacific Islanders), and Native Americans (including Alaskan natives). In identifying communication disorders and deviations in diverse populations, the SLP must be careful not to confuse a dialect with a communication disorder. According to a paper drafted by the Committee on the Status of Racial Minorities (1985), "It is apparent that the assessment and remediation of many aspects of speech, language, and hearing minority language speakers require specific background and skills. This is not only logical and sound clinical practice, but it is the consensus set forth by federal mandates...." The report further indicated that state regulations are being developed to acknowledge the need for specific competencies to serve minority language populations. In California, for example, school districts are being encouraged by the education agency to require resource specialists, speech-language pathologists, and school psychologists to pass a state-administered oral and written examination on Hispanic culture, the Spanish language, and assessment methodology before they conduct assessments for Spanish-speaking children with limited English proficiency.

Harris (1985) discussed the importance of the clinician's investing time and effort to learn about the culture of the population that he or she serves. Harris, who was codirector of the Native American Research and Training Center, University of Arizona, stated

To appropriately measure and evaluate the English performance of minority language children on measures of speech and language, the examiner must be familiar with the behavioral characteristics of that group as they relate to language learning and language use. The level to which the particular child employs the traditional linguistic/cultural practices of his ethnic/minority group must be determined in order to assess his performance in an appropriate manner.

For example, requesting an Apache child to answer incessant questions, especially to answer in English, may put the child into a cultural conflict in which his or her resulting behavior (silence) may not be indicative of potential or knowledge but rather of cultural integrity.

This is not to say that school SLPs should not evaluate and provide services to children who have limited English proficiency and who have speech, language, or hearing handicaps. Interim strategies may be employed, such as utilizing interpreters or translators; establishing interdisciplinary teams, including a bilingual professional (for example, special education teacher or psychologist); or establishing cooperatives among school districts to hire an itinerant or consultant bilingual SLP or audiologist (Committee on the Status of Racial Minorities, 1985).

In regard to social dialects (Black English, Standard English, Appalachian English, Southern English, New York dialect, Spanish-influenced English), it is the position of the American Speech-Language-Hearing Association (1985) that…no dialectal variety of English is a disorder or a pathological form of speech or language…(however) it is indeed possible for dialect speakers to have linguistic disorders within the dialect. An essential step toward making accurate assessments of communicative disorders is to distinguish between those aspects of linguistic variation that represent the diversity of the English language from those that represent speech, language, and hearing disorders.

ATTENTION DEFICIT AND CENTRAL AUDITORY PROCESSING DISORDERS

In order to benefit fully from the classroom situation, children have to be able to hear the teacher's message and understand what it means. Children who exhibit problems related to attention deficit and central auditory processing disorders are at risk for failure due to their inability to effectively process the information that is presented to them. They may have difficulty discriminating sounds, attending to spoken messages, making associations, recalling sequences of information, and processing the information they hear. Determining the existence of problems related to an auditory processing disorder is a complex task. There are several assessment and diagnostic tools that can be used to assess auditory processing skills. The speech-language pathologist should be a key member of the evaluation and planning team for this student.

The SLP can stress the importance of listening skills for the learning situation. In addition to providing direct instruction, clinicians can provide teachers with valuable information about techniques they can use to help students with these problems function more effectively in the classroom. Clark (1980) recommends a number of strategies that teachers can use for increasing listening potential. First and foremost, teachers must gain the student's attention and reduce distractions. It is advisable to provide preferential seating so that the student has the advantage of hearing the teacher's instructions and comments. Teachers must monitor their speaking delivery style and provide instructional transitions, giving students the opportunity to benefit from their awareness of the teaching moment. Efforts should be made to block out auditory distractions, use visual and written teaching aids, and avoid auditory exhaustion. Frequent checks should be made of the student's concentration and comprehension. Teachers should take steps to encourage participation and provide support or reinforcement during learning activities.

SEVERE COMMUNICATION DISABILITIES

Millions of Americans demonstrate severe communication disabilities. The federal laws have mandated the provision of services to children with severe and profound disabilities. Children with severe disabilities must be educated to the extent that their limitations allow. There is wide variation in the degree of disabilities demonstrated and capabilities of children who are impaired. Therefore SLPs, teachers, and other school personnel must evaluate each child and plan an intervention program specific to that child's strengths and needs.

Some children with severe mental retardation or developmental delays do not begin to use words until the age of five or six, whereas others may learn to communicate by pointing and gesturing. Others with severe and profound deficits may never learn to communicate meaningfully. Early intervention, parent education, and interdisciplinary collaboration are important factors in a program for children with severe and profound mental retardation and developmental disabilities.

Some students have neuromuscular, neurological, or physical disabilities that are so severe that they are unable to use speech as a primary method of communication. They may even be unable to use standard augmentative communication techniques such as gestures, facial expressions, and writing. The disabilities may be the result of congenital conditions, acquired disabilities, or progressive neurological diseases. These students may have been diagnosed as having cerebral palsy, multiple sclerosis, oral or facial deformities, developmental verbal apraxia, autism, or dysarthria. They may also have central processing disorders or severe expressive aphasia. Children who acquire traumatic brain injuries or spinal cord injuries may have reduced communication skills. Many students who are unable to communicate verbally or vocally have normal or near normal receptive language abilities and normal nonverbal intelligence.

To treat children such as these, the SLP works closely with the family, regular and special education teachers, physical and occupational therapists, psychologists, and health professionals. The National Joint Committee for the Communicative Needs of Persons with Severe Disabilities developed a number of recommendations for serving individuals with severe disabilities. The committee was comprised of professionals representing a wide variety of disciplines including speech-language pathologists, special educators, occupational therapists, and physical therapists. Their recommendations included several principal tenets clinicians might use to guide their decision making for facilitating and enhancing communication among persons with severe disabilities: (1) communication is a social behavior;

(2) effective communicative acts can be produced in a variety of modes; (3) appropriate communicative functions are those that are useful in enabling individuals with disabilities to participate productively in interactions with other people; (4) effective intervention must also include efforts to modify the physical and social elements of environments in ways that ensure that these environments will invite, accept, and respond to the communicative acts of persons with severe disabilities; (5) effective intervention must fully utilize the naturally occurring interactive contexts (e.g., educational, living, leisure, and work) that are experienced by persons with severe disabilities; and (6) service delivery must involve family members or guardians and professional and paraprofessional personnel (National Joint Committee for the Communicative Needs of Persons with Severe Disabilities, 1993).

Intervention goals generally emphasize development of self-help skills and social and adaptive behavior. It is important to select activities that are representative of common situations which may occur in the pupil's experiences.

The speech and language services provided depend on the needs of each child. Vanderheiden and Yoder (1986) list numerous responsibilities SLPs may undertake when treating persons with severe expressive communication disorders:

- Assessing, describing, documenting, and evaluating the communication needs
- Evaluating and assisting in the selection communication aids and techniques
- Developing speech and vocal communication to the fullest extent possible
- Evaluating and selecting the symbols for use with the selected techniques
- Developing and evaluating the effectiveness of intervention procedures to teach skills and strategies necessary to utilize augmentative communication in an optimal manner
- Integrating assessment and program procedures with family members and other professional team members
- Training persons who interact with the individual
- Coordinating augmentative communication services

The speech and language services provided depend on the diagnosis of each child. The most advantageous method or methods of communication are determined and may include gestural systems if appropriate, symbol systems, and orthographic or pictorial systems. Depending on the mode of communication selected, the process may include augmentative communication devices such as communication boards, computerized devices, speech output devices, synthetic voice instruments, word processors, and other electronic and mechanical apparatuses.

AUTISM

Autism is a neurological disability that interferes with the normal development of effective reasoning, social interaction, and communication skills. Some refer to autism as "the ultimate learning disability." Persons with autism experience difficulty understanding what they see, hear, and sense. They are unable to communicate effectively with others and relate to the world outside of the self.

IDEA required that school districts take steps to identify and serve students with autism. Because communication skills are so greatly affected by this disability, the SLP plays an important role in assessing and planning intervention for students with autism. Clinicians should be familiar with the characteristics of autism and accepted procedures for evaluating students. Several complex characteristics are associated with this devastating disability. Children exhibit severe delays in development of communication skills and understanding of social relationships. They are unable to recognize and respond to the behavior and communication of others. They experience problems with judgment and recognition of simple cause and effect. Their responses to sensations of touch, sight, and sound may be inconsistent response (oversensitivity or undersensitivity). Students demonstrate variable patterns of intellectual functioning; individuals may show high level skills in one domain and low performance in another. Activities and interests are restricted and they may repeat body movements and routines. Many of these characteristics are also symptomatic of other severe disabilities. Therefore, it is important that the diagnosis of autism be made by a team of healthcare and special education professionals who are familiar with the characteristics of autism.

Development of treatment strategies for this group of individuals is still in its infancy. Although the literature about intervention is growing rapidly, a definitive set of answers regarding the most effective methodologies has not yet been generated. It is generally recommended that intervention stress the development of functional communication and learning skills to encourage safety and independence. Clinicians should use intervention techniques that emphasize development of pragmatic language skills, work within a highly structured format, stress generalization of skills to various situations outside of the therapy or classroom context, use augmentative communication strategies, and incorporate the family into treatment planning and implementation.

HEARING IMPAIRMENTS

The educational audiologist should oversee management of hearing loss. Most school districts do not employ audiologists. They must rely on services provided on a shared or contractual basis. In the absence of a staff audiologist, the speech-language pathologist has greater understanding of hearing loss than any other professionals in the school setting. There are several aspects of care for these children for which the SLP may be responsible including making medical and audiological referrals when indicated, facilitating acquisition and use of assistive listening strategies and devices, developing teachers' awareness and understanding of hearing loss, making recommendations for general education programming, developing speech and language skills, and monitoring the student's hearing aids.

It is important for educators and parents to understand the problems children will experience if their hearing is impaired. Even mild hearing loss can greatly impact upon school success. Flexer (1999) states that "all hearing losses involve educational issues and some also involve medical issues." In the absence of the educational audiologist, the SLP is the most appropriate person for conveying this information to other educational staff members and to the family.

Flexer, Wray, and Ireland (1989) suggest that speech-language pathologists need to be aware of three areas which are critical to classroom success for children with hearing impairments: hearing and the impact of hearing loss on classroom performance; the use of sound enhancement technology for habilitation and environmental access for persons who are hearing impaired; and, the use of educational management strategies which emphasize hearing rather than minimize it. They offer the following list of hearing-oriented topics to assist the speech-language pathologist in delivering adequate services and answering pertinent questions posed by teachers who have children who are hearing impaired in their classrooms:

Hearing

- Classrooms are auditory-verbal environments with "listening" serving as the basis for classroom performance.
- Hearing loss occurs along a broad continuum ranging from a mild hearing loss to profoundly hearing-impaired; not as two discrete groupings of normally hearing or deaf. In fact, about 92 percent to 94 percent of hearing impaired persons are functionally hard-of-hearing and not deaf.
- Hearing loss, whether mild or profound in nature, negatively impacts on verbal language, reading, writing, and academic performance.
- Speech may be audible to someone with a hearing loss, but not necessarily intelligible enough to hear one word as distinct from another.

FM Equipment

- Persons with hearing losses need the signal of choice to be ten times more intense than background sounds in order for speech to be intelligible. This is an impossible classroom listening situation.
- Appropriately fit sound enhancement equipment, typically FM units (in addition to wearable hearing aids), are necessary for any hearing impaired child with any degree of hearing loss to function in a mainstreamed classroom because this equipment improves the Signal-to-Noise ratio.
- FM equipment must be fit by an audiologist who is mindful of: (1) The acoustic characteristics of the equipment; (2) Methods of coupling equipment to personal hearing aids; (3) Psychosocial issues of visual deviance; (4) Multiple equipment settings to allow flexibility in various listening environments.
- FM equipment must be functioning and teachers must be comfortable with its use, or it is of no value.
- The Ling 5 Sound Test is one method by which the classroom teacher can screen equipment function.

Educational Management Strategies Which Focus on Hearing

- Auditory skills training and development should be implemented during all therapy and classroom activities.
- "Listen," as a cue word used by all staff, can alert the hearing-impaired child to upcoming instructions.
- Teachers are encouraged to repeat or rephrase comments from other students in the classroom.
- Pre- and posttutoring programs can provide necessary redundancy of instructional information.

Anderson (1991) provides a summary of the relationship of the degree of long term hearing loss to the psychosocial and educational needs of children (see Appendix D). She describes problems and barriers that may be encountered and recommends educational strategies for treating children with varying hearing losses. She suggests that special education programming may be appropriate to meet the needs of individuals with any and all degrees of hearing loss. When making educational decisions, the special education placement team should consider the full range of service delivery options. This would include integrating the child into the regular education classroom and providing teacher in-service and supportive services. With adequate training and comprehensive support services, the regular education classroom teacher can have increased awareness of the impact of hearing impairment on a student's classroom function, and learn to adequately meet the student's needs.

In some school districts, SLPs take responsibility for teaching students with hearing impairments to communicate. The Listen Foundation (1991) describes five approaches that are frequently used: (1) The *auditory-verbal* method teaches children to use their residual hearing to learn spoken language. Integration into the hearing world is stressed. Appropriately fitted hearing aids and assistive listening devices are essential; (2) The *auditory-oral* approach is similar. It also uses aided hearing. Intervention is usually presented individually or in small groups and also teaches lip reading; (3) The *oral* approach introduces hearing during specific auditory lessons, and places emphasis on lip reading and written communication; (4) *Total communication* provides the child with a variety of communication methods simultaneously including signs, fingerspelling, lip reading, speech, and use of residual hearing; (5) *Manual communication* does not consider spoken language as a necessary component for communication. It considers sign language as the natural language of all deaf persons.

Parents should be provided with a clear explanation of all of these methods and invited to participate in the selection of a teaching method. Of course, before the SLP undertakes implementing a particular method, he or she should understand the philosophical basis and implementation techniques.

Children with hearing impairments should be monitored by an audiologist to ensure that they see a physician when necessary and that they are properly fitted for hearing aids and assistive listening devices. Lesner (1991) recommends that the SLP maintain records on the students' hearing aids (Figure 9.6). She also developed a protocol SLPs can follow to determine if students' hearing aids are functioning properly (Figure 9.7).

BRAIN INJURY

Each year, over one million American children and youths sustain a traumatic brain injury (TBI) as a result of motor vehicle accidents, falls, sports injuries, and abuse. Years ago, many of these children would have died. However, due to decreased emergency response time and improved medical treatment, lives are now being saved. Approximately 165,000 of the children injured will have to be hospitalized and 16,000 to 20,000 will suffer from severe or moderate symptoms as a result of their injuries (Savage, 1991).

Traumatic brain injury may affect children's capabilities in a broad number of areas including physical, cognitive, communicative, behavioral, and social skills. While many

FIGURE 9.6   Hearing Aid Data Sheet

STUDENT: _____	DATE: _____	
SCHOOL: _____		
Hearing Aid Information	*Right Ear*	*Left Ear*
Make/Model	_____	_____
Serial Number	_____	_____
Date of Manufacture	_____	_____
Battery Size	_____	_____
Battery Type	_____	_____
Volume Control Setting	_____	_____
Tone Control Setting	_____	_____
Output Control Setting	_____	_____
Compression Control Setting	_____	_____
OTHER:	_____	_____

*Developed by Sharon A. Lesner, The University of Akron. Reprinted with permission.

problems exist with this population following injury, the cognitive-communicative impairments experienced appear to be the main barriers to successful reintegration into home, school, and community.

Treatment after brain injury may be ongoing for years. Students' behaviors may change drastically in that time period. Consequently, more frequent evaluations and revisions of the IEP are required. During the 3team planning meeting, the SLP can provide a few representative examples of the deficits the student brain injury may exhibit, the resulting behaviors teachers might observe in the classroom situation, and the cognitive-communicative intervention strategies which would be effective for developing communicative skills. Information such as this can be helpful when jointly planning the treatment plan for the student.

The chart in Table 9.3 illustrates a few representative examples of the deficits students with TBI may exhibit, the resulting behaviors teachers might observe in the classroom situation, and the cognitive-communication intervention strategies which would be effective for developing communication skills (Blosser and DePompei, 1994). Information such as this can be helpful when collaborating with teachers and parents or planning the IEP.

BEHAVIOR DISORDERS

Schools have been wrestling with their role in the education and treatment of students with behavior disorders. In fact, the most recent reauthorization of IDEA provides schools with

FIGURE 9.7   Protocol for Hearing Aid Checks

VISUAL INSPECTION
1. Clean case with no cracks
2. Clean microphone opening
3. Volume control moves smoothly
4. No signs of moisture in the tubing or earhook
5. Earhook securely attached to hearing aid
6. No breaks or cracks in earhook
7. Tubing securely attached to hearing aid
8. Tubing is not yellowed, hardened, brittle, or broken
9. MTO switch set correctly
10. Volume control set correctly
11. Tone control set correctly
12. Well-fitting earmold
13. Earmold condition satisfactory (not cracked or chipped)
14. Clean earmold bore

Battery Check
1. Battery positioned correctly
2. Clean, noncorroded battery contacts
3. Battery appropriately charged (1.1 volts+)

Listening check while you listen with a hearing aid stethoscope
1. Sufficient output
2. No tinny, muffled, or raspy output
3. No scratchy or crackling sound when volume control is moved
4. No hum or buzz
5. No intermittent sound when case is rotated
6. Quality of the "Five Sound Test"

Listening check while the student listens
1. Lack of feedback when the hearing aid is in the student's ear
2. All sounds of the "Five Sound Test" are detected

---

*Developed by Sharon A. Lesner, The University of Akron. Reprinted with permission.

mandates for evaluating and providing services to this group of students. The SLP should be a member of the evaluation team. Oftentimes behavior disorders are manifested by problems with communication—either understanding the language of others or effectively communicating emotions, needs, wants, and positions. Many times students with emotional or behavior disabilities exhibit intelligible communication but have complex comprehension or pragmatic difficulties. Their performance may be affected by medication they are taking. The SLP can play a very meaningful role in helping student, teachers, and parents understand how to improve communication interactions.

TABLE 9.3   Cognitive-Communicative Impairments, Representative Classroom Behaviors, and Recommended Cognitive-Communicative Intervention Strategies (Blosser and DePompei, 1992)

COGNITIVE-COMMUNICATIVE IMPAIRMENTS	BEHAVIOR	COGNITIVE-COMMUNICATIVE STRATEGY
Word retrieval errors	Answers contain a high use of "this," "that," "those things," "whatchamacallits." Difficulty providing answers on fill-in-the-blank tests.	*WORD RECALL:* Teach the student association skills and to give definitions of words he or she cannot recall. Teach memory strategies (rehearsal, association, visualizations, etc.).
Verbal problem-solving ability is reduced	In algebra class, the student may arrive at a correct answer but not be able to recite the steps followed to solve the problem.	*PROBLEM SOLVING:* Teach inductive and deductive reasoning at appropriate age levels.
Poor reasoning skills	After behaving inappropriately, the student is unable to discuss actions with teacher.	*REASONING:* Privately (not during classroom situations or in front of peers) ask the student to explain answers and provide reasons.
Reduced ability to use abstractness in conversation (ambiguity, satire, inferences, drawing conclusions)	Says things that classmates interpret as satirical, funny, or bizarre although they were not intended to be that way.	*SEMANTICS:* Teach the student common phrases used for satire, idioms, puns, etc.
Delayed responses	When called upon to give the answer, the student will not answer immediately, appearing not to know the answer.	*PROCESSING:* Allow extra time for the student to discuss and explain. Avoid asking too many questions.
Unable to describe events in appropriate detail and sequence	When relating an experience, details are out of order, confused, or overlapping.	*SEQUENCING:* Teach sequencing skills. Direct the context of the student's responses.
Inadequate labeling or vocabulary to convey clear messages	Inappropriately labels tools in industrial arts class.	*SEMANTICS:* Teach the student vocabulary associated with specific areas and classroom activities.

ABUSED CHILDREN

An unfortunate condition that seems to be more widespread is that of the battered or neglected child, who may also have communication problems. The maltreatment of children usually falls into one or more of four general areas: physical abuse, neglect, emotional maltreatment, sexual abuse.

Some forms of abuse and neglect are easily recognized, such as beatings that leave facial bruises or being repeatedly locked out of the home for long periods of time. The more subtle forms of abuse may include verbal abuse, poor supervision, or overly strict discipline. What is the school clinician's role in regard to abused and neglected children? First, the SLP should be alert to the signs of abuse. It is important to keep in mind that abuse occurs among the rich and well educated as well as among the impoverished. The next step is to report your suspicions to the principal, backed up with as much evidence as possible. Your suspicions may be wrong, but you may also be saving a life. Children who are maltreated often exhibit learning disabilities. They show symptoms such as distractibility, inappropriate behaviors, poor memory skills, and inattentiveness. These symptoms are often blamed on the emotional distress the child may be experiencing due to the abuse. When symptoms such as these are noticed, the child should be referred for a multifactored evaluation, including speech-language and hearing testing. The behaviors may actually be related to brain damage caused by physical abuse.

VOCATIONAL HIGH SCHOOL AND SECONDARY TRANSITIONAL PROGRAM

The interest in preparing adolescents in high schools and vocational high schools for jobs in the outside world provides a unique challenge to SLPs. The number of SLPs providing services in vocational schools is not known at this time; however, the number is probably quite small. By the same token, it is not known how many adolescents with speech, language, and hearing problems are in vocational schools. A vocational high school is usually jointly operated by a group of existing school districts. In some cases, if the school district is a large one both in numbers and in size, the vocational high school may serve only one school district. Students often retain membership in the "home" school district but may attend classes at the vocational school for all or part of the school day.

The curriculum of the vocational high school may include basic academic classes such as English, American history, and government. It would also contain classes related to the students' vocational choices and laboratory classes during which the theory and training are applied to actual job projects. Upon graduation, the students receive a diploma from the home school and a vocational certificate from the vocational school.

Because the purpose of a vocational school is to prepare a student for a specific vocation, the needs and the motivations of students in this kind of setting differ from those of students in the regular high school. Awareness of the psychology of this age group is important to the school clinician. A strong desire to be accepted by peers and not to be different from them sometimes underlies a resistance to therapy. A good working relationship with the vocational instructor can do much to encourage students enrolled in therapy to maintain good attendance.

Regardless of how severe the communication deficit may be, it is of secondary importance to the student at this age level. The intervention program should be based on the student's personal and vocational vocabulary. Remedial sessions can be developed around such topics as computing, food preparation, getting a job, and other subjects of interest. In addition to a remedial program, a speech-improvement program may fulfill the needs of many of the students. For example, students preparing for their rotation assignments as assistants to area dentists can be introduced to the following topics: (1) selecting correct word choices; (2) eliminating slang; (3) speaking clearly with the appropriate volume and rate; and (4) eliminating syntactical errors.

Programs may also include in-service training programs for both students and staff members. Topics for vocational instructors include information on speech, language, and hearing problems and the recognition of them. In-service topics for students include speech, language, and hearing behavior in the young child for the students enrolled in the child-care program as well as the effects of prolonged and sudden loud noise on students working in shop areas, such as auto mechanics, industrial, carpentry, and agricultural shop areas.

Clinicians may initiate a hearing-conservation program. Staff members and students involved in noisy laboratory and shop classes should be made aware of the ramifications of noise pollution and the effects on the hearing of the persons involved. The clinician may arrange for decibel readings to be conducted in the suspected loud-noise areas. Measures may be taken to make ear protectors available in the school supply store for students and instructors.

High schools may also have transitional programs. In this type of program the student moves from school to the workforce, with activities focused on exploring employment opportunities, assessing vocational potentials, vocational training, and job placement. For students in the secondary transitional programs who have communication handicaps or limited communication skills, the services of the SLP are utilized. The school staff often carries out the programs with the cooperation of potential employers.

WORKING WITH GROUPS OF CHILDREN

In a sense, all therapy is group therapy. A dyadic group (group of two) in speech, language, and hearing consists of the clinician and the student. Therapy groups in the schools consist of the clinician and from two to five students, or in special instances, more students. The purpose of a therapy group is to help the student in such a way that in the future he or she becomes independent of the relationship. The clinician is in a leadership role whether he or she uses an indirect approach or a direct approach. The clinician is a facilitator who is aware of the feelings, values, and tensions of the participants. The clinician may play the role of an impartial judge in the event of friction. He or she keeps the group members moving toward the completion of the tasks at hand. Group sessions permit the development of interactive, social communication skills. Practice and drill routines do not give children the same type of practice for using new communication skills readily in social and interpersonal situations.

The clinician must be able to create the kind of environment in which the student is able to learn to use new skills and change existing behaviors. A group situation provides a greater possibility for this than does a one-on-one relationship between the SLP and the student.

Care must be taken that your group therapy doesn't become individual therapy with one child speaking and the other children in the group simply listening, watching, and waiting for their turn. Passive participation has no therapeutic value. In groups structured like this, group interaction is limited if it exists at all.

Leith (1984) describes a much more interactive and effective model of group interaction. Referred to as "the shaping group," each student is actively involved in the activity. The children elicit responses from one another and provide the modeling, corrections, and feedback. They learn to judge other group members' productions as correct or incorrect and apply the reinforcement. In this model, there is constant interaction and learning is an ongoing process.

There is no rule that says all therapy sessions must take place around a table. Working in front of a mirror, a flannel board, or a chalkboard will help group members to become better participants. It has been said that learning is movement. If this is true, the clinician who sits on a chair without ever moving, and the children who remain in their places during the entire session day after day, may not be making the best possible use of the therapy time.

COUNSELING

Counseling is an important factor in a holistic approach to therapy. The SLP in the school system counsels both students and parents in communication problems. Some of the counseling is geared toward the prevention of problems. For example, the SLP may give a talk to the families on the nature of speech, language, and hearing problems or the development of speech and language in infants and children. Or the counseling may be directly with the student, entailing self-perception, acceptance of the problem, understanding of the problem, relationship to peers, information about the specific disorder, reluctance to talk, and feelings about the problem.

The school clinician should be alert to any signs that would indicate that the student may require psychological or psychiatric treatment. Even the faintest doubt about seeking further professional help should be pursued.

Many school clinicians have found that fears and apprehensions surrounding many types of speech disorders are based on misinformation or no information. Much of the anxiety for both students and their parents can be alleviated by factual and general information. The student's negative feelings about the problem may also be allayed by the attitude of the clinician, who says, not only by words but also by actions, "I'm here to help you; we can work on this together."

Although SLPs are not trained as counselors, there is no question about their knowledge of their professional field and the fact that they have been doing counseling. Without counseling, therapy alone would be ineffective. Recognizing that there are some children whose emotional problems may go beyond the communication problem, the school SLP seeks consultation and possible referrals of such children to other agencies and services specifically designed to deal with them.

PREVENTION OF COMMUNICATION PROBLEMS

It is the responsibility of the profession to include not only the treatment but also the prevention of communicative disorders. Included in one of the areas of prevention is the early detection and treatment of young children. Public Law 99-457 mandated assistance to pre-school children, ages birth to five. As discussed previously, services may be provided by a number of disciplines and should be coordinated. Family involvement is essential.

What does this mean to the school SLP? Essentially, it means that if you are employed as a school clinician in a state that includes in its laws the detection and treatment of young children, the responsibility of servicing these children will be with the local healthcare or education agencies. Because of financial restraints few school systems have this type of program; however, the detection and treatment of young children with disabilities are often being provided by local community voluntary agencies and by private agencies and healthcare programs.

The school SLP has a stake in encouraging and assisting these agencies in early detection and remediation. The earlier that handicapping conditions are identified, the better chance there is of remediation. And eventually fewer of these children will turn up in the caseload of the school clinician. Communication deviations that go untreated may develop into communication disorders and cause these children difficulties with the acquisition of such academic skills as reading, spelling, writing, and mathematics.

The SLP may intervene by providing information about speech and language development, environmental factors that influence development, and techniques to facilitate and stimulate speech and language development. Talks to groups of parents, early childhood educators such as day-care workers, preschool and nursery school teachers, members of the health professions, elementary school teachers and administrators, student groups, community organizations, and other professional groups, will help individuals understand how they may prevent and ameliorate speech, hearing, and language problems in children. Information may also be disseminated through newspaper articles, radio and television appearances, and other media. In a school or preschool the SLP may also provide demonstration lessons for the teachers.

DISCUSSION QUESTIONS AND PROJECTS

1. Collect samples of Individualized Education Programs and Individualized Family Service Intervention Plans used in various school systems. Compare and contrast IEPs and IFSPs. How are they alike? How are they different?

2. If you are working with a client in your university-based clinic, develop an IEP, IFSP, or ITP for that client.

3. Prepare a lesson plan for two of the students listed below. Be sure to show how you will incorporate information and materials from the school curriculum into your plan. Each speech-language goal should be related to some aspect of the classroom or a school subject.

   Students: an eight year old girl from Vietnam with limited English proficiency; a 3-year old child with cerebral palsy; a fifth grader with severe dysfluency; a third grader with a language learning disability that affects reading comprehension; a five year old with delayed articulation; a high school junior with cognitive-communicative impairments as a result of a TBI.

4. Describe steps you could take to motivate a student who is not interested in participating in your therapy program any longer.

5. With a fellow classmate, enact a discussion you might carry on with a classroom teacher to explain a student's communication impairment, the impact of the impairment on the learning process, and recommendations of how the two of you might work collaboratively to facilitate generalization of communication skills within the classroom. Role-play your discussion for your classmates (one person assume the role of the SLP).

6. Prepare an in-service presentation for the teachers of a student with an emotional disability.

7. Plan a lesson for the fourth grade students on your caseload with multiple articulation problems. Base your lesson on a social studies unit.

8. What behavioral signs would alert you to the possibility that a student is being physically abused? What steps are required of the educators in your state if they discover abuse?

9. Plan a presentation for high school students who have had children. What might you tell them to encourage them to help their children develop appropriate communication skills?

10. Develop a lesson plan for a group of students in the vocational education program who are studying cosmotology and/or auto mechanics. Build a vocabulary list. Construct a list of recommendations to help them prepare for a job interview.

11. Survey your classmates to determine the existence of various learning styles.

■ ■ ■ ■ ■

CHAPTER TEN

WORKING WITH OTHERS: COLLABORATION AND CONSULTATION

In Chapter 8, we looked at a collaborative/consultative model of service delivery and intervention. This model reinforces the importance of working closely with other individuals who are involved in the lives, education, and rehabilitation of school children. To implement this model effectively, it is important to understand the roles and responsibilities of family members, administrators, teaching personnel, and nonteaching staff who interact directly with the speech-language pathologist in order to help children with communication impairments. In other words, what can we expect from various individuals and what can they expect from us?

The school SLP works not only with school-based personnel but also with staff from community health and rehabilitation facilities. In fact, federal legislation mandates that schools and community agencies work closely together to provide services to children with disabilities and to their families. In some cases, services are purchased from agencies outside of the school district if they are not available in the local education agency.

Parents and/or guardians are encouraged to take leading roles in the planning of speech, language, and hearing services for their children. Although interactions with parents are not new for school clinicians, the importance cannot be emphasized enough. It is helpful to understand problems that interfere with interactions with families and strategies for forming meaningful relationships with them.

The school speech-language pathologist is also a consultant to the community and a source of information on speech, language, and hearing disorders and services.

The roles of the director of special education, elementary and secondary supervisors, superintendent, assistant superintendents, and board of education have already been discussed in Chapter 3. In this chapter, we will examine the roles, responsibilities, and working relationships we can establish with other individuals who are involved with school children.

THE IMPORTANCE OF COLLABORATING AND CONSULTING WITH OTHERS

In each situation and environment a child enters, there are demands for communication. Therefore, it is important for individuals with whom children interact to learn the importance of communication for success, to recognize communication delays and disorders, and to play important roles in facilitating speech-language development and modification if problems exist.

The service delivery options presented in Chapter 8 have, as a major component, collaborative-consultative services. In this service delivery model, the clinician, family members, and other professionals work together as a team to develop plans and strategies for helping children with communication impairments. They may also join forces to prevent communication problems from occurring. The child is the central focus of planning and problem solving and each team member brings to the situation his or her own unique expertise and contribution. This transdisciplinary model advocates teaching specific techniques to a variety of professionals with whom the student interacts (Orelove & Sobsey, 1996).

Idol, Paolucci-Whitcomb, and Nevin (1986) define collaborative-consultation as "an interactive process that enables teams of people with diverse expertise to generate creative solutions to mutually defined problems. The outcome is enhanced and altered from the original solutions that any team member would produce independently." Pershey (1998) reviewed numerous sources of information on collaborative models of speech-language service delivery. Several articles focused on the coordination of language intervention with reading and language arts instruction.

As the collaborative-consultative model has been more frequently applied, communication disorders professionals have begun to expand the purposes for which it can be applied (Pershey, 1998). The collaborative-consultative model can be used to:

- Determine the severity of the communication impairment
- Assess the impact the communication impairment has on the student's academic and social performance
- Define a student's communicative needs for various educational and social situations
- Observe a student's communicative abilities under specific circumstances
- Develop strategies for stabilizing the new skills the student is learning in therapy
- Monitor the student's progress after dismissal from a direct service program

Several professionals (Blosser & Kratcoski, 1997; Wiig & Secord, 1991; Marvin, 1990; Damico & Nye, 1990) have described the role of the speech-language pathologist as a collaborative-consultant for children with various communication disorders. To be successful in this role, the SLP must have a solid theoretical foundation in communication development and disorders; must be able to identify childrens' strengths and needs; must be able to develop prescriptive techniques; must understand the school curriculum and the learning process; and should be able to relate these aspects of communication to oral and written language.

The essentials of programs that are successful involve cooperation, communication, and joint planning and programming. Professionals focus on how they can best combine their talents, expertise, and schedules to facilitate a comprehensive program for children.

ATTITUDES

The functions of the school SLP are ideally carried out as an equal member of the educational team. To provide the best possible treatment for pupils with communication impairments, the school speech-language pathologist must work cooperatively with students' families and with other professionals in the education community. Sometimes, this involves providing information and support. Oftentimes, it means receiving information and support. But most often, it entails both.

The attitudes others have toward the speech-language-hearing program are crucial to its success. Equally important is the attitude SLPs display in relation to working cooperatively with other individuals to improve students' communication skills. In most situations, the reactions and quality of cooperation of individuals are determined by what the situation signifies to them. People possess varying degrees of difference in their understanding and attitude toward children with communication difficulties and toward the services of the speech-language-hearing pathologist. There may be a lack of clarity about the roles and responsibilities of the SLP leading to confusion and misinterpretation. This confusion may limit the effectiveness with which the SLP can function in school districts or individual school buildings. A concerted effort must be made to ensure that parents and other professionals are informed of and clearly recognize the functions of the speech-language pathologist within the school setting.

While educators may be favorable toward the speech and language program, they may not have extensive enough understanding to provide assistance for the youngster. They may not understand the nature of communication disorders or the impact of communication impairments on academic performance. They may be unclear about the role and responsibility of the SLP or how to work in collaboration with the clinician. More importantly, they may be unaware of how to create favorable conditions for reinforcing speech and language skills or facilitating change and carryover.

There are many school clinicians that are doing a good job of collaborating and consulting with other individuals to build support and understanding of their school therapy programs. Their interactions lead to more comprehensive and effective services for students. Successful clinicians generally have good communication and interaction with parents and school professionals.

INTERVENTION ASSISTANCE TEAMS

To promote collaborative planning, many school systems have organized Intervention Assistance Teams. The teams are generally comprised of the child's teacher, a school administrator such as the principal, the school psychologist, a special education teacher, and other professionals who have knowledge of the child's skills and needs. This includes the speech-language pathologist and audiologist.

The implementation of this model varies from school to school and state to state. In some schools, the Intervention Assistance Team serves as a resource or counseling committee. Intervention Assistance Teams can provide help to teachers who are puzzled by a child's behavior and are looking for suggestions and strategies. Teachers bring problems to the committee and receive recommendations of strategies that may work. Meeting time is often spent asking probing questions or reviewing classroom work. These activities give insights into the child's problems and needs. This often occurs prior to a formal referral for a multifactored assessment.

In another version of the Intervention Assistant Team model, the team members and the child's parents make decisions regarding assessment procedures needed and intervention strategies to be used. Specific responsibilities are assigned and timetables for implementing procedures and evaluating progress are established.

To implement an Intervention Assistance Team, the following questions must be addressed: Which children will be served by the team? Who will participate on the team? How will it operate? How will the team's effectiveness be evaluated? To be most effective, team members must be prepared for the job they are to do. Goals and expectations of what can be accomplished must be realistic. It is wise to keep minutes of team meetings. These can then be used to document assistance as well as to serve as a guide for implementing recommendations in the months following the meeting.

THE PRINCIPAL

The building principal is a key person for the success of the speech-language pathology program. This individual's attitude regarding the importance of communication in the learning process can make or break a program. Without the understanding and cooperation of the principal it would be extremely difficult to carry out an effective program. The principal is the chief administrator of the building, and in a sense, the school SLP is responsible to that person while in that building. The school SLP is a staff member of that particular building in the same way that other teachers are staff members.

What can the school clinician expect from the principal? First, the principal is legally and educationally responsible for each child enrolled in the school. Therefore, it is important for the principal and speech-language clinician to work closely together to ensure the delivery of quality services. Principals can be instrumental in creating an educational environment that promotes collaboration among members of the teaching staff, including the SLP. This can be accomplished by providing the staff with time to work together on projects, attend professional development seminars, or form peer-mentoring relationships. In addition, collaboration can be promoted by providing the technological supports for communication such as internet access, E-mail, and teleconferencing opportunities (Pershey, 1998).

The principal is often the representative of the local education agency in the development of individualized education programs (IEPs) for children and may serve as the coordinator of the placement team.

The principal is responsible for arranging for adequate working space and facilitating the procurement of equipment and supplies. The principal acquaints the clinician with the policies, rules, regulations, and all procedures in that school.

Personnel in the principal's office may help the SLP integrate the goals of the speech-language program into the total school curriculum. In some situations, the principal may assist the clinician in scheduling screening and testing programs and in setting up the caseload and schedule for children to be seen in therapy.

The principal can be expected to visit the therapy sessions and observe. Indeed, a wise clinician will invite the principal to observe therapy sessions and will encourage questions.

The interpretation of the program to other members of the school staff, the parents, and the community is ongoing. The principal may arrange opportunities for the clinician to interpret the program to the staff and the parents as well as to professional and lay groups in the community. The principal is the liaison between the school and the community and between the school clinician and the school staff. When a parent, a classroom teacher, or a member of the community has a question regarding the speech, language, and hearing program, that person will ask the principal, who may answer the query or refer it to the school SLP.

On the other side of the coin, the school clinician has some important responsibilities to the principal. Providing information about the program to the principal is one of the most important factors in maintaining a good relationship. The clinician will want to confer with the principal regarding major aspects of the screening, assessment, and intervention program. For example, the clinician should provide information to the principal on screening policies and procedures, grades and numbers of children to be screened, plans and time scheduled for follow-up testing, criteria for case selection, scheduling policies and procedures, and plans for developing intervention goals jointly with parents and teachers. The principal needs to know the children on the active caseload, the children dismissed from therapy, and the children being monitored indirectly. It is helpful to identify children by name, age, grade, communication problem, room number, and teacher, and to provide a brief statement of progress.

It is advisable to furnish the principal with written reports both periodically and systematically. Some information is valuable if submitted on a monthly basis; other information can be submitted semiannually or annually. Any plans for in-service programs for teachers and group meetings with parents and local professionals should be discussed with the principal prior to inception. Written reports or correspondence pertaining to a child in that school should be shown to and approved by the principal prior to sending them to parents or other professional personnel. Reporting information to the principal in this manner will help keep your program activities visible and it will keep the principal aware of the important role you play in the school.

If the clinician is itinerant, more than one building and more than one principal will be involved; therefore, the clinician needs to know the policies and procedures in each school. Because clinicians often work in several buildings and with several principals at one time, it is good practice to keep all the principals informed in a general way about the programs in the other schools. This practice serves to keep the principals well informed about the total program in the school system, facilitates cooperation and coordination among schools, and helps keep the clinician's workload well balanced. Care should be taken not to share private information from one building to the next and never gossip about colleagues.

THE CLASSROOM TEACHER

In the speech-language pathologist's role as a collaborator and consultant to the classroom teacher, several areas should be considered:

- The strengths and needs of the student with the communication handicap
- The academic and social demands placed upon him or her in the classroom
- The student's interaction with peers
- The teacher's interest in and capability for collaborating and providing assistance

This means that the SLP must understand the education process in addition to having competency in the communication disorders profession. It also means that the SLP must know what is going on in the classroom as well as making sure that the classroom teacher understands the speech-language intervention program and the role of the speech-language pathologist.

In most school systems there is an administrator for curriculum development. With assistance from teachers, principals, directors of special services, or other administrators, this person is responsible for the selection of textbooks and instructional supplies and materials. The business of educators is the selection of what will be taught, at what level, and in what sequence. That which is taught is the curriculum. Teachers organize the curriculum into instructional units, each made up of lesson plans.

One of the ways in which the speech-language program can be integrated into the curriculum is for the SLP to participate on the school's curriculum committee, either as a member or in an advisory capacity. In this way the pathologist can be perceived by the rest of the staff as someone who contributes to students' learning program. As a communication specialist the pathologist can provide information on pragmatics, communication in the classroom, how to help the children follow directions, how to encourage children to ask questions, and how teachers can become better communicators in the classroom. The pathologist can offer suggestions on how the teaching of improved communication skills can be integrated into language arts, social studies, science, art, physical education, math, reading, spelling, and writing.

The speech-language program should be fully integrated into the curriculum. It is essential that the classroom teacher understands the program, but it is equally important that the speech clinician understands what is going on in the classroom. It is not enough to give lip service to the idea of integrating the program into the educational framework; it must be put into practice. How can this be accomplished? The answer is not a simple one, but let us first consider some of the things the school pathologist can expect of the classroom teacher; then let us look at some of the expectations of the classroom teacher in regard to the clinician.

The school SLP can expect the teacher to provide a classroom environment that will encourage communication and will not exclude the child with the stuttering or articulation problem or the child who is hearing impaired. A teacher who shows kindness and understanding toward the child with a disability is not only assisting that child but also is showing other children in the classroom how to treat individuals who are disabled. Sometimes it takes more time and patience to deal with children who are disabled, but the rewards in terms of the child's performance are many. The teacher in the classroom takes the lead by establishing the emotional climate, and the children learn by example.

The classroom teacher is also a teacher of speech and language by example. If you doubt this, watch a group of children "playing school" sometime. Teachers provide the models for communication and children imitate the teachers. Teachers must have an awareness of their use of language, quality of speech, rate and volume of speech, and use of slang or dialect.

The SLP can expect the teacher to help identify children in the classroom with speech, language, or hearing problems. Some children with communication problems are not spotted during a routine screening, and teachers who see children on a day-to-day basis will have more opportunity to identify the children and refer them to the SLP.

The clinician can expect the classroom teacher to send the children to therapy at the time scheduled. The SLP will need to supply the teacher with a schedule, and both teacher and clinician should stick to it. The SLP can also expect the teacher to inform him or her of any changes in schedules that would necessitate absence from therapy.

One of the most important areas of cooperation between the SLP and the classroom teacher is the generalization stage—when speech and language behavior learned in therapy is brought into the classroom. For this to be accomplished it will be necessary for the SLP to keep the teacher well informed about the child's goals in therapy, progress in therapy, and steps in development of new patterns. This must be done not in general terms but in very specific ones. The teacher needs precise information on the child's problem and what is being done in therapy before there can be a carryover into classroom activities. The teacher can provide the SLP with information concerning how well the child is able to utilize the new speech or language patterns in the classroom.

When confronted with the idea of helping the child with communication problems in the classroom, the teacher's reaction is apt to be "I don't have time to work with Billy on his speech when I have 25 other children in the room." The SLP's role in this situation is to give the teacher specific suggestions on how this can be accomplished as a part of the curriculum. This of course means that the clinician will have to be well acquainted with classroom procedures, practices, and activities. It also means the SLP will have to know what can be expected of children of that age and on that grade level. This will happen if there is a continuous pattern of sharing ideas and information between the SLP and the classroom teacher.

We have considered what the SLP can expect of the classroom teacher. Now let us look at the other side of the coin—what the teacher can expect of the clinician.

If you are new in the school, starting off on the right foot is important. Being friendly and open with teachers, showing an interest in what they are doing in their classrooms, and showing a willingness to give them information are all steps that can be taken to help build trust and understanding. There are many ways in which this can be accomplished. One way is to plan to eat lunch with the teachers in the teachers' lunchroom. Another is to participate in some of the social activities. Because clinicians deal with many teachers in different schools it is not wise to become identified with cliques and associate only with a very small group. Outside the school you will have your own circle of friends, but inside the school be friendly with everyone.

If you have a schedule, keep to it, and if you make changes in it, as you surely will, be sure to tell the classroom teachers who are affected. If you send a child back to the classroom late, you will have no basis for complaint if the teacher fails to send a child to you on time. Share information with teachers through informal conferences, arranged conferences held periodically, invitations to observe therapy sessions, and observation in classrooms. Always make arrangements in advance for conferences and observations. The principal can often help make arrangements for any of these activities.

Information can also be transmitted in written form. Short descriptions or definitions of the various speech, language, or hearing problems or any aspects of the program will help teachers understand the program better. *Short* is emphasized because realistically teachers are not going to take the time to read long treatises.

In working with classroom teachers, the school SLP is a partner in effecting the best possible services for the child who has a communication disability. The more help that is given to the teacher, the more opportunity there will be for integrating the speech, language, and hearing program into the schools.

As schools strive to improve their inclusive practices, teachers are increasingly faced with the task of integrating children with special needs into regular classrooms. Providing in-service programs or arranging university courses for credit are excellent ways of supplying teachers with information about children with communication disorders.

What are some of the things that classroom teachers will need to know about communication and communication disorders? Following is a list of topics that might be included in an in-service program:

- The mission and goals of the speech and language program in the school, including the preventive, diagnostic, and remedial aspects. Describe policies and procedures for case identification, selection, enrollment, and dismissal.
- Normal patterns and milestones for speech, language, and hearing development.
- A brief description of the major types of communication impairments to be expected in the school-age population (i.e., articulation, delayed language development and language/learning disorders, fluency, voice disorders) and impairments associated with specific disability conditions including autism, developmental disabilities, emotional disturbances, traumatic brain injury, organic disorders, and the like. Briefly describe the characteristics, range of severity, possible causes and related factors, diagnosis and assessment procedures, criteria for selection, intervention strategies, impact on school performance, and the role of the classroom teacher for each disorder category.
- The importance of hearing for learning and information related to hearing problems including the anatomy of the ear, nature of sound, types of hearing loss, causes of hearing loss, identification and measurement of hearing loss, role of the classroom teacher, rehabilitation and habilitation of hearing deficiencies, hearing aids and assistive listening devices.
- The relationship of speech, language, and hearing to the educational/learning process.
- Medical and dental intervention where applicable for specific disorders such as cleft palate.
- The roles of other professionals in treatment such as physicians, physical therapists, occupational therapist, psychologists, and counselors.
- Treatment techniques and intervention strategies that can be successfully implemented in the classroom.
- Aspects of the curriculum where focus can be placed on improving students' communication skills and where communication goals can be integrated.
- Assistive devices and augmentative communication systems used to facilitate communication in students with severe impairments.

Figure 10.1 shows an observation form developed to facilitate teachers' awareness and understanding of their own classroom communication style. It can be given to teachers (or others) for self-evaluation or used as an observation tool. Analyzing the results jointly with the teacher can lead to meaningful discussion about how to modify communication style in order to meet a particular child's needs. For example, if Johnny cannot process language at

FIGURE 10.1   Communication Style Observation Form

INSTRUCTIONS

During communication interactions with (_____), pay close attention to your own communication manner and style. As completely as possible, describe the characteristics of your communication manner and style in the categories listed below. In consultation with a speech-language pathologist, determine those characteristics which can potentially pose difficulty for the student. Place a minus sign (–) next to them. Place a plus sign (+) beside those behaviors which can be used to promote the use of good communication skills.

1. _____   Average rate of speech

2. _____   Typical length and complexity of sentences

3. _____   Use of sarcasm, humor, and puns

4. _____   Word choice (simple, difficult, technical)

5. _____   Attentiveness to students during conversations

6. _____   Organization of conversations

7. _____   Use of hand and body gestures

8. _____   Use of objects to help make explanations

9. _____   Manner of responding to students' questions

10. _____   Manner of giving directions and instructions

11. _____   Patience while waiting for someone else to talk or answer

12. _____   Ability to understand students with communication impairments

---

a fast rate and the math teacher, Mr. Butler speaks very quickly, Johnny will be at a disadvantage for learning math. Therefore, a reasonable and doable modification for Mr. Butler would be to slow his rate of speech when presenting important information or new concepts to his class. Figure 10.2 outlines numerous communication strategies which can be recommended to teachers who are interested in modifying their communication styles in order to accommodate a child in their classroom who has a communication impairment.

SPECIAL EDUCATION TEACHERS

Speech-language pathologists and audiologists relate to all the providers of special instructional services in the schools. This includes teachers of children who present emotional disturbances, specific learning disabilities, cultural and linguistic diversity, developmental disabilities, physical impairments, visual impairments, and hearing impairments. Instructional services are available to children in all of these groups and more as mandated by public laws. The collaborative team should be comprised of those educators who have the greatest expertise in the areas of need defined for each particular student.

FIGURE 10.2   Recommended Strategies for Modifying Communication Styles to Accommodate the Needs of Children with Communication Impairments

Following is a list of communication strategies that teachers and others can use while interacting with a child who demonstrates a communication impairment.

Based on the results of formal and informal assessment procedures, indicate those strategies which will facilitate development of communication skills or correct speech and language productions.

For example, when GIVING INSTRUCTIONS AND DIRECTIONS, it is recommended that the communication partner make attempts to modify his or her communication style by reducing the length of complexity of the utterance, reducing the rate of utterance, repeating the instructions, altering the mode of instruction delivery, or giving prompts and assistance.

GIVING INSTRUCTIONS AND DIRECTIONS

_____   Reduce length of instructions

_____   Reduce complexity of instructions

_____   Reduce rate of delivery

_____   Repeat instructions more than once

_____   Alter mode of instruction delivery

_____   Give prompts and assistance

_____   Vary voice and intonation patterns to emphasize key words

EXPLAINING NEW CONCEPTS AND VOCABULARY

_____   Give definitions for terms

_____   Show visual representations of concepts and vocabulary

_____   Present only a limited number of new concepts at a given time

_____   Ask questions to verify comprehension

READING TO THE STUDENT

_____   Reduce rate

_____   Reduce complexity

_____   Reduce length

_____   Determine comprehension through questioning

_____   Redirect student's attention to important details and facts

PRACTICING MEMORY SKILLS

_____   Encourage the student to categorize information and make associations

_____   Provide opportunities for rehearsing information

_____   Encourage the student to visualize information

FIGURE 10.2　Continued

PRACTICING HIGHER-LEVEL THINKING AND COMMUNICATING

_____ Provide opportunities for problem solving
_____ Provide opportunities for decision making
_____ Provide opportunities for making judgments
_____ Ask questions to elicit solutions, judgment, decisions

ANNOUNCING AND CLARIFYING THE TOPIC OF DISCUSSION

_____ Introduce the topic to be discussed
_____ Restate the topic frequently throughout the conversation

ATTENDING TO STUDENT'S BEHAVIORS, QUERIES, COMMENTS

_____ Reinforce queries and comments
_____ Inform the student if the message is not understandable
_____ Request repetition of utterances not understood

RELAYING IMPORTANT INFORMATION TO STUDENTS

_____ Avoid sarcasm, idiomatic expressions, puns, humor
_____ Reduce rate, complexity, length of utterance
_____ Use or reduce gestures dependent on student's responses and needs
_____ Incorporate visual cues and imagery for clarification
_____ Permit ample time for student response
_____ Introduce alternative and/or augmentative communication systems if necessary
_____ Arrange the physical environment to reduce distractions, eliminate barriers, and invite communication
_____ Invite questions
_____ Present information in clusters and groups
_____ Introduce information with attention-getting words
_____ Select materials appropriate for skills, age, interest levels

Because the laws do not clearly define the areas of professional specialization which must be involved in the delivery of services to particular groups of children, confusion sometimes arises concerning the professional scopes of practices. This is especially evident between SLPs and learning disabilities specialists because many children with learning disabilities demonstrate problems processing and producing spoken or written language. Their deficits negatively affect learning and result in academic problems in subject areas such as reading, spelling, writing, mathematics, and other academic and social areas that require adequate language abilities.

The working relationship between the SLP and other special educators is dependent on the local school and the individual professionals involved, including the principal and the classroom teacher. The SLP has the academic background, interest, and competence in language development and communication disorders.

Using the continuum of service delivery options, cooperation between special educators may be provided under different plans. The service delivery options are not mutually exclusive. The SLP may function as a member of the diagnostic team during the initial evaluation procedures or on an ongoing service-delivery basis. Specific remediation may be provided to children placed in full-time special classes or in regular education classes. The SLP may function as the resource room professional or as a consultant to the other specialists in relation to general or specific problems. Obviously, different service delivery models would depend on each local school system's situation. The possibilities have not been fully exploited, and the creativity of the SLP may be utilized in determining innovative approaches to helping pupils with language-learning disabilities.

In some school districts, SLPs function as resource teachers for children with language-learning disabilities. To function successfully, communication specialists must have a theoretical background in language development. They must be able to identify and develop prescriptive techniques for problems related to phonology, syntax, and semantics; and they should be able to relate these aspects of linguistics to all levels of oral and written language. In addition, the speech pathologist must be a generalist as well as a specialist. In other words, the speech pathologist must know much about the learning process.

FOSTERING EFFECTIVE INVOLVEMENT THROUGH MENTORING

Current "best practice" philosophies for service delivery in health care and education settings support increased inclusion and involvement of families and teachers in the planning, assessment, and treatment of individuals with disabilities. Federal legislation has consistently supported these philosophies by mandating equal responsibility for families and professionals in planning programs. As a result of these important steps, service providers in all types of settings are being called on to have more frequent and regular contacts with families and educators of individuals they serve. They are seeking methods for working with families that are proved to be effective. They are looking for strategies that will result in the clarification of the roles and responsibilities others can play in intervention and education.

Families and teachers need support services and guidance in order to play meaningful roles. Everyone involved in the student's education should learn to interact effectively to obtain appropriate services and optimal opportunities for the student. It would be especially helpful for the family to learn about the legal rights of students with disabilities and how to access financial assistance when needed. To accomplish these difficult feats, family members and educators must first have a good understanding of communication disabilities. They must become skilled at interacting with service providers and other professionals at all levels. And, most importantly, they have to feel positive about their role and efforts.

Mentoring offers a viable approach for preparing families and educators to play an important role in communication development and intervention of youngsters with speech and language disabilities. What is a mentor?

> The origin of the term "mentor" dates to the time of Homer, specifically to *The Odyssey*. Homer describes his hero, Odysseus, preparing to set out on an epic voyage, though his son, Telemachus, must remain behind. Odysseus asks a trusted friend, Mentor, to guide and counsel Telemachus in his absence. From this ancient literary figure, mentor has come to mean one who helps guide a protege through a developmental process, whether that process is the transition from childhood to adulthood or from student to professional. Because of the complexity of this task, mentors are variously considered to be teachers, counselors, friends, role models, and more.

The mentoring process can be described as a relationship in which a person of greater rank or expertise takes a personal interest in the professional and personal development of a younger person and provides experiences for the protege that have an unusually beneficial impact on the protege's performance. Mentors have been described as advocates, teachers, counselors, role models, guides, facilitators, friends, and critics. Research has shown that mentors have a significant and positive impact of professional development and achievement. Mentoring has been used successfully in business and educational settings to assist teachers, professors, students, and employees so they succeed and make effective contributions.

Proteges have derived many benefits from participating in mentoring relationships in these settings. Mentors can help proteges avoid obstacles, develop contacts, and gain insight into organizational systems. Proteges show the effects of learning at a faster pace and more thoroughly than their nonmentored counterparts. Newcomers understand the norms and rituals associated with being in a particular environment. They develop insights into acceptable and appropriate behavior for specific situations. Proteges gain understanding of expectations and patterns of interaction. Feelings of isolation are mitigated. They learn to access restricted information and key persons. They learn about important facts and operational policies and procedures. Perhaps most importantly, individuals who have been mentored report higher levels of (job) satisfaction and enjoyment. To summarize, persons who are mentored develop those skills, forms of knowledge, attitudes, and values necessary to successfully and effectively carry out their occupational role.

Why Mentor Families and Educators?

Mentoring offers promise as an effective technique for developing the competencies and skills of people who are significant in the student's life. Creating mentor relationships can provide potential solutions to the needs, problems, and concerns families and educators experience. Just as employees in the work setting or professors in academe stand to make greater gains by being mentored, so do others stand a better chance of developing the skills they need for living with and effectively helping their child.

Similar to employee proteges in work settings, many benefits can be derived by implementing a mentoring approach for preparing families and teachers. The presentation of important information can be timed to parallel the needs to adapt to difficult and ever-changing situations. Family members can be introduced to the norms, rituals, policies, and procedures associated with medical, rehabilitation, or educational settings. Opportunities can be seized for developing the insights into acceptable and appropriate behavior for interacting with particular service providers in difficult situations. Others can gain familiarity with terminology, expectations, and patterns of interaction necessary for various situations. Feelings of isolation can be reduced because closer relationships generally form between proteges and mentors. Hopefully, those who are mentored will assume leadership roles providing guidance to other families and professionals.

How Mentoring Differs From Other Types of Education and Counseling

Working with families of persons with disabilities is not new. Service providers have always held conferences with family members to explain students' disabilities and the treatment program. They have conducted in-service programs to improve family members' understanding of the treatment process. Many have invited family members to observe treatment and be a part of therapy. In response to federal mandates and accreditation standards, programs have established formal family education and counseling programs designed to provide information and improve the skills of family members and educators.

These efforts tend to be "generic" in nature. Often the actual interaction time with family members is somewhat restricted. The explanation and exploration of important topics is limited. Service providers often "talk to" or "teach information to" their audiences. Efforts may range from providing brief introductory explanations to supplying written materials. The information disseminated is not always tailored to meet the family's individual needs and situation. While efforts of this type are a good beginning, they may not always go far enough in preparing the family to independently meet the challenges that lie ahead. Brief interactions such as these are good beginnings; but they are not sufficient preparation to enable the family to make a real contribution in the intervention process.

Mentoring is different because the mentor and protege form a different type of relationship with one another, one that is much closer and much more interactive. The mentor-protege relationship is dynamic and changes overtime as the protege gains confidence, skill, and independence.

Mentoring Activities

There are a number of mentoring activities that can be used with families and educators. These include informal contact, interactive dialogue, role modeling, direct assistance, demonstration, observation and feedback, and assistance with long-term planning. The activities are discussed in the following section. Brief examples of when these activities can be implemented are provided.

Informal contact.   This strategy can be implemented with the family when they come to the school or participate in school activities. Educators can be reached at different times throughout the daily routine. Consider it an opportunity to impart important information whenever you engage in brief conversations with others.

Situations such as these are good opportunities for initiating and developing mentoring relationships. Mentors can use comments and questions to initiate relationships and discussions with those they identify as candidates to be proteges. Comments such as "call me if you need anything" and "let me know if I can give you any information" can open the door to dynamic interaction and communication if conveyed with sincerity. Following are several questions framed to elicit discussion: "What would you like to know about your Jane's speech problem?"; "What do you understand about John's disability and needs?"; "What do you understand about her capabilities and strengths?"; "Is there anything bothering you right now about your son's program or your responsibilities?"; "Do you need help or assistance?"; "How does Sam's dysfluency interfere with his relationship with other family members?"; "Are you interested in learning the techniques and strategies we use in therapy?"

The family should be advised about the best times and means of making contact so that calls are not perceived as interruptions. Otherwise, communication breakdowns may occur if requests for assistance are made during busy or inappropriate times. Even though encounters of this nature may be brief, they afford mentors opportunities for developing the family's awareness of the environment, promoting confidence in the staff's skills, offering words of encouragement, passing along critical information, and providing general suggestions to increase understanding. Examples of information that can be conveyed during initial informal contacts are listed below:

- Information about the speech and language disorder
- Medical aspects associated with the problem
- The stages of physical and behavioral development of communication skills
- How treatment will progress
- The potential impact of the communication disorder on the youngster's learning, behavioral, physical, and emotional skills
- Qualifications, roles, and responsibilities of various staff personnel
- Procedures for developing the IEP
- Services available and procedures for accessing additional services
- Support organizations and resource centers available in the community

Interactive Dialogue. Every contact with the family and teachers should be viewed as important and an opportunity for developing their awareness and skills. Mentors need to make special efforts to reduce anxieties and increase confidence and capabilities. Strive to make each contact and interaction meaningful. Seek others' ideas, opinions, and feedback. Involve them in planning treatment activities.

After treatment sessions, service providers often make general comments such as "he did really well today" or "she was really trying hard." In mentoring relationships, comments would also be directed toward the performance or involvement of the educator or family member. For example, "today we read stories in therapy. I'd like you to try reading these two stories at home (provide specific verbal and written instructions) and let me know how he does for you."

Mentors can help family members adjust to their responsibilities and develop a more positive outlook by discussing concerns with them as they arise. Be sure to let them know how a particular activity relates to a class activity or household chore. Discuss their impressions of the reasons the student is successful or not. Invite them to make suggestions or recommendations for improving or changing an activity.

Interactive dialogue can be used to promote understanding and skills in the following ways:

- To reinforce positive efforts
- To stimulate thinking about future intervention issues
- To teach others how to monitor the student's behavior for subtle positive or negative changes in performance
- To provide information about preparing or structuring the home environment to promote good communication
- To obtain information about the family's goals for the student and home routines that might be valuable for planning future treatment or services
- To suggest ways of incorporating specific treatment techniques and strategies into the home and classroom environments
- To explain mystifying terminology and confusing procedures
- To better understand the others' concerns and needs
- To answer questions that arise
- To provide encouragement and motivation when progress seems slow or limited

Role modeling. Perhaps one of the most valuable and effective mentoring techniques is role modeling. Much can be learned from observing the mentor in action. Other than rare events like an open house when families are invited to visit the school, opportunities are generally limited for getting an "up close and personal" look at a professional in action. Teachers don't often take time to go to the therapy room to observe the SLP. However, there are opportunities for role modeling when the SLP goes into the classroom.

Mentors can use role modeling during the following activities:

- Team planning meetings
- Classroom and treatment sessions
- Phone calls (for example, to establish contact with another service provider or agency; transmit or exchange information about the person's program or needs; inquire about available services; seek assistance; or look for answers to difficult questions)

Demonstration. Similar to role modeling, demonstration also provides opportunities to "see how it's done." It goes a step further, however, and enables the proteges to practice techniques under the guidance and supervision of the mentor. Demonstration is a more purposeful activity than role modeling.

Demonstration is particularly useful for teaching significant others to execute treatment strategies in the home and school environment. One of the primary goals of involving other people directly in the treatment process is to help them develop and refine the skills needed to encourage and teach the student more effectively. It also enables them to develop confidence about their efforts and skills. To implement this approach, plan functional therapy activities based on expectations and demands of the school situation. This approach makes it easier to involve other people and it makes treatment more relevant. Discuss the purpose and design of specific tasks planned for the day. Demonstrate the clinical techniques while the teacher or parent is watching, including ways to praise or reinforce the student's positive behaviors and make changes to elicit improved responses and behaviors. After demonstrating the activity, ask the person to conduct the same activity with the student. If the technique is not demonstrated in the proper way, the mentor again demonstrates, adding suggestions. The family should also be asked to critique their own performance of the task and ideas for making changes. For some, just a little guidance and encouragement is enough, for others more reinforcement is needed. The extent of reinforcement needed is as diverse as the personalities and cultures represented. Mentors have to evaluate each protege to determine individual needs for instruction, explanation, and reinforcement. The suggestions made should be matched to the protege's ability, tools, and technology available.

Demonstration can be particularly effective in many of the same situations as presented for role modeling. Mentors should cue proteges to listen for the way the mentor elicits a response or identifies the steps followed while performing a specific therapy task.

Observation and Feedback. A key factor in the mentorship process is providing meaningful feedback to the protege as quickly as possible after the completion of a task or activity. In this way, the performance will still be fresh in each person's mind and the protege will still be enthusiastic and receptive to suggestions. This conference time should be viewed as a time to recall the experience with the protege and exchange information as well as to provide guidance.

Allow time to express fears, frustrations, and feelings of success. Provide feedback; it enhances learning. Therefore, positive interaction is a must. Positive relationships do not just happen; they need to be cultivated. This is not always an easy task. The mentor must be very sensitive to the other person's level of understanding, communication style, feelings, hopes, and attitudes. Awareness of these factors will help the mentor formulate and deliver comments.

For example, after observing a teacher interact with the student, the mentor can comment on his or her perception of how the conversation went. Reinforcement can be given for positive interactions. Suggestions for rewording or rephrasing comments can be made if misunderstandings occurred.

As the mentor-protege relationship is refined, it will be easier for the mentor to deliver feedback and for the protege to receive it. With the goals in mind of transferring responsibility for case management, it is essential for the others to learn to recognize when they are doing well and when their efforts are not as successful as they could be. Observing the teacher in action and providing feedback during times such as those listed below will provide opportunity for them to refine their skills and build their confidence.

Mentors can observe and provide feedback when they observe others in the following situations:

- Conducting therapy activities
- Talking about the student's disability and discussing the impact on learning and treatment strategies
- Making recommendations during an IEP meeting
- Conveying their thoughts, concerns, and recommendations during a team planning meeting
- Interacting with staff personnel to ask questions, relate experiences, or express concerns
- Conversing with the individual student, or giving instructions
- Inquiring about desired services or procedures
- Interpreting reports about the student's skills and capabilities

Plan for the Future.   Key proteges should be given guidance as they plan for the student's future. Issues of concern should be addressed and either brought to solution or recommendations made for seeking additional assistance. Many families ask service providers to clarify the "next step" they will need to take. Planning together will help alleviate future shocks. Here are some steps that can be taken:

- Provide referral lists and information about community services
- Help establish networks with families with similar needs and concerns
- Determine roles all family members can play (immediate as well as extended family) in caretaking, transportation, implementing treatment, and providing respite for primary caregivers

Selecting Mentors and Proteges

It is unrealistic to think that all service providers can serve as mentors or all families can be mentored. Disposition, willingness, personality, knowledge, and experience are important factors for consideration. A high level of energy is generally devoted to mentoring relationships. Therefore, mentors as well as proteges have to be committed to effectively working together. Professionals who have a proven record of commitment to working with students with disabilities make excellent mentors. They demonstrate an attitude of willingness to help as well as learn from others. As the protege shows progress, the mentor will need to modify his or her role, thus building independence and confidence.

Mentor Responsibilities

One does not implement this model without advance preparation. Here are some helpful hints for success:

- Remain available to talk and meet when needed
- Develop and maintain a resource library with materials about communication disorders
- Prepare instructional materials explaining how families can be active in developing the IEP or transition plan

- Conduct workshops and training sessions about topics such as understanding the evaluation process, how language relates to reading, and inclusion
- Promote networking among people with similar needs and interests
- Prepare and distribute a calendar illustrating the focus of treatment sessions and inviting others to visit
- Establish a hotline or web address for quick responses to questions that arise
- Prepare a listing of opportunities such as camps, schools, and classes
- Prepare a directory of agencies and services available in a community
- Prepare a calendar of upcoming workshops, meetings, and classes that would be of interest.

The schedules and demands of all that are involved will dictate the amount of effort and time that can be devoted to the mentoring relationship. Mentoring means assisting, not assessing. The mentor facilitates the protege's learning rather than controls it. The mentor functions as a teacher and role model and promotes growth through encouraging self-reliance. The most important aspect of mentoring is establishing a cooperative spirit between the family member and service providers. The speech-language pathologist engaged in a mentoring approach is able to help establish the spirit needed. How does one go about mentoring? There are a number of mentoring techniques depending on the circumstances, time frame, expertise, goals, unique personalities, and relationships that evolve. Try these techniques as you interact with other professionals and family members.

THE EDUCATIONAL AUDIOLOGIST

The most evident interrelationship between specialists in education to children with hearing impairments and members of the speech-language profession is in audiology. Educational audiology, a comparatively new specialization in the field of communication disorders, was born out of a need for improved services for the children with hearing impairments in the school.

The adverse effects of hearing loss on school children has been well documented (Flexer, 1999). Hearing loss causes delay in the development of receptive and expressive communication skills (speech and language). As a result, youngsters experience learning problems and experience poor academic achievement. Children's inability to understand the speech of others and to speak clearly often results in social isolation and poor self-concept.

The educational audiologist plays a primary role in identifying children who have impaired hearing through mass screening programs and/or teacher or parent referrals. The children who fail screening tests are given a comprehensive audiological assessment. Air and bone conduction pure-tone tests are administered as well as speech-reception and speech-discrimination tests. Immittance or impedance testing evaluates the function of the middle ear and can provide valuable information about the presence or absence of middle-ear pathology (for example, otitis media).

Additional evaluative and/or therapeutic recommendations may be made by the audiologist if indicated by the tests. If audiological and medical evaluations reveal that amplification is necessary, the educational audiologist helps the parents to obtain the aid or assistive device. Parents are taught to monitor the child's behavior and hearing ability to ensure their acceptance and proper use.

In addition to parent counseling, it is necessary to provide classroom teachers with information to help them deal with students who are hearing impaired. The educational audiologist participates in multidisciplinary team meetings. The audiologist also monitors classroom acoustics, measures noise levels, makes recommendations for sound treatment, and calibrates audiological equipment. Ideally, all these functions are performed by the educational audiologist. Unfortunately, they are in short supply and often must spread themselves very thin.

The quality of educational services provided for youngsters who are hearing impaired creates some concern. Case management must be comprehensive to ensure optimum coordination of services. The educational audiologist appears to be in the best position to be a case manager if the optimization of residual hearing is the starting point for learning. Moreover, the classroom teacher typically monitors hearing aids even though the educational audiologist is the best-equipped person for this function.

Direct services provided for the child with a hearing impairment in the classroom are often termed aural habilitation and are essential if the child is to develop skills that will enhance learning opportunities. Other areas of concern include the availability of counseling for parents and for the child as well as consultative services for teachers, administrators, and other resource personnel. All services provided for the child should be coordinated (Flexer, 1999).

There are many possible areas for cooperation between the SLP and the educational audiologist. The SLP is specifically prepared to provide a program of language and speech intervention and is the person best qualified to do so. As information is obtained from the audiologist concerning the child's need for auditory development, it can be incorporated into the speech and language program. Because most audiologists service a wide geographical area, they are not in a specific building with the same regularity as the SLP. Thus, the clinician is considered to be the critical link between the student in the classroom and comprehensive audiological services.

The SLP may work with the educational audiologist in the evaluation of the child with a hearing disability. Consultation with classroom teachers and visits to the classroom may be scheduled by both the SLP and the educational audiologist in an effort to better assess the needs of the student.

To summarize, it may be said that to provide the child with a hearing impairment with the best possible services, the SLP and the educational audiologist must work together in the evaluation, habilitation, and psychosocial adjustment of the child.

School SLPs would do well to encourage the employment of educational audiologists who are—by training or experience—familiar either with schools or the process of education. Educational audiologists must utilize their clinical knowledge and awareness of the educational and communicative needs of the child with a hearing impairment in the classroom.

Although the number of educational audiologists employed in the schools is increasing, there are still many schools with partial or limited audiological services. The school SLP may be playing a larger role in the delivery of services in these situations. Without an educational audiologist in the school system the task of caring for the child with a hearing impairment falls to the SLP.

The school clinician's role is to provide appropriate components of supplemental services directly to hearing-impaired children. The SLP serves as a hearing consultant to teachers, administrators, and resource specialists, helping them make reasonable accommodations to meet the special needs of the child in the integrated class setting. He or she is a member of the interdisciplinary team and develops new components of comprehensive hearing services within the school district.

SPEECH-LANGUAGE PATHOLOGY ASSISTANTS

The involvement of speech-language pathology assistants is becoming a more common component in service delivery in schools as well as health care settings. The use of assistants has increased in recent years as professionals have sought mechanisms for expanding service delivery options while containing costs (ASHA, 1999). As caseloads grow in size and diversity, there is a need to broaden the services that are offered. SLP assistants perform tasks that are prescribed, directed, and supervised by ASHA-certified speech-language pathologists. Thus, assistants support clinical services provided by the SLP. By incorporating an assistant into the intervention services, many SLPs have been able to focus their attention on more complex treatment issues rather than the day-to-day operational activities such as filing, preparing clinical materials, recording data, and so on. While the SLP's relationship with the assistant is usually in a supervisory capacity, it is clear that by working as a team the value of services can be expanded to better serve the needs of youngsters. The Code of Ethics of the American Speech-Language-Hearing Association (1995) clearly deals with the issue of supportive personnel and their supervision in "Principle of Ethics II: Individuals shall honor their responsibility to achieve and maintain the highest level of professional competence." (Refer to the Code of Ethics printed in Chapter 2.)

In the school setting, support personnel have been referred to by different titles (e.g., speech-language pathology assistants, communication aides, paraprofessionals, speech aides, teacher's aides, classroom aides, educational associates, and volunteer aides). Sometimes, they are paid employees or they may be volunteers. In some states, they are licensed. The background and educational levels and amount of training may vary, depending on the requirements of the state and local school district. Speech-language pathology assistants may receive training provided through on-the-job training, formal course work, workshops, observation, supervised field experiences, or any combination of these activities. Some universities and community colleges have training programs leading to state certification of assistants. Appropriate areas of training may include:

- Normal processes in speech, language, and hearing
- Disorders of speech, language, and hearing
- Behavior management skills
- Discrimination skills including, but not limited to, the discrimination of correct and incorrect verbal responses along with the dimensions of speech sound production, voice parameters, fluency, syntax, and semantics
- Instructions for presenting stimuli to students, collecting data, reporting observations, and utilizing instructional materials

- Management of equipment and materials used in speech-language pathology programs
- Overview of professional ethics and their application to the assistant's activities

The American Speech-Language-Hearing Association has promoted greater understanding of the potential scope of responsibility of speech-language pathology assistants and issues surrounding the use of this group of support personnel. Some state licensure boards have also developed a set of criteria for the use of aides and assistants.

The use of assistants has spurred great debate in the profession over the years. Those who support the use of assistants believe it to be a good mechanism for expanding the delivery of services to an increasingly diverse client base. Administrators often see it as a way to be more cost efficient. Some SLPs fear that the use of speech-language pathology assistants will eventually lead to the replacement of qualified, licensed and/or certified practitioners. This will not happen as long as professionals continue to maintain responsibility for the types of work assistants are permitted to do. The public expects speech-language pathology services to be delivered by the highest qualified practitioner, and that is the speech-language pathologist who holds the appropriate credentials. ASHA guidelines and state licensure laws mandate just what those credentials are. Assistants can function only in supportive roles and must be supervised by qualified professionals. If properly integrated into the speech-language pathology program, assistants can be very beneficial. The use of assistants permits the SLP to perform those professional-level tasks that require expertise and clinical judgement while still enabling the completion of day-to-day tasks that may be necessary but time consuming.

Since 1995, ASHA published a document, "Guidelines for the Training, Credentialing, Use, and Supervision of Speech-Language Pathology Assistants" (ASHA, 1995). These guidelines included the definition of supportive personnel, qualifications, training, roles, and supervision.

The legal, ethical, and moral responsibility to the client for all services provided cannot be delegated; that is, they remain the responsibility of the professional personnel. Supportive personnel can be permitted to implement a variety of clinical tasks given that the speech-language pathologist responsible for those tasks provides sufficient training, direction, and supervision. Examples of tasks that assistants may perform under the supervision of a qualified speech-language pathologist are listed in the ASHA Guidelines:

- Conduct speech-language and hearing screenings
- Follow documented treatment plans or protocols including implementing reinforcement activities to strengthen skills previously introduced by the SLP
- Document patient/client progress; this may include observing the student in settings around the school including classrooms, cafeteria, and playground
- Assist during assessment
- Assist with informal documentation and other clerical duties
- Prepare, fabricate, and maintain clinical materials, equipment, and tools
- Program augmentative communication devices as prescribed by the clinician
- Add information to students' records as dictated by the SLP, including attendance and filing data
- Schedule activities, prepare charts, records, graphs, or otherwise display data
- Perform checks and maintenance of equipment

- Participate in research projects, in-service training, and public relations programs
- Escort children to and from the classroom and the therapy room

The SLP must maintain the primary responsibility for the speech/language program for students with communication disorders. By specifying those tasks that assistants are permitted to perform, the SLP clarifies the expectations of the job assignment for the assistant as well as for other personnel in the school system such as the principal. Instructions should be communicated to the assistant verbally and in writing. The clinician must establish a plan for observing how these activities are executed to confirm that the assistant is not overstepping his or her boundaries. The ASHA guidelines document also provides an extensive list of what assistants *cannot* do including:

- Performing standardized or nonstandardized diagnostic tests or evaluations
- Interpreting test results
- Provide counseling to the student or family
- Write, develop, or modify a student's individualized education plan
- Implement any aspects of the treatment plan without being supervised
- Select or discharge students from the speech-language program
- Share clinical or confidential information orally or in writing with anyone
- Make referrals
- Communicate with the student, family, or educators regarding any aspect of the student's status or service without being directed to do so by the supervisor
- Represent himself or herself as a speech-language pathologist

Supervision of a speech-language pathology assistant is an important responsibility and should not be entered into lightly. The use of assistants will be much more effective if you take this responsibility seriously and learn how to provide the guidance and supervision that is needed to ensure they execute their role appropriately. Supervision of support personnel must be regular, comprehensive, and documented to ensure that the student working with the assistant receives the highest quality services he or she needs. The amount of supervision should be based on the assignments and skills of the assistant. The ASHA 1995 speech-language pathology guidelines recommend supervising 30 percent of the assistants' weekly work for the first 90 workdays and 20 percent after the initial work period. Supervision includes on-site, in-view observation and guidance while an assigned activity is being performed. Care should be taken to follow stated guidelines because funding is often linked to the qualifications of the person providing services.

Speech-language pathologists in Broward County, Florida developed their own training and supervision plan for speech-language assistants (Goldstein & Ehren, 1999). They were especially interested in establishing a method for identifying individuals who were qualified for employment as speech-language pathology assistants and for evaluating the quality of their work.

Once a speech-language pathology assistant is employed, it becomes the SLP's responsibility to assure others that the assistant is doing the job appropriately. Evaluation protocols serve two purposes. They serve as a mechanism for clarifying expectations, and they enable supervisors to identify performance that is good as well as that which is problematic. A sample evaluation form is provided in Figure 10.3.

FIGURE 10.3   **Speech-Language Assistant Evaluation**

Assistant's Name _____   Date of Evaluation

School_____   Reviewer

Check Items   E = Excels   S = Satisfactory   NI = Needs Improvement
                  U = Unsatisfactory   NA = Not Applicable

	E	S	NI	U	NA
A. General: Record Keeping					
1. Knowledge of program goals.					
2. Ability to update standardized pupil information records.					
3. Knowledge of school organization and operation.					
4. Performs routine clerical duties.					
B. Work With Students					
1. Ability to work with individual students.					
2. Ability to work with small groups of students.					
3. Ability to assist students with SLP-planned activities.					
4. Knowledge and ability to prepare instructional materials and teaching aides.					
5. Knowledge and ability to use instructional materials and teaching aides.					
6. Ability to maintain control and discipline.					
7. Ability to manage behavior of students when SLP is not present.					
8. Awareness of students' therapy goals.					
9. Ability to describe students' performance.					
C. Work Habits and Personal Relations					
1. Performs adequate amount of work.					
2. Work is accurate.					
3. Maintenance, storage, and clean-up of materials.					
4. Initiative and resourcefulness.					

FIGURE 10.3 Continued

5. Neatness of work product.					
6. Attendance.					
7. Observation of work schedule.					
8. Compliance with rules, policies, and directives.					
9. Communication with students and school staff.					
10. Cooperative and flexible					
11. Exhibits positive attitude.					
12. Shows tact and good judgment.					
13. Accepts constructive criticism.					
14. Implemented appropriate suggestions for improvement.					
15. Understands assigned responsibilities.					
16. Performs effectively under stress and opposition.					
D. Overall Performance					

Paraprofessionals have been used effectively in the health, education, and human service fields for many years. The need for supportive personnel in our field undoubtedly will increase in the coming years. As professionals it is incumbent upon us to determine the competencies and preparation needed to perform the duties of a speech-language pathology assistant. We must then monitor and supervise them closely in order to ensure that, with their involvement, our services continue to be effectively and efficiently delivered.

THE PSYCHOLOGIST

The school psychologist is a member of the team of professional persons helping the child with communication impairments. The National Association of School Psychologists defines four major areas of practice including psychological and psychoeducational assessment, consultation, direct service, and planning/evaluation (Levinson & Murphy, 1999). The psychologist can provide valuable information regarding the student's cognitive and academic abilities. The psychologist assesses a student's eligibility for special education services as well as identifies and tests the effectiveness of interventions designed to solve academic, social, or behavioral difficulties. Psychologists' knowledge of learning and behavior theory is valuable in determining the optimal conditions for learning. Educators and the school clinician may make referrals to the psychologist to obtain additional information about educational diagnosis, school adjustment, personality, learning ability, or achievement. The child's speech, language, or hearing problem may be closely related to any of these factors, either as a result, a cause, or an accompanying factor.

The school clinician and the psychologist will find that a close working relationship is mutually beneficial. The school clinician will want to know the kinds of testing and diagnostic materials the psychologist uses. On the other hand, the clinician may be helpful to the psychologist in interpreting the child's communication problem so that the best possible tests may be used. In making a referral to the psychologist the clinician should ask specific questions regarding the kind of information being sought. The school clinician can also furnish the psychologist with helpful information that would facilitate working with the child.

The school psychologist's role differs from one school system to another, so the clinician should make a note of that role and find out what additional kinds of psychological help are available in the community.

THE SOCIAL WORKER

Social workers can contribute much to programming and transition planning for students with disabilities. The Council on Social Work Education (CSWE) describes the social work profession as "committed to the enhancement of human well-being and to the alleviation of poverty and oppression" (Hepworth et al., 1997, p. 4). The major role of the social worker is to help students and their families access support services. They facilitate interagency linkage among tax-supported and voluntary agencies. They may assist in gathering data needed to determine eligibility for special education services. The social worker pays particular attention to self-advocacy.

This professional's thorough knowledge of social agencies in an area can be of considerable aid to the school clinician. The social worker is a key person in helping families find places where they may receive needed help. The social worker may provide counseling, make home visits, and serve as the liaison between the school and the family. They can be particularly helpful in advocating for a person with disabilities as they transition from school to work or post-secondary education (Markward & Kurtz, 1999). When financial assistance is required for supplemental services, the social worker is the one who can be of assistance to the family in locating that aid. Not all school systems are fortunate enough to have a social worker on the staff, but if there is one, the school clinician should explore ways in which they may work cooperatively.

THE BILINGUAL EDUCATOR AND/OR ENGLISH-AS-A-SECOND-LANGUAGE (ESL) TEACHER

America is truly a multicultural nation. Across the country there are children in our schools who do not speak the same language as their teachers and classmates. They may speak a language other than English or a nonstandard dialect. They may be from families who have recently moved to the United States, have parents who do not speak English, or live in communities where a unique dialect is spoken. These children are classified as presenting cultural and linguistic diversity. Their traditions, values, attitudes, and beliefs may be different from their teachers and classmates. They often struggle in the school setting while trying to learn to communicate and participate in school activities.

Class placement and service to children in these groups varies widely. In communities where there are large numbers of children from different cultures, programs and protocols for meeting their needs may be established. The speech-language pathologist is often called on to assist these children in developing communication skills that will permit them to learn and benefit from the education setting. In these cases, SLPs should work cooperatively with the bilingual educators or English-as-a-Second-Language (ESL) teachers in the district to determine how to best assess and establish a plan for intervention.

In a discussion of considerations when working with multicultural populations, Damico and Nye (1990) stressed the importance of selecting individuals who can act as informants or interpreters during interviewing, testing, planning, and intervention procedures. Inclusion of a person who speaks the child's native language and understands the child's culture will help ensure that the program developed is appropriate and relevant for the student's needs.

Chamberlain and Landurand (1990) indicated several competencies that are preferred when selecting informants. These include proficiency in both English and the child's language, an understanding of the importance of maintaining confidentiality, and other cognitive, personality, and experience factors which would facilitate cooperation during the time that the person is acting as an interpreter or informant. If using informants or interpreters in these functions, it will be important to provide training for them so they clearly understand their role and duties (Damico and Nye, 1990).

THE GUIDANCE COUNSELOR AND VOCATIONAL REHABILITATION COUNSELOR

The guidance counselor works with students with adjustment or academic problems, helps students plan for future roles, and makes available to them information pertinent to their situation. This individual may also do individual counseling.

The guidance counselor is especially helpful in dealing with students in the junior high and high school. Students with communication problems are often known by the guidance counselor, so the school clinician may depend on this person for referrals, supplementary information, and cooperative intervention.

The vocational rehabilitation counselor is usually employed by a district or state agency. This individual assists students 16 years of age and older in overcoming handicaps that would prevent them from being employable at their highest potential. The vocational rehabilitation counselor, although not a member of the school staff, may work in conjunction with the school system.

THE SCHOOL NURSE

Depending on the size of the system, there may be a number of school nurses, only one, or one working part time. In some localities the school nurse may be part of the staff of the city, county, or district health department and work either part time or full time with the school. The new school clinician will want to know in which of these arrangements the school nurse functions.

The school nurse is a manager of medical and health information and is key to ensuring that the health component objectives of the IEP or ITP are implemented. The nurse maintains the health and medical records of the children in the school. Children with hearing loss, brain injury, cleft palate, cerebral palsy, and other physical problems are already known by the school nurse. The nurse is the one who arranges for medical intervention when it is needed, makes home visits, and knows the families. It goes without saying that the school nurse and the speech-language pathologist work closely together and need to share information on a continuing basis.

In some states, the school nurse is legally responsible for conducting hearing screenings. The nurse, the school clinician, and the educational audiologist may work together in organizing and administering the hearing-conservation program of detection, referral, and follow-up. Medical referrals and follow-ups involving family doctors, otologists, and other medical specialists may be carried out by the school nurse. Medical problems in addition to those connected with hearing loss would be included.

The school nurse is one of the best sources of information for the school clinician and should be one of the clinician's closest working allies.

THE PHYSICAL THERAPIST

By definition a trained physical therapist works in the general area of motor performance. The services may focus on correction, development, and/or prevention of motor-related problems. Physical therapists can assist in maximizing the students' physical functioning so they can participate in various daily living, leisure, and vocational activities. More physical therapists can be found working in hospitals or home health care agencies than in public schools. Often school systems contract with other agencies to provide physical therapy services. They no longer work under a doctor's prescription but often under medical referral. Physical therapists usually develop a written treatment plan for each patient, which is countersigned by a physician.

Physical therapists work with persons with ambulatory problems, focusing on the improved use of the lower extremities in sitting, standing, walking, and movement with and without aids.

The school SLP and the physical therapist may work together in serving children with orthopedic and neurologic problems, and on developmental programs for high-risk infants. Physical therapists may also provide information and assistance to SLPs in achieving good posture for optimal breath support and control and in the stabilization of extraneous movements for cerebral palsied children. In addition, physical therapists may evaluate motor abilities for students who are possible candidates for communication boards or augmentative communicative equipment.

The speech-language pathologist can provide the physical therapist with assistance in the establishment of methods of communication modes with their clients.

THE OCCUPATIONAL THERAPIST

Because the work of the occupational therapist covers such a wide range it is difficult to define that person's scope of activities. The profession of occupational therapy is concerned with human lives that have been disrupted by physical injury, accident, birth defects, aging, or emotional or developmental problems. The programs in occupational therapy are designed to enhance a person's development, restore independence, and prevent disabilities. The word *occupation* does not necessarily refer to the individual's employment but rather to being occupied in meaningful day-to-day activities, including work, leisure, and play. In the school setting, occupational therapists address sensory-motor, cognitive, and psychosocial skills and habits. Their intervention helps students learn to perform self-care, classroom, work, and play tasks in multiple contexts such as the classroom, gym, cafeteria, playground, work setting, and community at large (Shepherd & Inge, 1999).

Occupational therapists work in a variety of settings, and today an increasing number are employed in public school systems. The occupational therapist and the SLP will find many areas of cooperation that will enhance the disabled student's potential. These same areas, however, may also give rise to conflicts regarding professional responsibility as well as differences in therapeutic approaches. The answer to this problem seems to be the establishment of a truly cooperative working relationship. Each profession has unique skills, and the recognition and respect for each other's expertise will serve to help the handicapped individual.

Occupational therapists may work with the severely disabled child, especially in the development of adaptive devices, such as conversation boards, that aid greater independence. They may work with children with visual-spatial perceptual problems or with children who are having trouble adjusting to handicaps. They may work with a child individually or with groups of students in such activities as role playing, games, work adjustment sessions, and discussion groups.

THE HEALTH AND PHYSICAL EDUCATION TEACHER

One staff member who may be in as close of contact with pupils as the classroom teacher is the health and physical education (HPE) teacher. This individual sees students in an environment where movement is stressed, where pupils are engaged in activities in which they may be more relaxed, and where talking may be more spontaneous. School SLPs may be able to work with the HPE teacher in generalized activities for the pupil with an articulation problem. The HPE teacher can also help the pupil with a voice problem who yells too much. The HPE teacher is competent in teaching relaxation strategies and may help the children who are dysfluent or who present motor disorders. The HPE teacher on the elementary or secondary level can be a valuable resource person for the SLP.

NON-TEACHING SUPPORT PERSONNEL

In every school building, there are many non-teaching support personnel with whom speech-language pathologists, audiologists, and students interact. This includes the clerical staff, cafeteria workers, bus drivers, gardeners, custodians, and volunteers who make the school function.

These individuals, who often know the students in different ways than do the teachers, are important people without whom the school could not run smoothly. The SLP can rely on them for information on where to get things and where to find things as well as information on the school buildings, equipment, and classroom housekeeping. The custodian may be the only one who knows that in the back of a storage closet there are some textbooks, workbooks, chairs, or a portable chalkboard that the clinician could use.

All of these individuals can contribute something to the success of a school therapy program even if it is just a positive comment now and then. Their work and contributions to the operation of the school should be acknowledged. They will provide you with more efficient and effective services if you take the time to share information about your program with them. Oftentimes these individuals live in the school district community and will promote your program to their neighbors if they understand what it is that you do. In addition, they interact with children on a daily basis and can provide compliments and reinforcement to children on your caseload.

WORKING WITH FAMILY

Throughout this book references are made regarding the importance of working with the family. State and federal legislation have mandated the inclusion of parents and/or guardians in the planning and intervention process. This is not a new role for the SLP; most have always worked with the parents of children on their caseloads and the parents of children at risk. In this section the term *family* shall be used to include parents, guardians, and significant other family members who can contribute to the program designed for a child.

Involving families can facilitate development of meaningful intervention goals, better implementation of recommendations, and effective transfer of skills from the therapy room to daily life. Families are the constants in the child's life. Clinicians, teachers, and other service providers enter temporarily. It is for this reason that families should be considered equal partners in the assessment and intervention process. The treatment plan should be designed to foster families' decision-making skills as well as their capabilities for providing their child with assistance. Professionals need to recognize the individuality of clients and families and modify services to meet those needs. This means that services must be delivered in contexts which are considered "normal" for the youngster. All services should be coordinated so that the family and youngster are not stressed by having to go in too many directions at one time.

While there is not one set of rules on how the school SLP should work with families, the beginning clinician might find it helpful to have some general ideas. Most clinicians develop their own "style" of working with family members as they gain confidence and experience.

The first and most important thing to remember is that parents are people. The basic ingredients for effectively working with people are understanding and respect. The inexperienced clinician sometimes approaches parents with a preconceived idea of how they are going to react and behave and, therefore, expects resistance. At the same time the parents may anticipate the clinician's role as that of the "expert" who has at hand all the information and know-how to "cure" their child's problem. Obviously, then, everyone gets off on the wrong foot. If the clinician approaches the parents in a friendly open way and lets them see her or him as a person whose task is to apply the most appropriate principles of rehabilitation (or habilitation) to the situation, the clinician will set the stage for the next step in the process. It is the clinician's responsibility to establish the ground rules and create the climate for a positive working relationship.

The climate that is established for the parent conference can help formulate the foundation needed for success. Make sure parents are seated comfortably. Avoid leaving spaces between parents and other professionals. This will make them feel isolated and as though they are not a part of the team. Be sure there are no obstructions such as desks between you and the parents. This creates a barrier to open communication. Equip the conference setting with adult-size chairs. There is nothing more uncomfortable than trying to have a serious conversation with your knees up against your chin. Check to be sure that chairs are arranged neatly so that a conversation can be conducted. Ensure that lighting is adequate, not too bright or too dim. Draw the drapes if the sunlight is directly on your face or that of the parents'.

Parent Groups

In schools it is common for clinicians to work with parents in a group as well as individually. Parent groups may be organized by the school clinician as support groups or by the parents themselves as a result of the need for more information about their child's disability. Many parents are interested in assuming a greater amount of involvement in the treatment program. The professional in this kind of relationship assumes the role of a resource or support person. Parents should be encouraged to express both positive and negative feelings without being judged about what they say or how they say it. Parents of children with disabilities often have feelings of guilt, as if something they did or didn't do caused the child's handicap. Professionals need to understand this response and help parents use the group situation as an opportunity for change, growth, and personal development. The use of the words ought and should are best dropped from the SLP vocabulary when dealing with anxious parents.

Parents can be the most reliable sources of information concerning the child's speech, language, and hearing behavior. For example, if a parent insists that his or her child cannot follow simple directions or stammers when playing with an older sibling, accept his or her word for it. Subsequent observation will often prove the parent correct.

Involving Siblings

Brothers and sisters may experience several emotions related to their sibling's communication problems. They may be embarrassed about the way people react when they cannot understand the child. Some siblings feel the need to defend or translate for their brother or sister. All members of the family can play a positive role in the treatment of a communication problem if they understand the nature of the disorder and the ways they can help. Be sure to make brothers and sisters feel welcome to visit the therapy room. Describe the speech and language problem. Explain simple tricks for increasing their understanding of unintelligible speech. Show them how to model good speech patterns, how to stimulate correct productions, or how to help with homework assignments. Stress the need for patience and understanding. By providing the sibling with positive ways to respond, the likelihood of embarrassment and teasing will be reduced.

Changing Family Patterns

Family patterns are changing in the modern world. There are many single parent families or divorced and remarried parents in families in which children are "his," "hers," and "ours." Many children are cared for on a daily basis by someone other than a parent, others are "latchkey" children who care for themselves and/or their siblings many hours each day. Some children are negatively affected by family situations such as these while others don't seem troubled. The speech-language clinician needs to be sensitive to the child's emotional well-being.

Unique family situations that are new to the school clinician, such as abuse, neglect, or poverty, may arise. One can never be prepared for all circumstances. However, situations such as these will be easier to handle if you strive to increase your knowledge about them and learn recommended strategies and solutions. The school clinician should keep in mind that children who come to school hungry, malnourished, inadequately clothed, or frightened have difficulty learning and concentrating on tasks such as speech and language production. Make no assumptions about a child's worth or capabilities or a parent's love and interest in his or her child based on the family's income. Many poor families have homes that are rich in love.

INVOLVING THE STUDENT

Too often, children with impairments are treated as inanimate objects. Other people talk about them and decide how to teach them or how to "fix" their communication problems. They are eliminated from the decision-making process. This approach does not enable us to understand if the student feels the communication impairment is important or not. It also prohibits us from gaining insights about the student's interest or motivation for improving communication skills. Some students can even provide their recommendations about how to structure therapy to benefit them the most.

Reports in the professional literature have demonstrated that families, educators, and others are being included in the decision-making process more frequently. We often read recommendations that the patient/client should be included, but anecdotal reports from clinicians appear to indicate that this recommendation is not commonly practiced. Perhaps that limitation results from a lack of clinician awareness of how to involve the client meaningfully in program planning and decision making.

What kind of information can we obtain from the children we serve? When people participate in planning a treatment program, they are likely to be more actively engaged in the success of the program. The student has expectations and opinions about what his or her treatment should be. Intervention will be much more effective if the treatment meets the client's expectations and if motivation is high. The plan that is developed should reflect the client's goals and special needs regardless of age. Students' comments should lead to specific recommendations to be incorporated into the treatment plan.

According to IDEA, students are supposed to be a part of the team, especially when transition services are discussed. The regulations state that the coordinated set of activities developed for the transition plan must be based on the student's needs, taking into account the student's preferences and interests. This directive has sound implications for servicing all clients regardless of age. There is nothing "magical" about the age of 14 (the time period when transition plans are developed for children). Children of other ages and adult clients have opinions and expectations that will impact on their commitment and performance in treatment.

Individuals who have a sense of control over their own destiny generally are more successful at the tasks they attempt. It is vital that service providers do everything possible to encourage the development of the client's ability to understand his or her communication disability and participate meaningully in the treatment process.

The IEP meeting is one opportunity for soliciting youngster's opinions about strengths, needs, preferences, and interests. If that opportunity is not possible due to barriers such as time constraints, cost, conflicting schedules, and so on, the clinician can take other opportunities to obtain relevant information. In the initial weeks of enrollment in a therapy program, the youngster's opinion can be sought through dialogue and questioning to obtain information that would contribute to determining treatment priorities and procedures to be used for the coming year. Ideally these questions would be asked during a team planning conference attended by the child, parents, key teachers, speech-language pathologist, other specialists, and administrators. If that is not possible, the SLP can ask the questions during a therapy session. The student's responses can then be considered and incorporated into future treatment plans, thus increasing the quality of the treatment plan and the student's motivation to perform.

Some youngsters may find it difficult to participate in the team process. They may be reluctant to be in a meeting with several adults. They may be too shy to say what is on their minds. They may not be able to find the words to clearly express their thoughts, feelings, and opinions. In addition, they may not feel like doing so in such a forum. Youngsters can be prepared for making contributions ahead of time through coaching. Or, their opinions can be sought during one to one discussions with the parent or speech-language pathologist.

Ultimately the goal is for students to have control and manage their own intervention program including selecting goals and identifying treatment procedures.

Efforts should be made to provide the student with a clear understanding of the communication impairment and how it affects their performance academically and socially. The student should be asked to contribute ideas for developing a treatment plan that can effectively meet his or her personal needs. Of course, the quality and quantity of a student's involvement as a member of the collaborative team will depend on how the involvement is sought and on the student's capability for understanding the problems and for providing information. The level of involvement should be commensurate with the student's cognitive and social maturity.

SATISFACTION WITH SERVICES

It is reasonable to believe that children, like adults, have opinions and expectations about the situations in which they participate. Manufacturers of children's products such as toys and food often seek children's opinions via simple questionnaires and surveys. Clinical experiences and anecdotal evidence shows that clinicians have been less likely to sample children's likes and dislikes or satisfaction with the services they receive. Perhaps we assume that we already know what's good for the children we serve. The consumer satisfaction tools that have been devised to sample satisfaction with speech-language pathology services have not been geared to our young consumers. However, the principles that apply to meeting the needs of our adult consumers apply equally to meeting the needs of the young children and adolescents we serve. Blosser and Park (1996) developed a "Kids are Consumers Too" satisfaction survey to sample youngsters' opinions about speech and language services. The survey questions can be found in Figure 10.4. Responses to questions such as these could be used to guide the improvement of services.

WORKING WITH PHYSICIANS IN THE COMMUNITY

A good relationship with the physicians in the community enhances the speech, language, and hearing program. School clinicians should take every opportunity to establish such relationships by conducting their programs in a professional manner, following established local protocol in referral procedures, writing letters and reports that are professional in content and style, and giving talks to local medical groups if invited to do so.

A competent school clinician never oversteps professional bounds by giving medical advice or advice that could be construed as medical in nature. For example, the school clinician may think that a child's persistent husky voice may be the result of either vocal abuse or vocal nodules, or possibly a combination of both conditions. After collecting as much information as possible from parents, teachers, and the child, the clinician must follow local referral policies established by the school system. These policies will differ from school system to school system. In some places all medical referrals are done through the school nurse, the school social worker, or some designated administrator. The school policy may allow the clinician to discuss the contemplated referral with the parents, who then follow through by taking the child to the family physician. The referral is accompanied by a letter from the clinician and includes results of diagnostic procedures, general impressions, and specific questions, as well as any other helpful information. The clinician should also include a request for the results of the physician's diagnosis and suggestions. It is best to request that the physician's results be sent to the SLP, with a copy to the parents. When parents ask the clinician to suggest a physician because they don't have a family doctor, the acceptable policy is to give the family the names of at least three doctors from which they can choose.

Care should be taken when referring for a medical evaluation or opinion. In some circumstances the school system is required to pay for the evaluation; in others payment is the responsibility of the family. Each school district will have guidelines specifying the circumstances for making referrals to physicians and determining the responsible payer. Be sure to discuss and clarify this important information before recommending a visit to the doctor. While it is imperative to understand who will serve as the pay source, the decision to refer for a medical opinion should be based on the child's physical condition, not the pay source.

FIGURE 10.4   Kids are Consumers Too!

SATISFACTION SURVEY

Age:_____   Communication Problem: _____   articulation

Grade: _____   _____   language

Length of Time   _____   voice

Enrolled in Therapy: _____   _____   fluency

SLP (optional): _____   _____   other

School (optional): _____

Directions: Read each question. (If the child cannot read, SLP shold read to him or her.)

Place an X on the face that describes how you feel.

1. Do you know what you are learning in speech therapy class?

    Yes   Sometimes   No   Don't know

2. Do you sound as good as other children in your class when you talk?

    Yes   Sometimes   No   Don't know

3. Do you think the speech therapy room is interesting and a good place to learn?

    Yes   Sometimes   No   Don't know

4. Do you think you should come to speech therapy more often?

    Yes   Sometimes   No   Don't know

5. Do you like the activities you do when you come to speech therapy class?

    Yes   Sometimes   No   Don't know

(continued)

FIGURE 10.4   Continued

6. Do you think you can talk better with your family and friends becasue you come to speech therapy class?

Yes	Sometimes	No	Don't know

7. Do you tell your friends about what you do in speech therapy class?

Yes	Sometimes	No	Don't know

8. Do you tell your family about what you do in speech therapy class?

Yes	Sometimes	No	Don't know

9. Would you tell one of your friends to come to speech therapy if he or she had problems talking?

Yes	Sometimes	No	Don't know

10. Do you like having speech therapy?

Yes	Sometimes	No	Don't know

My two favorite activities were:

1. _____

2. _____

FIGURE 10.4   Continued

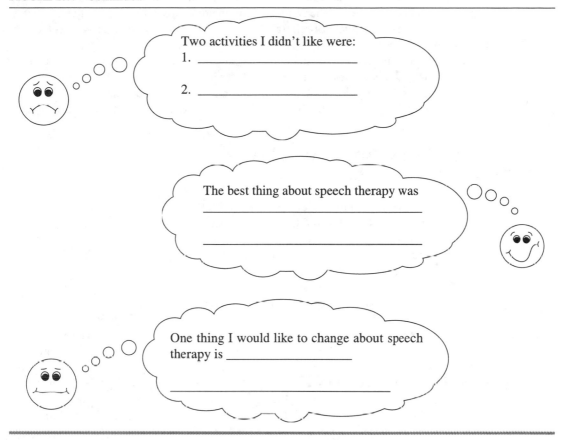

Nothing is more important than good health. The child who is ill or in need of medical attention cannot be expected to perform well in school. School clinicians should be alert to the child's physical condition. If there are any behaviors or symptoms that might be related to a health condition, the school clinician should discuss this with the school nurse and/or the principal. Proper referral steps should be taken to ensure the youngster's health and safety.

WORKING WITH DENTISTS

There are a number of areas of specialization within the dental profession, among them pedodontists, who are concerned with children's dental care; orthodontists, who are concerned with dental occlusion; and prosthodontists, who are concerned with designing and fitting appliances to compensate for aberrations within the oral structure. SLPs may make referrals to, or may be the recipient of referrals from, these dental specialists as well as the dentist in general practice within a community. The referrals may be children whose articulation problems are related to dental or oral cavity problems, such as cleft palate or other cranio-facial anomalies. Children with dysarthrias associated with cerebral palsy, as well as children with developmental disabilities, may require special handling by dentists. Thus the professional relationship between the dentist and the SLP requires cooperation.

WORKING WITH VOCATIONAL COUNSELORS AND EMPLOYERS

Schools are becoming more concerned about and involved in planning for the student's success after leaving school. From the time a student is around 14 years of age, the planning focuses on transition from school to post-secondary activities, either additional education or work. A variety of professionals can contribute to the vocational assessment and transition planning necessary to assist students.

The vocational evaluation process should be conducted by a qualified vocational evaluator who can help collect, synthesize, and interpret complex information (Leconte, 1999). High school educators are often charged with this responsibility. Vocational assessment and training strategies are a major component of transition planning. The SLP can be a valuable contributor to the discussion. However, oftentimes SLPs are not asked or do not volunteer to participate. Discussions should center around the type of communication that is required and expected for successful performance, strategies employers can use to ensure effective performance, and advance preparation of the students' communication skills including vocabulary, direction following, reading instructions, and conversing with customers and coworkers.

MAINTAINING ONGOING COMMUNICATION WITH COLLABORATIVE PARTNERS

How do SLPs bridge gaps in understanding? First, it must be emphasized that understanding is a two-sided coin and that although clinicians seek to be understood, they must also understand the roles and responsibilities of school administrators and personnel. Second, this is a continuous, ongoing process requiring a vigorous and assertive stance on the part of the SLP. Third, the responsibility for communicating with others about the profession should be shared with others including members or the state and national professional organizations.

Administrators and teachers may not invite us to tell them who we are or what we can do. The pathologist must take the initiative and invite others to learn more about our profession. An assertive, proactive approach is needed to gain administrative support. To accomplish this, administrators must first be educated about the profession and be encouraged to work with the SLP to facilitate effective service delivery. The SLP needs to establish a more visible position in the school so that administrative attention, understanding, and cooperation can be attained. The following School Personnel Education Program can be initiated in school buildings throughout the school district:

- Conduct a quality program. No program change or growth can occur unless quality is already in operation.
- Identify the key decision makers within the school district. Determine who needs to be "educated." This may include principals, teachers, curriculum directors, central office administration, school board members, and parents.
- Continually supply key administrators at the building, central administration and top administration levels with facts and information that will challenge them to act on behalf of the speech-language therapy program when decisions are being made.
- Increase the visibility of the speech-language therapy program districtwide:
  - Join school committees and attend building activities
  - Participate in prevention services and in-service activities
  - Host invitational days ("Board of Education Day"; "Principal's Day"; "Administrator's Day"; "Teacher's Day") and invite important people to observe therapy sessions
  - Establish a mechanism such as a newsletter for ongoing communication
  - Offer to speak at Board of Education meetings, parent groups, church groups and so on
  - Serve as a source of information to other educators regarding communication skills
  - Forward informative clippings and articles about communication disorders and their relationship to learning
- Inform administrators of your aspirations and goals for your program. Arrange for a meeting with district leaders to share your ideas about the program's strengths, weaknesses, and potentials.

The wise clinician will seize every opportunity possible to form working relationships with parents, students, and fellow professionals. Because there may be conflicting schedules and time is a precious commodity for all, it is essential for clinicians to be creative and use a wide range of mechanisms for exchanging information with others about communication disorders, program goals, and intervention strategies. These mechanisms can include face-to-face conferences, written communication (letters, reports, newsletters), audio and videotape recordings, discussion groups, in-service meetings, news articles, and observations.

Figure 10.5 shows a variety of mechanisms that can be used to form effective working relationships with specific constituency groups.

COMMUNITY INFORMATION PROGRAM

There are a number of advantages that will result from keeping the community informed about the speech-language pathology program in the schools. Begin by interpreting the program of prevention, assessment, and intervention. This will help remove any possible stigma attached to having a child enrolled in the program. It will also build a feeling of trust and confidence in the program and toward the school system in the community.

FIGURE 10.5   Methods for Communicating with Others

Listed below are several methods that can be used to form effective working relationships with others in order to develop awareness of the SLP program and cooperation for effective intervention.

STUDENTS
Visits to classrooms
Interactions throughout the building
Visual displays inside and outside the therapy room

STUDENTS' PARENTS
Discussion groups and training programs
Written communication (newsletters, progress reports, homework notes)
Conferences (face to face and telephone)
Observation days and school visits

TEACHERS AND SPECIAL EDUCATORS
Meetings and conferences to develop educational plans
Written communication (notes, letters, reports, newsletters, summarizing relevant articles)
In-service meetings
Audio and videotapes
Discussion groups
Informal interactions (lunch, school events, after school activities)

ADMINISTRATORS
In-service meetings
Meetings and conferences
Written communication (budget requests, annual reports, summaries of relevant professional literature, service statistics, thank you notes, state association newsletters, reports describing conferences attended)

COMMUNITY
Participation in school events
Speaking and/or membership in community organizations

LOCAL PROFESSIONALS
Networking through professional organizations
In-service meetings
Written communication (newsletters, letters, reports)

A community information program should not be a haphazard affair; it should be well planned and executed. It should not be a "one-shot" deal but rather continuous, consistent, and persistent. It should also be varied, informative, and interesting.

The school clinician may want to survey the types of media available within the community. The most commonly used are newspapers, radio, television, websites, service clubs, lectures and presentations, and displays.

The clinician may wish to make arrangements with the local newspaper to run a series of articles. Topics of interest include: characteristics of communication problems, how parents can help children learn to talk, helpful suggestions for families of children with fluency problems or hearing impairments, and the importance of early referral. Many other topics will be of interest to parents and community members.

In preparing articles for release in the local newspapers, it is best to inquire of the editor how long the article should be and then stick to the length suggested. If an article submitted is too long the editor is likely to trim it and may inadvertently cut out an important part. Most editors like to have articles submitted, but they should be well written and interesting. The school clinician can usually obtain from a member of the newspaper staff the pertinent facts on style and length for that publication. If pictures are used and they contain any children, it is an absolute must to first obtain written consent from the parents.

Some school systems have community information or public relations offices. The person responsible for internal and external communication for the district can often assist the clinician in preparing articles for publication or contacting the appropriate person at the news office.

Radio interviews or other types of programs are a good way of getting information across to the public. Local radio stations often welcome suggestions on programs of special interest. Clinicians can utilize such timely events as "Better Speech and Hearing Month" in May to focus attention on the needs of persons with speech, language, and hearing disorders. The same can be said of television programs. Often local television stations have programs during which various personalities are interviewed. Or the television station may cooperate in preparing a program on various aspects of the speech, language, and hearing program.

Talks to community service clubs, professional organizations, and other groups can yield innumerable benefits. Many of these groups sponsor special projects or programs as part of their community service activities. Another effective way of informing the community about the program is through displays at health fairs and similar events. Public libraries are often willing to add to their shelves books of interest to parents of handicapped children. The school clinician can make suggestions for specific books, which could then be made available to the public.

DISCUSSION QUESTIONS AND PROJECTS

1. Invite an elementary principal in to talk to the class on how he or she views the speech, language, and hearing program.

2. Interview a learning disabilities teacher on how he or she works with the school SLP.

3. List ways the SLP in the school can work with the classroom teacher on the teaching of reading. How would you implement these strategies?

4. How would the SLP in the schools schedule time for collaboration?

5. Plan an in-service session or a group meeting for elementary-school principals to acquaint them with the speech, language, and hearing program.

6. Do a survey of the health and rehabilitation agencies in your community. What are their referral policies and their criteria for accepting clients?

7. Ask a practicing school pathologist what the policies are concerning medical referrals in that school system.

8. Write a brief article about a speech-language or hearing topic that could be submitted to a local newspaper or radio.

9. Role-play the following situations with your classmates. What would you say? How would you respond?

   ■ Parents ask whether having their child's tonsils removed will help his speech problem.
   ■ Parents ask how long Johnny will be enrolled in therapy in order to cure his fluency problem.
   ■ Parents ask how they can stop the neighborhood children from teasing their child because she "can't talk right."
   ■ A parent asks if her smoking during her pregnancy caused her child to be learning disabled.

STUDENT TEACHING

Student teaching is sometimes regarded with trepidation by the prospective student teacher, probably because like all new experiences it contains the element of the unknown. The unknown is usually anticipated with a mixture of fear, curiosity, and excitement. The actual experience may bear out what was anticipated, and it may also contain some surprises. The following comments from student teachers provide insights for contemplation, not only for prospective student teachers but for school and university supervisors as well.

The thought that occupied my mind as I drove home after my first day of being a student teacher, was, "How will I ever make it?" How am I going to remember everything I need to know about all of the disorders? How will I write so many reports? I foresaw weeks ahead of writing lesson plans and thinking up activities. And now, here I am fifteen weeks later. I can look back to that first day and laugh when I think of how my ideas have changed. It doesn't seem possible that I could have experienced all that I did. My student teaching was in all aspects a total learning situation.

Student teaching has been a great experience and has been more of a benefit, not only from the professional point of view, but also from the personal point of view, than I ever imagined it would be. There has been a lot of hard work and a lot of time invested, but the satisfaction, rewards, and learning that this has created has made it all worthwhile.

I suddenly realized that I didn't need to be unsure, for I could handle the situations that I feared, adequately and surprisingly well.

I feel much more confident being out in the schools since I am no longer regarded as a "student." When the teachers ask my opinion about various children, their confidence in me boosts my confidence in myself.

I feel the most important lessons I learned from my student teaching experience were learned through my own mistakes. I had a very excellent school supervisor who allowed me to experiment and try new things on my own. When I failed, I learned a great deal. Instead of telling me my ideas were inappropriate, she allowed me to find out for myself through my own mistakes.

As a student teacher I have grown to understand the daily routine, unexpected problems and hassles a school clinician must go through and accept. I have also experienced the rewards an SLP gains when a child achieves progress and success. Being able to take over many of the responsibilities has opened my eyes and allowed me to see how fulfilling it is to be able to help children improve their communication skills.

One mistake I feel that I made at the beginning of student teaching was in failure to ask questions about everything that was going on around me. I don't know if I was afraid to ask them or if I didn't know which questions to ask but either way it was a mistake. I think I went in with the attitude that I was "supposed" to know everything. This is, of course, the wrong attitude to have. The whole purpose of student teaching is to learn and what better way to learn than by asking questions?

My supervising clinician was very helpful when I asked questions. She gave me her professional opinions and/or referred me to other professional sources. Although she informed me of reasons why some therapy sessions were less successful, she did not fail to commend the progress she saw and my success in therapy.

Student teaching has shown me how a school can function, how to deal with faculty, staff and parents, and possible procedures to follow in making referrals and recommendations.

What is the purpose of student teaching in speech-language pathology and why is it a necessary and important part of the preparation of school SLPs? Student teaching provides hands-on experiences that are not available at the university clinic or other settings.

THE STUDENT TEACHING TRIAD

Basically, three persons are directly involved in the process of student teaching. The first is the student teacher who is doing his or her practicum in an off-campus school system; the second is the pathologist employed by the school system, who is directly responsible for the day-to-day supervision of the student intern; the third is the university supervisor.

Too often the roles and responsibilities of the various participants in the student teaching process are not clearly defined and these individuals are put in a situation of not knowing what is expected of them, what to do, or how to do it. Following is a list of the roles, qualifications, and responsibilities of the persons involved in the clinical practicum in the schools. This is by no means a complete list, and others may wish to add to it or delete from it (Neidecker, 1976).

I. Qualifications of the University Supervisor
   a. Shall have a master's degree in speech pathology and/or audiology.
   b. Shall have ASHA Certificate of Clinical Competence in speech-language pathology and/or audiology.
   c. Shall have had experience as a full-time public school pathologist for a minimum of three years.
   d. Shall be a competent speech-language pathologist.
   e. Shall have had experience in teaching on a university speech pathology and audiology staff.

f. Shall demonstrate ability in supervision techniques, evaluation methods, counseling, and in-service training.

g. Shall have knowledge of school administration; general and special education policies and laws; physical planning of speech-language and hearing facilities; the process of developing programs for children with speech, language, and hearing disabilities; available social and welfare agencies and services; and the practice and psychology of management techniques.

h. Shall be aware of the current issues facing educators and contemporary trends in education.

i. Shall have the following personal characteristics:
1. Shall be an effective communicator.
2. Shall be objective, flexible, and able to adapt to change.
3. Shall have the capacity for self-evaluation and the ability to profit from mistakes.

II. Responsibilities of the University Supervisor

a. Shall be responsible for establishing criteria in regard to the time when a student is ready for practicum in the public schools.

b. Shall be responsible, in part, for selection of the cooperating pathologist.

c. Shall assume that the university still has the ultimate responsibility for the student's practicum experience.

d. Shall be responsible for conducting in-service training for cooperating pathologists.

e. Shall act as consultant to the cooperating pathologist.
1. Shall provide time for conferences to keep the cooperating pathologist informed of the university program and policies.
2. Shall provide written materials concerning the university policies and procedures.
3. Shall provide information on the background of the student teacher, both general and specific.
4. Shall be able to provide a wide variety of resource materials, approaches, and techniques which are based on sound theory, successful therapy, or documented research.

f. Shall establish goals with the student teacher which are realistic and easily understandable.
1. Shall prepare informational material about the expectations of the student teacher and policies of the university regarding the school practicum.
2. Shall observe the student teacher during the practicum.
3. Shall confer with the student teacher each time a visit is made to the school.
4. Shall provide opportunity for the students to give feedback on their practicum experiences both during and after the practicum experience, either in writing or through conferences.

g. Shall promote communication between the university and the public school setting.

h. Shall act as mediator between the student teacher and school administration.

i. Shall act as mediator between the cooperating pathologist and the student teacher.

j. Shall participate in conferences with the student teacher and the cooperating pathologist individually and collectively.

k. Shall establish that the responsibility for the student teacher's practicum is shared equally by the university supervisor and the cooperating clinician, but that the daily supervision of the student is the responsibility of the cooperating pathologist.

l. Shall be able to demonstrate therapy for both the student and the cooperating pathologist during the therapy session.

m. Shall share with the cooperating clinician in making the final evaluation of the student teacher.

III. Qualifications of the Cooperating Clinician

    a. Shall have had at least three years experience in the public schools as a speech, language, and hearing pathologist.

    b. Shall have the appropriate credentials as a speech-language pathologist in the schools.

    c. Shall be recognized by colleagues as a competent professional person.

    d. Shall be willing to work with a student teacher.

IV. Responsibilities of the Cooperating Clinician to the Student Teacher

    a. Shall be responsible for the day-to-day supervision of the student teacher.

    b. Shall acquaint the student teacher with available materials and equipment for screening and diagnostic procedures.

    c. Shall acquaint the student teacher with materials available for therapy.

    d. Shall encourage the student teacher to create and develop his or her own materials.

    e. Shall supplement the student teacher's background information through reading lists and other references.

    f. Shall provide the student teacher with information regarding the school system in reference to school policy, location of schools, the community, dismissal and fire drill procedures, and other appropriate information.

    g. Shall provide the student teacher with opportunities to:

        1. Observe the cooperating pathologist doing therapy.

        2. Assist in screening and diagnostic programs.

        3. Plan for and evaluate therapy sessions.

        4. Visit classrooms where children with speech, hearing, and language impairments are enrolled.

        5. Meet other school personnel informally and also confer with them about specific children.

        6. Write progress reports, case history reports, letters, therapy logs, and individual educational programs.

        7. Become familiar with the reporting, recording, filing and retrieval systems used by the cooperating pathologist.

    h. Shall provide feedback to the student teacher regarding strengths and weaknesses. The feedback shall be done on a regular basis and may take the form of verbal communication, written communication, tape recordings, video taping and/or demonstration therapy.

    i. Shall encourage the student teacher to develop behavioral objectives regarding him or herself and the children with whom he or she works.

    j. Shall encourage and assist the student teacher to utilize supportive personnel and aids when available.

    k. Shall encourage the student teacher to become increasingly independent in thinking and problem solving.

V. Responsibilities of the Cooperating Clinician to the University Supervisor

    a. Shall inform the university supervisor immediately of any problems that arise.

    b. Shall be aware of and assist the student teacher in fulfilling university requirements.

    c. Shall provide the university supervisor with feedback concerning the student teacher's progress.

VI. Qualifications of the Student Teacher

    a. Shall, after completion of practicum, be no more than one quarter or semester away from completing the degree program in speech-language pathology and/or audiology at an accredited university.

    b. Shall have completed the required clinical practicum.

    c. Shall have had observation experience in a school setting prior to school practicum.

    d. Shall demonstrate physical, mental, and emotional stability.

    e. Shall possess acceptable speech and language patterns and adequate hearing.

VII. Responsibilities of the Student Teacher

    a. Shall be aware of and adhere to the Code of Ethics of the American Speech-Language-Hearing Association.

    b. Shall be aware of and carry out the university requirements during school practicum.

    c. Shall adhere to the policies and practices of the school to which assigned.

    d. Shall comply with the directives of the cooperating pathologist as to working in the school therapy program.

    e. Shall expect to be treated as a professional person and act accordingly.

    f. Shall demonstrate ability to be dependable and assume responsibility while realizing that the cooperating clinician is legally responsible for the children being treated.

    g. Shall contribute to the fullest extent to the school therapy program based on academic background and university clinical practice.

    h. Shall demonstrate ability to establish and maintain appropriate interpersonal relationships with school personnel.

    i. Shall demonstrate ability to establish and maintain appropriate rapport with children.

    j. Shall demonstrate ability to evaluate self in therapy and a willingness to accept and utilize constructive criticism.

    k. Shall be aware of the criteria for evaluating the practicum experience.

    l. Shall recognize status as a learner and regard the practicum as a learning situation from which much is to be gained.

    m. Shall expect the practicum experience to assist in the development of skills enabling one to function as an independent professional person.

    n. Shall demonstrate interest in continued professional growth by making use of resource centers, attending in-service meetings, workshops, and professional meetings.

THE STUDENT TEACHING PROGRAM

Universities have many ways of carrying out the student teaching program in speech, language, and hearing. Obviously, there are many different patterns that are followed successfully depending on conditions and factors present in local areas and on the philosophy of the university concerned. There are, however, some commonalities that we will consider.

Schedules.   It is important that the student teacher submit a day-by-day schedule to the university supervisor. Because many school therapy programs are on intermittent program schedules, several centers may be involved in the student teacher's assignment. Important also is the obligation of the student teacher to keep the university supervisor informed of the hours he or she will be at the schools, as well as times when therapy may not be going on as a result of interruptions to the school's daily schedule.

Log of Clinical Clock Hours.   In addition to fulfilling the university's requirements for daily attendance, the student clinician must also consider the future possibility of verification of clinical clock hours for certification by the American Speech-Language-Hearing Association, licensing in various states, and certification by state departments of education. Most universities use a weekly reporting system, and the forms used to record this information vary. Besides the identifying information, the forms should include places to record the age range of the children; the various types of communication problems; and the amount of time actually spent in diagnosis, audiometric testing, screening, and group and individual therapy sessions. The student teacher and the cooperating pathologist should sign the completed form. A summary form may be filled out at the conclusion of student teaching.

Lesson Plans.   A daily written plan of intervention for each child with whom the student teacher works is a necessary tool of therapy. The plan should include both long- and short-range goals for each child, procedures, materials used, and evaluation of the therapy session. The evaluation is done by both the cooperating pathologist and the student teacher and may include the progress of each child, the effectiveness of the procedures and the materials used, and the effectiveness of the approach used by the student teacher. There is no one universally accepted form for a lesson plan, but most forms include the same basic elements.

Seminars.   It is common practice to hold seminars for the student teachers on a periodic basis. These seminars may be held weekly or less often, depending on the philosophy of the university. Frequently, the seminar time may be used for discussions and sharing of information and problems; speakers may be invited to discuss pertinent issues, panels may be utilized to familiarize student teachers with current information, demonstration therapy or diagnosis may be carried out, visits may be made to agencies or centers, and one seminar may be devoted to an explanation of school policies and practices. It is valuable for student teachers in speech, language, and hearing pathology to attend at least several seminars that include all student teachers in a school system.

Evaluations.   Assuming that self-evaluation and evaluation by supervisors is an ongoing procedure, it also may be useful to have a more formal type of written evaluation at the midpoint and at the conclusion of student teaching. The form used for these evaluative procedures should be in the hands of the student teachers during the first week of student teaching, or even prior to it, so that they know exactly what will be expected of them.

The midpoint evaluation should let the student teacher know his or her weak points, strengths, areas needing improvement, and how these improvements may occur. The student teacher then has the responsibility to act on the suggestions.

The final evaluation may be an evaluation of the student teacher during that experience, and it may also contain the perceived professional potential of that individual. It is important to differentiate between these two items. No student teacher emerges from the experience a "finished product," and this should be conveyed in the final evaluation report.

ASHA CERTIFICATION REQUIREMENTS

The American Speech-Language-Hearing Association has set standards in regard to the supervision of student clinicians on both the graduate and undergraduate levels. They have specified that in states where credential requirements and/or state licensure requirements differ from ASHA certification standards, the supervised clinical experiences, including student teaching, must be supervised by ASHA certified personnel (CCC) in order to satisfy ASHA requirements.

At this writing, in some states, there are discrepancies among state requirements, state licensure requirements, and ASHA certification requirements. Student teachers seeking ASHA certification should be aware of these discrepancies. The university supervisor with ASHA certification (CCC) is ethically bound to inform the student in student teaching and other clinical practice that the experience obtained under non-ASHA-certified personnel cannot be applied to ASHA certification (ASHA, 1991).

ADDITIONAL GUIDELINES FOR STUDENT TEACHERS

Student clinicians should know something about the community in which they are doing their teaching. Knowing the socioeconomic backgrounds of the families in the school districts helps student teachers to understand better the children with whom they will be working. This may be especially important for student teachers whose own backgrounds are different from those of their prospective clients.

There are additional requirements for student teaching that many university training centers have found productive and valuable in assisting student teachers to become full-fledged, competent professional persons. One is a checklist of experiences the prospective student teacher has had before the teaching experience. Such a checklist submitted to the cooperating pathologist is helpful in acquainting that person with the student teacher's capabilities. It might include information on any experience in child care such as baby-sitting or teaching church school; observational experience; clinical practicum experience; diagnostic experience; academic experience; and experience with tape recorders, audiometers, assistive listening devices, video tape machines, duplicating machines, and computers and augmentative devices.

Each university training center has developed its own requirements and often includes policies regarding the behavior of student teachers. The following partial list was adapted from the Student Teaching Handbook at Bowling Green State University (Weinberger, 1991).

A. Student teachers should not be used as substitute therapists nor should they be used to perform such activities as playground, cafeteria, or recess duties.

B. Dress and grooming of student teachers should be consistent with the standards of the schools to which they have been assigned.

C. Many school speech-language pathologists visit several schools during the course of their work week. Policies on transportation for student teachers among schools and to and from the school system should be clearly understood and adhered to prior to starting the student teaching assignment. Most student teachers provide their own transportation.

D. Outside activities such as jobs or coursework are discouraged during the student teaching experience. Student teaching is a full-time job and the stakes are high for a successful performance.

E. Under no circumstances should a student teacher administer corporal punishment to a child or serve as a witness.

F. Student teachers should not become involved in strikes, boycotts, work stoppages, or riots. In fact, it is not advisable for a student teacher to report for work should any of these things occur (Weinberger, 1991).

It goes without saying that student teachers should be well versed on the university's policies and keep in mind that during the student teaching or field experience they are guests of the school system.

COMPETENCY-BASED EVALUATION OF THE STUDENT TEACHER

Competency-based evaluation systems can be used to evaluate the student teaching experience. Glaser et al. (1998) developed a form comprised of competencies which was field-tested on student teachers and supervising clinicians (see Figure 11.1). The results indicated that the two groups favored the competency-based form to that of the traditional numerical form to evaluate knowledge, skill, and value objectives.

The procedures are as follows:

At the beginning of the semester, the university supervisor distributes the competency-based forms to both the supervising clinician (the public school speech-language pathologist to which the student is assigned in the schools) and the student teachers. The university supervisor meets with the supervising clinician and student teachers to discuss the use of the form. At this time, several aspects of the competency-based form are explained:

1. An explanation of a minimal competency is given. This is the minimal requirement that the student must meet by the end of the student teaching experience.

FIGURE 11.1   Miami University

COMPETENCY BASED OBJECTIVES FOR STUDENT TEACHING
IN SPEECH-LANGUAGE PATHOLOGY AND AUDIOLOGY

[ ] MIDTERM   [ ] FINAL

Student's Name: _____

Cooperating Therapist: _____

School District: _____

Semester: _____

Competencies student teachers will demonstrate by the end of student teaching:

RATING KEY:

C–Competent—Is proficient for level of training   NI–Needs improvement   NA–Not applicable

E–Emerging—Making appropriate progress   NE–Not showing effort

PROFESSIONALISM—DEMONSTRATES A PROFESSIONAL ATTITUDE AND WORK ETHIC BY:

C   E   NI   NE   NA   1. Effectively balancing work and personal responsibilities

C   E   NI   NE   NA   2. Attending professional meetings

C   E   NI   NE   NA   3. Exhibiting interest and enthusiasm about his/her work

C   E   NI   NE   NA   4. Interacting appropriately with cooperating therapist

C   E   NI   NE   NA   5. Arriving at school on time

C   E   NI   NE   NA   6. Regular attendance

C   E   NI   NE   NA   7. Showing initiative

C   E   NI   NE   NA   8. Being dependable

C   E   NI   NE   NA   9. Dressing appropriately

C   E   NI   NE   NA   10. Utilizing appropriate vocal quality, rate and intonation

LAWS AND STANDARDS

C   E   NI   NE   NA   1. Explain IDEA (Individual with Disabilities Education Act)

C   E   NI   NE   NA   2. Participate in Intervention Assistance Team (IAT)

C   E   NI   NE   NA   3. Participate in MFE/IEP Team/Annual Review

C   E   NI   NE   NA   4. Prepare Individualized Education Plans (IEP)

(continued)

FIGURE 11.1 Continued

LAWS AND STANDARDS

C	E	NI	NE	NA	5. Utilize diagnostic information to determine present levels of performance
C	E	NI	NE	NA	6. Utilize diagnostic information to determine annual goals
C	E	NI	NE	NA	7. Utilize diagnostic information to write measurable objectives

DAILY PLANNING PROCEDURES

C	E	NI	NE	NA	1. Write lesson plans in advance
C	E	NI	NE	NA	2. Write plans to meet IEP objectives for:
C	E	NI	NE	NA	■ individual/small group
C	E	NI	NE	NA	■ classroom
C	E	NI	NE	NA	3. Plan therapy that addresses multiple goals in a session
C	E	NI	NE	NA	4. Collaborate effectively with other school personnel
C	E	NI	NE	NA	5. Use information and evaluations from previous therapy sessions
C	E	NI	NE	NA	6. Utilize a variety of materials appropriate to client's interests, abilities, age level, and curriculum
C	E	NI	NE	NA	7. Manipulate equipment and materials before therapy sessions

DIAGNOSIS

C	E	NI	NE	NA	1. Informally assess the need for further testing
C	E	NI	NE	NA	2. Select appropriate diagnostic instruments and procedures
					3. Effectively complete:
C	E	NI	NE	NA	a. an oral-facial examination
C	E	NI	NE	NA	b. diagnostic tests for articulation/phonology
C	E	NI	NE	NA	c. diagnostic tests for language
C	E	NI	NE	NA	d. a spontaneous language sample analysis
C	E	NI	NE	NA	e. a diagnostic assessment for voice
C	E	NI	NE	NA	f. a diagnostic assessment for fluency

FIGURE 11.1 Continued

C	E	NI	NE	NA	g. hearing screening/thresholds
C	E	NI	NE	NA	h. classroom observation/teacher consultation
C	E	NI	NE	NA	i. a parent checklist or interview
C	E	NI	NE	NA	j. other _____
					4. Interpret and communicate diagnostic results:
C	E	NI	NE	NA	▪ verbal
C	E	Ni	NE	NA	▪ written

SCHEDULING

C	E	NI	NE	NA	1. Select caseload based upon eligibility criteria established by school district
C	E	NI	NE	NA	2. Schedule therapy program in relation to total school schedule
C	E	NI	NE	NA	3. Communicate with parents and school personnel about therapy schedule

THERAPY

C	E	NI	NE	NA	1. Establish and maintain good rapport with client
C	E	NI	NE	NA	2. Provide the rationale for selection of specific therapy techniques
					3. Employ therapy procedures appropriate to child's:
C	E	NI	NE	NA	▪ age level
C	E	NI	NE	NA	▪ ability level
C	E	NI	NE	NA	▪ curriculum
					4. Give directions clearly to
C	E	NI	NE	NA	▪ individual/small group
C	E	NI	NE	NA	▪ classroom
					5. Handle child's behavior effectively in
C	E	NI	NE	NA	▪ individual/small group
C	E	NI	NE	NA	▪ classroom

(continued)

FIGURE 11.1   Continued

C	E	NI	NE	NA	6. Begin and end therapy on time
C	E	NI	NE	NA	7. Provide for carry-over to classroom and home
C	E	NI	NE	NA	8. Communicate goals, therapy techniques and progress to parents
C	E	NI	NE	NA	9. Communicate goals, therapy techniques and progress to teacher

ARTICULATION THERAPY

C	E	NI	NE	NA	1. Conduct articulation/phonology therapy techniques appropriate to child's needs.
C	E	NI	NE	NA	2. Conduct therapy consistent with goals
C	E	NI	NE	NA	3. Discriminate correct/incorrect sound production with 85 percent agreement with cooperating therapist
C	E	NI	NE	NA	4. Provide appropriate type and level of cue
C	E	NI	NE	NA	5. Implement oral-motor exercises
C	E	NI	NE	NA	6. Obtain maximum number of responses per therapy session
C	E	NI	NE	NA	7. Provide appropriate reinforcement
C	E	NI	NE	NA	8. Be flexible in therapy situations
C	E	NI	NE	NA	9. Evaluate the pupil's performance with respect to moving on to the next therapy step
C	E	NI	NE	NA	10. Record progress on a consistent basis for a specific goal

LANGUAGE THERAPY

C	E	NI	NE	NA	1. Conduct language therapy techniques appropriate to child's needs
C	E	NI	NE	NA	2. Recognize correct/incorrect language productions with 85 percent agreement with the cooperating therapist
C	E	NI	NE	NA	3. Provide appropriate level of models and prompts
C	E	NI	NE	NA	4. Obtain appropriate number of responses per therapy session
C	E	NI	NE	NA	5. Utilize a variety of appropriate activities
C	E	NI	NE	NA	6. Record progress on a consistent basis for a specific goal

FIGURE 11.1 Continued

FLUENCY THERAPY

C	E	NI	NE	NA	1. Provide information and consultation to teachers and parents
C	E	NI	NE	NA	2. Conduct fluency therapy appropriate to child's needs
C	E	NI	NE	NA	3. Be flexible in therapy situations
C	E	NI	NE	NA	4. Record progress on a consistent basis for a specific goal

---

VOICE THERAPY

C	E	NI	NE	NA	1. Conduct appropriate therapy techniques
C	E	NI	NE	NA	2. Conduct therapy consistent with goals
C	E	NI	NE	NA	3. Counsel pupils/parents /teacher about vocal hygiene
C	E	NI	NE	NA	4. Discriminate appropriate voice production
C	E	NI	NE	NA	5. Be flexible in therapy situations
C	E	NI	NE	NA	6. Provide appropriate reinforcement
C	E	NI	NE	NA	7. Provide student with self-evaluation and self-management techniques for appropriate vocal behavior
C	E	NI	NE	NA	8. Explain the steps of making a medical referral
C	E	NI	NE	NA	9. Record progress on consistent basis on a specific goal

---

SELF-EVALUATION

C	E	NI	NE	NA	1. Evaluate therapy through audio/videotapes or reflective journals
C	E	NI	NE	NA	2. Follow through on suggestions from the cooperating therapist
C	E	NI	NE	NA	3. Set personal objectives for change as a result of self-evaluation

---

AUGMENTATIVE/ALTERNATIVE COMMUNICATION SYSTEMS

C	E	NI	NE	NA	1. Identify a variety of systems (sign, communication board, electronic devices hearing aids, and so on.)
C	E	NI	NE	NA	2. Collaborate with students, peers, teachers/family in order to select vocabulary

(continued)

FIGURE 11.1 Continued

C	E	NI	NE	NA	3. Prepare and/or program systems appropriate to child's level of functioning
C	E	NI	NE	NA	4. Train student, teacher, family in use of communication systems

FEEDING/ORAL MOTOR THERAPY

C	E	NI	NE	NA	1. Collaborate with support personnel on diagnostic results and intervention strategies
C	E	NI	NE	NA	2. Implement strategies (positioning, textures, cues, and safety precautions)
C	E	NI	NE	NA	3. Implement oral motor exercises
C	E	NI	NE	NA	4. Record progress and adopt plans as needed

OBSERVATION

C	E	NI	NE	NA	1. Gain knowledge about a range of disabilities by working with or observing students with a variety of speech/language disorders.
C	E	NI	NE	NA	2. Gain knowledge about a range of related professions by working with or observing professionals in related fields

COMMENTS

Glaser, Ann Johnson; Prudhomme, Marie; Rogero, Elaine (1998). "Competency-Based Objectives for Student Teaching in Speech-Language-Pathology & Audiology." Miami University. Institute for Speech Pathology.

2. Several practice and skill areas are evaluated including: professionalism, knowledge of laws and standards, daily planning procedures, diagnostics, scheduling, therapy procedures, implementation of articulation, language, voice, and fluency therapy, self evaluation, augmentative/alternative communication systems, feeding/oral motor therapy, and skill at observing.
3. The student's performance is determined to be "competent," "needs improvement," "emerging," "not showing effort," or "not applicable." A competency is achieved if the student demonstrates a skill with acceptable accuracy by the end of the term.
4. At midterm, the supervising clinician reviews the evaluation form with the student teacher and discusses the student's strengths and weaknesses in various areas.
5. At the end of the term, the supervising clinician completes the competency-based objective evaluation form and discusses the results with the student again.

In conjunction with the competency-based objectives form, a traditional numerical rating form was used at both midterm and at the end of the semester. The numerical form, which utilized a scale from 1 to 7, rates the same skills evaluated on the competency-based form with the exception of those skills that could not be rated on a 1–7 basis, that is, the entire laws and standard section.

GUIDELINES FOR THE COOPERATING CLINICIAN

In a chapter dealing with student teaching it is appropriate to include information useful to the person who plans and directs the student internship. That person is the cooperating clinician in the schools.

An article by Hess (1976) contains many excellent suggestions. According to Hess,

It is vital for the cooperating clinician working with a student clinician to realize the importance of student teaching. The student deserves the chance to be involved in a worthwhile program, and it will be worthwhile if he or she is met with leadership, an opportunity for growth, and a well-planned program.

Hess discusses the responsibilities of the cooperating clinician in the first week of student teaching. They are:

1. Communicate with the student clinician before the first week, by telephone call or letter, or an invitation to visit the school ahead of time.
2. On the first day provide orientation for the student by having a meeting between the program director, other school pathologists, and student teachers to discuss school policies, complete necessary forms, map out routes to the schools, and generally to minimize anxieties. He or she could also be informed of time schedules of the various schools, as well as the school calendar.
3. During the first week the student teacher should be given a tour of the school buildings and should be introduced to the principal and secretary of each building to which he or she has been assigned, as well as to the teachers, school counselor, nurse, and psychologist.
4. The cooperating pathologist should prepare the children enrolled in therapy for the arrival of the student teacher in such a way that they understand that person's role in relation to them.
5. The cooperating pathologist and the student teacher should discuss the university's materials, requirements, and suggestions so they are mutually understood.
6. The major goals for the student teaching program, as well as assignments and weekly goals, should be discussed. The cooperating pathologist should discuss what is expected of the student teacher and encourage the student to express his or her own expectations.
7. The student teacher should be made aware of rules, regulations, and policies of individual schools, the school system as a whole, and of the speech-language and hearing program in the state.

8. The first week of student teaching should include the opportunity to observe therapy sessions and to become acquainted with the children. During the first week the student teacher may assist with segments of the therapy sessions.

9. If the student teacher is assigned at the beginning of the school year he or she may assist in the screening programs.

According to Hess, the assigned weeks of student teaching should be utilized effectively and efficiently, but the student teacher should not be overloaded.

There are numerous school activities the student clinician can take part in during the weeks of student teaching. It is important for the cooperating clinician to have a list of priorities or activities that seem most valuable for the student. The list can be compiled from various sources: university information, other clinicians, published articles, and discussions with the student clinician. The student should have the opportunity to take part in as many phases as possible of the school therapy program. Besides learning to organize and carry out a therapy program, the student clinician will want to become familiar with related activities. For instance, it is helpful for the student to attend meetings of the clinicians as well as those meetings held in the individual schools.

The cooperating clinician should discuss with the student clinician how to begin and how to terminate the school year. The clinician will want to include the student in obtaining referrals for therapy and in conferences with teachers and parents. Furthermore, the cooperating clinician can discuss with the student clinician bulletin board ideas, newsletters for parents, parent conferences, and special therapy ideas that have proved successful. The student should learn to use the computer and any other office equipment that is applicable to the therapy program. Also the student clinician will want to have information about the many sources of therapy materials.

A WORD OF ADVICE TO STUDENT TEACHERS

Are you ready to start your student teaching? Here are some suggestions that might be helpful:

1. Work in harmony with your cooperating pathologist and university supervisor. Their job is to help you become a better speech-language pathologist and/or audiologist.

2. Be enthusiastic about your work and sincerely interested in the children with whom you will be working.

3. Keep healthy; get plenty of rest and eat the right foods.

4. Take advantage of every opportunity to become involved in the unique experiences a school has to offer.

5. Ask questions when you aren't sure, and ask questions even if you *are* sure.

6. Know what you can expect of children at various age and ability levels.

7. Be firm, fair, consistent, and compassionate in all your dealings with children. Every human being deserves respect.

8. Know the ground rules of the various schools and adhere to them.

9. When making professional decisions always ask yourself, "Is this in the best interests of the child?"
10. Enjoy your student teaching experience!

DISCUSSION QUESTIONS AND PROJECTS

1. Interview a current student teacher on his or her suggestions to beginning student teachers.

2. Invite a principal to talk to your class on what he or she expects of the student teacher.

3. What is the student teacher's role when a child must be punished for misbehavior?

4. What is the student teacher's role in relation to children in therapy? Defend your choice.
   a. A buddy
   b. Parental figure
   c. "One of the gang"
   d. Authority figure
   e. Permissive big brother or big sister
   f. Teacher
   g. Counselor
   h. One who "lays down the law"
   i. Referee

5. What do you hope to learn from student teaching?

6. Interview a school SLP on what he or she expects from a student teacher.

7. Ask a first-, second-, or third-grade child what he or she likes best about a favorite teacher. Ask a junior high and high school student the same question. Did you find any differences or similarities in their answers?

CHAPTER TWELVE

LIFE AFTER COLLEGE

Changes in the field of speech-language pathology are occurring rapidly. As Heraclitus once said, one may not step in the same river twice, not only because the river flows and changes, but also because the one who steps into it changes, too, and is never at any two moments identical.

What does this mean to you as a beginning SLP? And more specifically, what does it mean to those of you who will be employed in education? First, it means that this is an incredibly interesting time to be alive and working in the field of communications and education. You will need to be knowledgeable and involved in the world, not only the world of the therapy room and the classroom, but also the community beyond.

In this chapter we will look at some of the ways you will be able to keep abreast of current information through professional reading and continuing education programs. Your role as a researcher will also be examined. Collective bargaining and the school SLP is an issue of importance to you. We will also look at ways you may provide interviewers and prospective employers with information about your skills, knowledge, and attitudes in order to enhance your employment opportunities.

The importance of being familiar with state and federal laws is discussed. Due process procedures in the light of malpractice claims are described, and liability insurance is explained.

There *is* life after college. Welcome to a very interesting, challenging, and important profession. Be your best self and do your very best.

PROFESSIONAL PUBLICATIONS AND RESOURCES

As the role of the school SLP expands, there is a need to keep abreast of current information. This is particularly crucial for school clinicians working in remote areas or in areas where access to academic institutions, medical centers, or even libraries may be limited. There is no need to worry if these institutions are not near your home. Thankfully, we can connect with the top resources in the world through the Internet.

Throughout the United States, regional resource centers have established a statewide network system with regional centers that have among their services the collecting and distributing of special education materials as well as providing information about the materials. They also help school personnel create new materials when commercially produced products are not available. Announcements of services and materials available are made through newsletters and other forms of publication.

National and state associations publish professional journals that discuss state-of-the-art research and intervention. Each of the special interest divisions of ASHA maintains an E-mail listserv, offers continuing education opportunities, and publishes newsletters. It is difficult to keep up with all the written communication that crosses our desks. One possible way of accomplishing this daunting task is to schedule time for reading professional materials each week.

Public and university libraries have an interlibrary loan service whereby library materials are made available by one library to another for use by an individual. In addition to books, materials may include audiotape, videotape, film, and computer disks. The community public library can be of great assistance to the school clinician, and librarians are always helpful in obtaining materials. The school clinician may want to visit the library and find out what kinds of services are available.

The Internet provides access from your home or office to information from throughout the world 24 hours a day. Surfing the net can connect you to leading experts who specialize in diagnosis and treatment of communication disorders. Through listservs, chat rooms, and discussion groups you can pose complex questions and obtain answers from fellow SLPs. You can obtain research findings, intervention protocols, and clinical resources. Technology continues to change the way we learn and do business.

CONTINUING EDUCATION

Another way in which the SLP keeps up to date on professional matters is through continuing education in the form of workshops, short courses, seminars, miniseminars, in-service training courses, professional meetings highlighted by competent speakers, university courses, teleconferences, televised courses, and satellite or videotape presentations. Continuing education can be carried on in a structured program or on a more informal basis. Learning must be a lifelong process for an individual expecting to remain accountable and qualified. It is a process by which one keeps one's skills and knowledge up to date.

Continuing education is valuable to practitioners and to clinicians who have temporarily stepped out of their professional lives and wish to reenter at a later date. Continuing education is not the responsibility of any one institution or agency but should represent the coordinated efforts of a number of groups. Universities cannot offer courses in a geographical area unless there is an expressed need concerning the content area of such a course. For the university to plan for such courses, the need should be expressed to the university staff by the school clinicians. By the same token, universities should be willing to offer courses at a time that would be convenient to the school clinicians and in a location that would be accessible to them. Advances in technology have enabled universities and school systems to form partnerships to deliver advanced education via the web, television, videotapes or other forms of distribution. Many states have formed collaborative projects to enable school practitioners to get their master's degrees while still working full-time. The education "anywhere, anytime" concept has been very beneficial for that group of professionals.

Members and nonmembers of the American Speech-Language-Hearing Association who are holders of the Certificate of Clinical Competence may apply for an award called the ACE (Award for Continuing Education). Credits are earned through continuing education activities under ASHA-approved sponsors. A specific number of CE units are awarded to the participant for each instructional activity, and a national CE registry is maintained. Upon the completion of the required number of units, the ACE is awarded.

RESEARCH

It is doubtful that anyone would argue against the need for research about public school speech-language pathology programs. Neither is there any question that the public school is a fertile field for research in communication disorders. To add further emphasis, federal legislation has created pressure to find answers to questions about prevalence of speech-language disorders; impact on learning; treatment outcomes; comparison of delivery systems; efficacy of therapeutic methods; qualifications for service delivery; and other important issues.

Schools are unquestionably a fertile field for research. Unfortunately, school-based clinicians have produced little research in the past. There are a number of possible reasons given by school clinicians. Among them are lack of time, lack of funding, lack of support by school boards, lack of cooperation by university staff members, and lack of interest by journal publishers. The fear of performing statistical analyses, the lack of training in research methods, and the lack of rewards have also been suggested as reasons for the lack of research in the schools. Another reason may be that SLPs are simply more interested in being clinicians than researchers. This is understandable in light of their employment setting. On the other hand, school clinicians eagerly read journals and attend professional meetings in the hope of finding answers to questions.

A profession must be based on a body of knowledge, and this body of knowledge is accumulated by research. There must be interested individuals to pose questions and interested individuals to seek answers and solutions. Collaboration by researchers in universities, specialists in departments of education and special education on both the state and federal levels, and school SLPs is one of the best methods for generating research on the public school level.

Public schools provide a good base for research projects, and university personnel are a good source of information for consultation on research design.

Research projects that employ a single-subject design are especially appropriate for school SLPs. So is research on treatment outcomes, program management, and the relationship of communication disorders to learning. The clinician can carry out most types of research without schedule disruption and without ethical constraints on using school-age clients for research. School administrators should be advised and parents should be informed and must give their consent if the student is to be considered a "human subject" in the research project.

Longitudinal studies, in which a single subject or a group of subjects are followed for months or even years, are ideally suited for public school researchers in speech-language pathology. Examples of this type of study can be readily found in journals such as *Language, Speech and Hearing Services in the Schools* and the journal published by the National Students in Speech, Language, Hearing Association (NSSHLA).

The school clinician of the future will undoubtedly be involved in research on the local level, the state level, or as part of a national research project. The questions are everywhere, and the need to find answers is urgent. The questions of the school clinician in Mississippi may be the same ones asked by the clinician in Montana. Not only is the search for answers important, but also equally important is the need to exchange professional information.

COLLECTIVE BARGAINING AND THE SCHOOL SPEECH-LANGUAGE PATHOLOGIST

In school districts where there is a teachers union and collective bargaining, speech-language pathologists must determine in advance what will be their role and response during negotiations or strikes. Collective bargaining has a long history in the private sector and since 1962, when New York City teachers negotiated a collective bargaining agreement, it has become a significant factor in American education. Collective bargaining is an outgrowth of the desire to have a fair discussion in such issues as salary, fringe benefits, and working conditions.

Whether the American Federation of Teachers and the National Education Association call themselves labor unions or professional organizations is a moot point. If they bargain collectively with management they are functionally labor unions. The American Speech-Language-Hearing Association and the various state speech, language, and hearing associations are professional organizations because they do not negotiate salaries, contracts, and fringe benefits.

Many, but not all, states have collective bargaining laws and the laws differ from state to state. Your state labor relations board can give you information on your state's collective bargaining law. Whether you, as a speech-language pathologist, are considered management or labor will depend on your state's collective bargaining law. If your state classifies you as management, during a strike you may be called on to staff a classroom. If you are classified as labor, it is important to become involved in and work with the union or unit at the local level to make sure the issues and concerns important to you are brought to the bargaining table.

The decision of whether or not to affiliate with a local collective bargaining unit depends on the local situation. If you belong to the local unit of either AFT or NEA you must also belong to the state and national organization. Even if you choose not to join the locally designated unit, the law requires the unit to bargain for you regardless.

School speech-language pathologists are at a disadvantage primarily because they comprise a very small percentage of persons covered by the bargaining unit. During negotiations when concessions are made it would be easier for a unit to give up a demand affecting the few speech-language pathologists in favor of a demand affecting all the classroom teachers.

According to Dublinske (1986): It appears that speech-language pathologists can have the most impact in the collective bargaining process if:

- ASHA works with the NEA and AFT at the national level to make them aware of the general needs related to the working conditions of speech-language pathologists and audiologists employed in the schools

- State speech-language-hearing associations work with the NEA and AFT affiliates at the state level to make them aware of specific state needs and to work on state legislation that will improve working conditions
- Individual speech-language pathologists and audiologists get involved in the collective bargaining process at the local level

If speech-language pathologists and audiologists are going to be able to use the collective bargaining process to improve their working conditions it is important to become knowledgeable about their state's collective bargaining law and how negotiations are handled locally.

SLPs in the Broward County School District in Ft. Lauderdale, Florida worked through their union to bring their concerns about high caseloads to the superintendent's attention. Their actions resulted in changes in school organization and funding for SLP programs.

The bargaining unit can also be a good vehicle for informing colleagues about speech-language and hearing services that members should consider in their healthcare plans that are offered to employees. For example, you can be a good advocate for your profession by petitioning for coverage for hearing aids, therapy services after stroke, and services for children with developmental disabilities.

YOU AND THE LAW

Free and appropriate education for all children with disabilities has been mandated by federal legislation since 1976. The laws also described procedures for parents and other parties to appeal when they believe it is not being provided. The 1986 Public Law 99-372 provided for the recovery of attorney's fees when the parents prevailed. This legislation opened the door for the possible increase in the number of appeals generated. Due process hearings are the proceedings between the school and the family, presided over by a presumably impartial hearing officer. Often, prior to the due process hearing, the school district attempts to amicably resolve the misunderstandings.

How can the school SLP prepare for a due process hearing? A checklist of activities was compiled by staff members of the Montgomery County Public Schools, Rockville, Maryland (Clausen, Gould, Corley-Keith, Lebowitz, 1988). These activities include the following:

1. *Case Background.* Review student school files; review speech/language file, note the reason for referral; consult with pertinent staff (teachers, therapist, and others); compile a chronology of significant dates and events.
2. *Individual Education Program (IEP).* Check inclusion of and be familiar with: disability codes; model of service recommended and intensity of program; evaluative instruments, including validity and norms; data reported; strengths and needs; goals and objectives related to needs; mastery criteria; committee members, parent's presence; other special education services.
3. *Program Implementation.* Review therapy logs and note attendance, group composition, techniques and materials, and progress; review observations of student in educational program; note parent contacts, frequency, and content.

4. *Testimony.* Be prepared to summarize your credentials, educational background, and experience; discuss your knowledge of the case; discuss evaluative finds and the basis for recommendations; describe test characteristics, validity and normative data; discuss the program in relation to student needs; describe progress and how measured.

Some behavioral do's and dont's were also recommended. They suggested maintaining professionalism and formality at all times, taking notes on any points you hear that may help your case presenter, and stopping testimony until the question is resolved if there is an objection from either side. They also advise not to panic if you are placed under oath and not to talk except when testifying. Conversing with the hearing officer and discussing hearing issues with the opposing side during breaks should not occur.

Malpractice claims are a continuing risk for speech-language professionals. There are preventive measures such as maintaining good client relationships, careful documentation of therapy procedures, and knowledge of current state and federal regulations. But the best guide to avoiding malpractice claims is strict adherence to the American Speech-Language-Hearing Association's Code of Ethics (see Chapter 2.) The Code of Ethics not only serves as a model of behavior for you, as a professional person, but it also protects the consumer (in this case, the student) against dangerous practices of inexpert and injudicious individuals.

As a school speech-language pathologist, you may be the subject of a claim in a malpractice suit but you are much more likely to be called as an "expert witness" in a trial. An expert witness does not have direct knowledge of the case at hand but by virtue of education, research, or experience is qualified to testify.

YOUR ROLES AS AN ADVOCATE

As noted throughout the book, state and federal legislation greatly impacts the delivery of services to individuals who have communication impairments. This cannot be taken lightly. The laws affect the qualifications you need to do your job, the environment in which you work, the salary you earn, the students you see, and the service delivery options you can offer. This translates to a very important need to get involved in the political process through grassroots political advocacy. You can make an important contribution by talking with your legislative representatives about your profession and the people you serve.

Meeting with state or national legislators can seem like a frightening experience; but only for the first time. Once you have done it you will soon realize that they want to hear from you. They are interested in what you have to say. And they will listen to your message. After all, you have the power to vote them into or out of office.

ASHA and many state professional organizations have developed simple procedures to help you understand the process and feel comfortable in your role as an advocate for the communication sciences and disorders profession and for individuals with communication disabilities. Following is a summary of several steps ASHA recommends for making working with your legislators.

Lay the Groundwork. First identify whom your local, state, and national legislators are. You can obtain this information by reading the newspaper, contacting your Board of Elections, or checking the government websites. ASHA's website links to the congressional directory which lists the representatives for all states <http://congress.nw.dc.us/asha>.

Once you have identified the elected officials you want to contact, learn as much about them as possible including their political party, voting record on key issues, legislative committees, personal facts, and profession.

Contact Your Representative or Senator.   First decide if you can visit or if you simply want to write to your lawmaker. If you want to visit, make arrangements to do so. You can call for an appointment by contacting the U.S. Capitol Switchboard. Be ready to state the intended purpose of your visit in one or two brief statements. Select only one or two priority issues. ASHA or your state association will be able to suggest timely issues.

Most likely you'll be visiting with the legislator's congressional aide who is assigned to health or education issues. That individual will in turn communicate your message and opinion for the representative or senator. You may be surprised to see that the staffer is not much older than you and your fellow students. He or she is most likely working in the office as an intern trying to learn the political process.

If the legislator or aide cannot see you, ask the receptionist if you may stop by the office to drop off materials. This is generally acceptable.

Prepare for Your Meeting.   If your organization offers the opportunity, attend a briefing session to learn the key issues that legislators are dealing with at the time. Learn to discuss the issue and be familiar with how it affects the students you serve or you. Take written materials with you when you visit. It you are visiting with a group of colleagues, decide in advance who will act at the spokesperson. When it is time for the visit, be punctual and to the point.

Present Your Issues.   Make your issue clear. What is it you want the lawmakers to do? Do you want them to vote on a particular bill or sponsor a specific law? Then let them know that is what you are asking. Concentrate on only one or two issues. Be sure to listen to the lawmaker's opinion even if you disagree. Some examples of issues that professionals have brought to their legislators lately include: infant hearing screening, funding cutbacks, capping services to Medicare patients, and the like. If you are asked a question you can't answer, don't be embarrassed. Find the answer and phone or mail it to the person who asked it.

Follow Your Visit With a Thank-You.   Be sure to let the lawmaker and his or her aide know that you appreciate the time they allotted for your visit. Reemphasize your key points. Offer to provide additional information if they need it.

Go Political.   If you really enjoy the political arena, consider expanding your activities to contact more legislators or serve on a grassroots committee. If you really like the environment, consider running for office. Local, state, and national governments need individuals who are committed to important causes.

PROFESSIONAL LIABILITY INSURANCE

As the school speech-language clinician's caseload and role expands to include a wide variety of communication disorders and intervention tasks, the possibility of situations occurring for which the clinician may be held liable is increased. Though this may be a sad commentary on the state of our world today, it is nevertheless a reality. The school-based SLP and other educators are treating youngsters with complex disabilities such as dysphagia, traumatic brain injury, and severe emotional disorders. The increased complexity leads to increased risk because the intervention treatment may be more invasive or involve physical contact. Thus, it is important to maintain professional liability insurance in case such an event should occur. The decision to be covered by liability insurance as a protective measure is a purely personal one. It is also dependent upon the kind of working situation you are in. Check with your local school system to see if there is coverage through an educational agency. Another source of information is ASHA or your state speech-language-hearing association. Liability insurance for speech-language pathologists and audiologists would cover all professional activities but may not cover corporal punishment, transportation by private auto, and travel by aircraft or watercraft. Your personal insurance agent is also a source of information; you may already be covered under your own insurance plan.

Insurance for students is usually offered by universities at a nominal sum and is often treated the same as a course fee. It is incumbent upon the student to find out what is specifically covered. Student teachers may also be covered under their parent's insurance plans.

GETTING YOUR FIRST JOB

In this section of the chapter, we are indebted to Bowling Green State University, Bowling Green, Ohio, and to JoAnn Kroll, Director of Placement Services. This information is based on and has been adapted from the university's publication *Job Search: A Guide for Success in the Job Market*.

Where to Start

The job search for you, as a beginning SLP, may start any time during the last year of college. The best place to start is your university placement office. The service is available at most universities and is usually free to students and alumni. The first step in your job search will be to visit your university placement office to find out what specific services are available. Generally speaking, this is what they have to offer:

- Individual counseling
- Internet career search engines
- Vacancy listings
- Credential services
- On-campus interviews
- Placement seminars and guest speakers
- Resource center with information concerning employment strategies, career opportunities, alumni placement services, videotapes, and slide/sound presentations
- Mock interview training and critique sessions
- Staff referrals of qualified candidates

After you find out what services are available, which ones are applicable to you, and which ones you want to utilize, it is time to plan your strategy. Timing is important here.

You will want to visit the placement office after you have completed most of your academic work and clinical practice but before you start your student teaching.

The Credential File and Portfolio

School personnel administrators expect to see well-organized and up-to-date credential files on prospective SLPs. The credential file you accumulate must document your past achievements and support your candidacy for a position. It is important to begin early to complete the necessary forms required by your university's placement office and gather the appropriate letters of recommendation from faculty members and past employers. A complete credential file should include the following:

Letters of Recommendation.   Most university placement services (and school districts) use a standard reference form on which reference writers make statements regarding your professional or personal relationship and how long the writer has known you. There should be a description of your academic or career growth and potential, a review of your principal achievements, an estimate of future promise, a paragraph on your personal qualities, and a final summary paragraph. If you intend to use someone's name as a reference it is always necessary to request that person's permission in advance. The reference letter may be sent directly to the university placement office or to you. If it is sent to the placement office it is desirable to request a copy for your records. Always enclose self-addressed stamped envelopes. Some persons who provide references may prefer not to send a copy. If this is what your reference indicates, you may want to probe the reason to be sure that it is not because they won't be providing a reference that is less than positive.

Professors are often asked to provide references for many students just prior to graduation. When asking for a reference, allow ample time for the person to fit the writing into their schedule. Otherwise the reference may not be compelling enough to help you get the job. Select your references carefully. Think of people who know you in different ways and can provide different perspectives about your skills and experiences. A good combination would be your academic advisor, a supervisor from your student teaching or extern site, and your summer employer.

Student Teaching Evaluation.   An evaluation is made by the student teaching supervisors during the experience. This may also include the perceived professional potential of the student teacher in the final evaluation report.

Transcript of Grades.   This is obtained from the registrar of the university. Be sure you check to see if the district wants an "official" transcript. If so, you must request to have it sent out from the registrar's office.

Examples of Work.   One of the most successful "marketing tools" is the use of the student teaching portfolio. Your resume, samples of lesson plans, photographs of displays or bulletin boards, and statements verifying your participation in educational projects both before and during student teaching should be placed in the portfolio. Your student teaching supervisor can offer excellent recommendations concerning the content and layout of your portfolio.

Regardless of immediate or long-range plans, establishing a credential file at the university placement office is strongly advised for all students and alumni. Be sure you keep it up to date by informing the office of current professional addresses and positions and by periodically including letters of reference from employers.

The Interview

One of the keys to successful interviewing is advance preparation. It is also one of the best ways to combat nervousness during the interview. The beginning point of your preparation is to know yourself. Review your personal inventory and background thoroughly and always in light of the position you are seeking. Be prepared to answer questions regarding your education, grades, courses, jobs, extracurricular activities, goals, strengths, weaknesses, and other information. Keep in mind that the interviewer is wondering, "Why should I hire you?" In answering this question be prepared to give examples and illustrations of your abilities, skills, leadership, effectiveness, and potential.

Successful preparation for the interview also entails knowing the school system. Your placement office may be able to assist you. Other sources for general information include newspaper articles, the school district's website, school board minutes, parent teacher organizations, or your university education department. However, you should also be interested in learning about the speech-language pathology programs. You may obtain this information by contacting colleagues in the profession and by asking the interviewer questions. Pertinent questions would include the following: How many SLPs are presently on the school staff? How long has the program been in existence? What is the school population? How many buildings and grade levels do the speech-language pathologists in the district service? Will the clinician be assigned to a particular age or disability group of children? To whom is the speech-language clinician directly responsible?

Another important way to prepare for the interview is to practice. Role-play a mock interview with a friend, instructor, relative, fellow student, or a placement staff counselor. Pay especially close attention to questions that may deal with some weaknesses or problem areas in your background. Don't wait until you reach the interview to think about responding to a question concerning a weakness.

Another facet of interview preparation is appropriate dress. First impressions are often lasting impressions, and you must look as if you fit the role before an employer will let you act the role. How you dress is a statement about how you feel about the significance of the interview and whom you will be meeting. Careful attention to dress and grooming is a way of putting your best foot forward. When in doubt it is best to be conservative in your dress.

What can you expect the interviewer to be like? Because you really don't know in advance you will need to take your cues from the content of the interview. If the interviewer wants you to do most of the talking and wants to assess your ability to communicate and reason, this individual's style will be nondirective. If the interviewer is concerned with eliciting specific and precise responses, the style will be more formal and structured. Sometimes interviewers will create some stress to ascertain how the candidate will react. How you handle the interview is important. Avoid short responses, as they tell the interviewer little or nothing—or perhaps the wrong things—about you. Use this opportunity to capitalize on your assets. Use anecdotal information to demonstrate your strong points, for example, "During my spring vacation I helped the school clinician in my hometown with the preschool screening program. We screened over 500 children for speech, language, and hearing problems. She was pleased with my work and wrote a letter describing my contribution. The letter is in my portfolio and I would like to have you read it." This tells the interviewer not only that you were able to function well in a professional situation and that you have gained some experience but that you were also interested in improving your skills by spending your spring vacation doing so.

Be prepared for questions like these: What is your philosophy of education? How would you plan to work with the learning disabilities teacher? What do you think a speech, language, and hearing program can add to a school system?

Inappropriate behaviors elicit negative impressions during an interview. They include candidates who show up late, chew gum, smoke without permission, bring uninvited guests, have poor hygiene, are braggarts and liars, are overly aggressive or too shy, lack confidence and poise, fail to look the interviewer in the eye, show lack of interest and enthusiasm, and ask no questions or poor questions.

Follow-up on the interview is important. Write a thank-you letter, noting anything that was said that you want to reemphasize; thank the interviewer for the opportunity to discuss your mutual interests and clarify any questions or ambiguities from the meeting. If you are interested in this position restate your desire to work for this particular school system. If you are undecided, write a thank-you letter anyway.

The Resume

Another important tool is the resume, a written document that introduces your education, background, skills, and experience to the prospective employer. It is a document that is used not only for the first job but also for subsequent employment searches throughout your professional life. The resume, whether we like it or not, has become a cornerstone of the job-hunting process. Its worth is seldom questioned; its necessity is simply assumed. However, despite its importance as a marketing tool, many people express anxiety and frustration about preparing it.

A resume is neither an autobiography nor merely a listing of your employment history. When properly prepared, it is an advertisement that excites an employer's interest in a particular product—*you*. Because there are no absolutes in resume writing, you will ultimately decide how it looks and what it says. Its style, format, and length should be determined by your employment interests or target markets and your background and qualifications.

An effective resume can be prepared in different styles or formats and contain widely diverse information. Making the strongest presentation of your unique and individual qualifications will contribute to the kind of distinction that will set your resume apart from others. So although there are no absolute rules on what all resumes should contain—except who you are and how you can be contacted—the following general rules address issues of honesty, accuracy, neatness, grammar, layout, and content that should be carefully observed:

■ Do not exaggerate your accomplishments to give the impression that you have more experience than you actually do. Employers know the difference between a restaurant hostess and an executive vice president for customer relations.

- Be reasonably brief. You are writing a resume, not an autobiography. Tailor your information to fit the employer's needs.
- Be careful with your grammar and the design and layout of your resume. There is no excuse for sloppy writing and poor grammar.
- Be sure the font size and style are legible, not too small or too fancy.
- Do not include information that will work to your disadvantage. Negative or harmful information is best handled in a personal interview.
- Use strong action verbs to make your resume as impressive as possible. This is essential since employers will most often see your resume before they see you.
- Always present accurate information. Honesty really is the best policy.

A sample resume is provided for your review (Figure 12.1). It is designed to help you produce a document that strongly reflects your interests, qualifications, and potential. By itself, a resume cannot get you the job you want; yet without it, you most likely will not even get started.

Not all interviews result in a job offer. In some regions of the country the supply of SLPs exceeds the demand. The individual who is willing to be flexible about location has a much better chance of finding a job. ASHA publishes job openings routinely. And don't neglect the classified pages of the newspapers although these are unlikely to yield a great amount of information about positions in school systems. The newsletters of state speech, language, and hearing associations often list job openings in schools, and the state consultants in speech-language pathology know of job openings within that state. The names and addresses of the state consultants can be obtained by writing to the state department of public instruction, division of special education. They are located in or near states' capital cities. Information can be found in educational directories or on the state government webpages.

Begin now to build a network of persons who may be able to provide you with information concerning job possibilities. This will be valuable not only for your first job but also for subsequent job searches.

Discussing Salary and Benefits

Realizing that you will finally be earning a salary is perhaps one of the most exciting aspects of getting your first job. The salary discussion is a very difficult one for most individuals. If the information is not offered by the interviewer, the candidate often is perplexed about when and if the question of salary should be raised. Most employment consultants suggest waiting until the job is offered to you and you have discussed the expectations and responsibilities fully. It is at that time that the interviewer will generally make the offer and discuss the compensation. The salary in most school districts is linked to a candidate's degree or educational level and years of experience. In public education the information is available for review through public sources.

Be cautious; there is more to consider than money. Compensation includes salary, reimbursement for travel (mileage), and medical coverage. In some districts membership and licensure fees might be covered. Be sure to inquire about reimbursement for professional and continuing education. And of course, sick days and vacation days are also considered a part of the full compensation package.

FIGURE 12.1   Sample Resume

Marrisa Cheney

Current Address: Permanent Address:
302 Jackson Hall   179 Elm Street
Bowling Green State Univ.   Hudson, Ohio 44100
Bowling Green, Ohio 43403   (000) 000-0000
(000) 000-0000

PROFESSIONAL OBJECTIVE	This is really the most difficult section to write. Many people believe that listing a job objective on a resume is too limiting. However, if you have a clear objective that applies to many organizations, it is to your advantage to include it. You may also state your professional objective in your cover letter rather than on the resume. Include the job function desired and the type of organization. For example: Position as a speech-language pathologist in an inner-city, medium-size school system that will allow me to work with bicultural, speech, and language handicapped adolescents. Or: Position as a speech-language pathologist in a rural school system that will allow me to do diagnostic and remediation work with K–12 students, as well consultative and preventive work with preschoolers and their parents.
EDUCATION	List highest or most recent degree first. Include name of college(s), major(s) (minor optional), date(s) of graduation. Add any special emphasis in your studies, such as relevant courses or research projects. If your grade point average is noteworthy include it. College expenses earned can be included here.
EXPERIENCE AND WORK HISTORY	This is a summary of your work experience, highlighting your most recent or most relevant employment first. Include descriptions of your responsibilities, titles of positions held, names of companies or organizations, and dates you were employed. Summer employment, volunteer work, student teaching, and internships may be included. If you are a recent college graduate without experience, do not be concerned; you are in the majority. Stress the level of responsibility, achievement, and motivation you demonstrated in previous jobs. This section should be an active statement of what you *can* do. How you describe the experience is the key.
ACTIVITIES/ INTERESTS	Extracurricular involvement highlights your leadership skills, sociability, and energy level. Choose activities that support your professional objective by demonstrating your leadership or organizational skills. If you have many activities, select the ones in which you were most involved and describe your degree of responsibility. If you have limited activities, point out that you worked and include hours worked per week as well as the percentage of school expenses earned.
REFERENCES	It is not necessary to include names and addresses of references. If requested, these can be provided on a separate sheet or included on an application form. State either "Available upon request" or "Available upon request from (your university placement service address)."
OPTIONAL INFORMATION	This includes honors and awards, publications, professional association, research projects, study abroad, and personal information. It is illegal for an employer to solicit personal data (age, weight, height, marital status, number of children, or disability) unless a genuine occupational requirement exists. Include this information only if pertinent to the job you are seeking.

CAREER DECISIONS

Preparation for the profession of speech-language pathology is complex, yet rewarding. The coursework is difficult, there are multiple points along the way where you must demonstrate your capabilities such as on the national examination or comprehensive exams at the university. You must work long hours alone or on teams to prepare for clinic and student teaching. You should be very proud of your efforts on the journey.

Some students reach the end of the trail and can't wait to begin practicing. Others decide that the profession is not for them. They may feel frustrated and afraid to tell anyone, especially family members, professors, and student peers who have been supportive along the way. Some clinicians join the workforce and then decide their interests and talents lie elsewhere or they are not happy providing therapy on a day-to-day basis. All of these circumstances are normal. Life is too short to spend years dissatisfied with your work and where you are doing it.

Prior to accepting a job, have a talk with yourself. Decide if the position, responsibilities, caseload, location, people, duties, and culture are right for you. If the answer is no, feel comfortable exploring other opportunities. Your education and experiences have provided you with the tools and qualifications to do many things. Following is a list of representative options illustrating the careers that speech-language pathologists are qualified to pursue

- Develop, promote, copyedit, or sell products for use in the clinical, education, health care, or rehabilitation fields such as:
  - Clinical materials and equipment
  - Educational materials and resources
  - Assessment instruments and diagnostic tests
  - Augmentative communication devices
  - Voice recognition and production systems
  - Textbooks and reference books
  - Assistive listening devices
  - Intervention software
  - Accommodations for individuals with severe physical disabilities
- Contribute to the "Edutainment Industry"
  - Develop educational programming
  - Review or write scripts
  - Coach actors in dialogue, accents, communication mannerisms
- Work in related fields
  - Rehabilitation counseling
  - Job coaching
  - Academic advising
  - Clinical assistants and support staff
  - Clinical intake specialists
  - Technology support staff
  - Group home staff
  - Mentoring youth

- Assisting families of individuals with disabilities
- Scouting for individuals with disabilities
- Community outreach programs
- Employment search firms
- Consider a degree in a related field such as
  - Special education
  - General education
  - Early intervention
  - Vocational rehabilitation
  - Mental health
  - Public health
  - Medical fields
  - Education or health law
- Be creative—use your imagination!
  - Scan the want ads
  - Make suggestions to perspective employers

SETTING TIME ASIDE FOR YOURSELF

It is easy to get so absorbed in work and forget your own needs once you are no longer a student and begin to take on work, family, and financial responsibilities. Sometimes we forget to set aside time for ourselves. We don't appreciate the contributions we make. Reward yourself for your success and set aside time to reflect on the positive aspects of life or just have fun. Following are some ideas to get you started (adapted from a list that appeared in CEC Today, 1999).

- Take a class for fun
- Learn a new hobby
- Get together with a group of friends and go rollerskating or to a play
- Buy fresh flowers for several rooms in your home
- Pack a lunch and go with a friend to a park in a different city
- See a matinee performance of a musical or play at your local playhouse
- When you are visiting a new city for a conference, schedule a vacation day for sightseeing
- Rent a limousine with six friends for an evening of fine dining and entertainment
- Go out with coworkers and don't let anyone talk about work
- Keep a running list of funny things that have happened to you lately
- Visit the pet store
- See where $100.00 will take you
- Enjoy a spa day with a friend—get a massage and facial
- Learn a new sport; join a neighborhood team
- Sit by the fire and read a good book
- Volunteer for an organization of your choice
- Host a theme party
- Add 10 ideas to this list

BEST OF LUCK

We wish you the best of luck as you pursue your career path whether it be as a speech-language pathologist in the schools or another setting, as an administrator, as a professional in a related field, or as a parent. Continue to grow and learn and enjoy helping people with communication disorders to reach their full potential.

DISCUSSION QUESTIONS AND PROJECTS

1. Look on ASHA's website. Note the range of information available and the wide variety of topics listed. Read two position statements.

2. Find out which universities, organizations, or other facilities in your state are ASHA-approved sponsors of continuing education programs leading toward the ACE. Do you think continuing education should be mandatory?

3. Do you think it is feasible for school SLPs to conduct research studies? What is the rationale for your answer?

4. Using the resume format in this chapter, prepare your resume.

5. Discuss the benefits list with a teacher in a local school district. Determine the benefits offer in that district.

6. Start assembling your credential portfolio.

7. Write a brief statement of your philosophy of speech-language pathology service delivery. Discuss it with your classmates.

■ ■ ■ ■ ■

CLASSIFICATION OF PROCEDURES AND COMMUNICATION DISORDERS

SPEECH-LANGUAGE PATHOLOGY AND AUDIOLOGY DIAGNOSES

The disorders section is designed to provide codes for communication diagnoses established by speech-language pathologists and audiologists. These codes are consistent with ASHA definitions approved in 1981 (*Asha,* November 1982, p. 949). Whenever more than one disorder is ascribed to a communicatively impaired individual, all disorders should be reflected in a listing of codes for that individual. The auditory disorders classification does include the traditional "mixed" classification as well as a more specific combination disorders such as middle ear plus cochlear disorders.

The coding system permits entry of time of onset at the second integer to the right of the decimal: .___1 unknown time of onset; .___2 prelingual time of onset; .___ 3 postlingual time of onset; or .___4 not applicable (noting time of onset is not appropriate or necessary).

For example, a motor speech disorder-dysarthria (131.1) is coded as 131.11 for unknown time of onset, 131.12 for prelingual onset 131.13 for postlingual onset and 131.14 if time of onset is not applicable. A conductive hearing loss, right ear (230.1) is coded 230.11 for unknown time of onset, 230.12 for prelingual onset, 230.13 for postlingual onset, and 230.14 if time of onset is not applicable.

SPEECH-LANGUAGE PATHOLOGY AND AUDIOLOGY PROCEDURES

01.0 **Hearing Screening** A pass-fail procedure to identify individuals who require further hearing evaluation.

02.0 **Speech Screening** A procedure to identify individuals who require further speech evaluation.

03.0 **Language Screening** A procedure to identify individuals who require further language evaluation.

04.0 **Dysphagia Screening** A procedure to identify individuals who require specific assessment to determine the presence or absence of a swallowing disorder.

05.0   **Follow-Up Procedure**   A procedure needed to complete an assessment. May refer to repetition of a test, continuation of a previous evaluation, or procedure to establish validity of a previous test.

0.60   **Consultation**   A procedure to provide professional expertise which may include, but is not ligmited to: conferring with other professionals during case staffings and team conferences, or in individual communication, providing information to business and industry and public and private agencies; and engaging in program development or supervision activities. Expert testimony is also a form of consultation.

07.0   **Counseling**   A procedure to facilitate the client's recovery from or adjustment to a communication impairment. Specific purposes of counseling may be to provide the client and his or her family or significant others with information and support, make appropriate referrals to other professionals, and to help the client to develop problem-solving strategies to enhance the rehabilitation process.

08.0   **Aural Rehabilitation Assessment**   A procedure to assess the impact of hearing loss on communication which may include but is not limited to, speech reading, auditory training, and counseling.

09.0   **Aural Rehabilitation**   A procedure to improve the communicative abilities of a hearing impaired individual. This procedure may include but is not limited to, speech reading, auditory training, and counseling.

10.0   **Product Dispensing**   A procedure by which a prosthetic device (e.g., hearing aid, assistive listening device, and/or augmentative communication device) is prepared and dispensed.

11.0   **Product Repair/Modification**   A procedure to restore or adjust a product used to facilitate an individual's communication abilities.

AUDIOLOGIC PROCEDURES

20.0   **Basic Audiologic Assessment**   A procedure to determine the status of the peripheral auditory system. This procedure may include, but is not limited to, the following: case history, developmentally appropriate behavior tests, acoustic immittance tests, communication handicap inventories, speech-language screening, interpretation of audiometric test results, written report preparation, and counseling.

21.0   **Comprehensive Audiologic Assessment**   A procedure to determine the status of the auditory system that cannot be determined by basic audiologic assessment (20.0) and/or to establish the site of the auditory disorder. This procedure may include items contained in the basic assessment in addition to electrophysiologic measurements (e.g., auditory evoked potentials, electronystagmography, tests of auditory adaptation, specialized speech tests, tests for nonorganic hearing etiology, written report preparation, and counseling).

22.0   **Electrophysiologic Assessment**   A procedure to determine or monitor the status of a physiologic system(s), e.g., auditory evoked potentials, electronystagmography, electrocochleography.

23.0   **Hearing Aid Assessment**   A procedure to determine the appropriateness and design of individual amplification systems. This procedure may include, but is not limited to, assessment of an individual's performance with different hearing aids, assistive listening devices, and/or tinnitus management devices, cochlear implant management, and counseling.

24.0   Hearing Aid Fitting/Orientation   A procedure to assist an individual in achieving maximum understanding of, and performance with, their individualized amplification system. This procedure may include electracoustic performance evaluation of the system.

25.0   Occupational Hearing Conversation Service

    25.1   Environmental Acoustical Survey: A procedure to determine sound levels in settings where noise levels may be injurious to hearing or interfere with communication.

    25.2   Occupational Audiometric Threshold Test: A pure-tone air conduction threshold procedure to identify the presence or absence of a hearing loss.

    25.3   Audiogram Review: A procedure to determine change in hearing status and need for monitoring, follow-up, and/or referral.

26.0   Unlisted Audiologic Procedure   Any audiologic procedure which is not listed above. Describe by report.

SPEECH-LANGUAGE PATHOLOGY PROCEDURES

30.0   Specific Assessment   A procedure to assess a specific aspect of speech, voice, language systems, and/or oral and pharyngeal sensorimotor competencies. Includes case history, assessment, written report preparation, and patient/family conference. Specific assessment is appropriate when the patient has a preliminary diagnoses. The assessment is usually completed for purposes of consultation reevaluation.

    30.1   Language

    30.2   Speech Articulation

    30.3   Speech Rate, Rhythm, Fluency

    30.4   Voice

    30.5   Resonance

    30.6   Oral/Pharyngeal Dysfunction

    30.7   Cognitive/Communication

31.0   Comprehensive Assessment   A procedure for detailed analysis of speech, voice, language systems and/or oral and pharyngeal sensorimotor competencies; may include evaluation of comprehension and expression, structure and function, behavioral relationships, and adaptation. Includes initial interview and patient history, diagnostic procedure, patient/family conference, and written report preparation.

32.0   Prosthetic/Adaptive Device Assessment   A procedure to determine the appropriateness of augmentative communication systems and devices, oral or laryngeal prostheses, and artificial larynges.

33.0   Treatment   A procedure to apply intervention strategies that improve, alter, augment or compensate for comprehension, speech, voice, language, and pharyngeal sensorimotor competencies.

34.0   Speech-Language Instruction   A procedure to teach various communication strategies with the primary goal of providing assistance in academic subject areas.

35.0 Communication Instruction (Speech Enhancement) A procedure designed to improve the communication abilities of an individual who does not exhibit a disorder. Includes instruction in public speaking and elimination of foreign dialect.

36.0 Unlisted Speech-Language Procedure Any speech-language pathology procedure which is not listed above. Describe by report.

SPEECH, LANGUAGE, AND RELATED DIAGNOSES

100.0 Speech And Language Within Normal Limits
101.0 Communication Variation
    101.1 Language
    101.2 Speech
    101.3 Voice
    101.4 Rate, Rhythm, Fluency
111.0 Language Disorder
    111.1 Spoken Language Comprehension Disorder
        111.1 Phonologic
        111.2 Morphologic
        111.3 Syntactic
        111.4 Semantic
        111.5 Pragmatic
        111.6 Mixed or Undifferentiated
112.0 Spoken Language Production Disorder
    112.1 Phonologic
    112.2 Morphologic
    112.3 Syntactic
    112.4 Semantic
    112.5 Pragmatic
    112.6 Mixed or Undifferentiated
113.0 Written Language Comprehension Disorder (Reading)
114.0 Written Language Production Disorder (Writing)
115.0 Arithmetic-Calculation Disorder (Dyscalculia)
116.0 Nonspoken Communication Recognition Disorder
117.0 Nonspoken Communication Production Disorder
120.0 Cognitive/Communicative Disorder
130.0 Speech Articulation Disorder
131.0 Motor Speech Disorder
    131.1 Dysarthria
    131.2 Dyspraxia
    131.3 Dysarthria and Dyspraxia
132.0 Structurally-Based Speech Disorder
    132.1 Facial
    132.2 Labial
    132.3 Dental
    132.4 Mandibular

132.5 **Lingual**

132.6 **Palatal**

132.7 **Pharyngeal**

132.8 **Mixed**

133.0 **Developmental Articulation Disorder**

134.0 **Other Speech Disorder**

140.0 **Speech Rate, Rhythm, or Fluency Disorder**

140.1 **Stuttering**

140.2 **Cluttering**

140.3 **Dysprosody**

150.0 **Voice Disorder**

150.1 **Motor-Vocal**

150.2 **Structural (e.g., Laryngectomy)**

150.3 **Functional**

150.4 **Mixed**

160.0 **Resonance Disorder**

160.1 **Motor-Vocal**

160.2 **Structural**

160.3 **Functional**

160.4 **Mixed**

170.0 **Oral/Pharyngeal Dysfunction**

171.0 **Dysphagia**

171.1 **Oral Prepatory Phase (Chewing, Biting, Feeding)**

171.2 **Oral Phase (Sucking, Bolus Manipulation, Swallowing)**

171.3 **Pharyngeal Phase (Aerodigestive Dysfunction)**

172.0 **Tongue Thrust**

173.0 **Oral Tics**

180.0 **Unlisted Category**

190.0 **Results Not Conclusive**

190.1 **Could Not Test**

190.2 **Could Not Determine**

AUDITORY AND OTHER DIAGNOSES

200.0 **Hearing Within Normal Limits**

200.1 **Undifferentiated**

200.2 **Right**

200.3 **Left**

200.4 **Bilateral**

210.0 **Middle Ear Dysfunction, Hearing Within Normal Limits**

210.1 **Right**

210.2 **Left**

210.3 **Bilateral**

220.0 Hearing Loss, Type Undetermined
    220.1 Undifferentiated
    220.2 Right
    220.3 Left
    220.4 Bilateral
230.0 Conductive Hearing Loss
    230.1 Right
    230.2 Left
    230.3 Bilateral
240.0 Sensorineural Hearing Loss
    240.1 Right
    240.2 Left
    240.3 Bilateral
241.0 Sensorineural Hearing Loss, Cochlear
    241.1 Right
    241.2 Left
    241.3 Bilateral
242.0 Sensorineural Hearing Loss, Retrocochlear
    242.1 Right
    242.2 Left
    242.3 Bilateral
243.0 Sensorineural Hearing Loss, Combined Cochlear And Retrocochlear
    243.1 Right
    243.2 Left
    243.3 Bilateral
250.0 Mixed Hearing Loss
    250.1 Right
    250.2 Left
    250.3 Bilateral
251.0 Mixed Hearing Loss, Conductive And Cochlear
    251.1 Right
    251.2 Left
    251.3 Bilateral
260.0 Central Auditory Disorder
270.0 Pseudohypacusis
    270.1 Right
    270.2 Left
    270.3 Bilateral
280.0 Vestibular Function
    280.1 Within Normal
    280.2 Peripheral Disorder
    280.3 Central Disorder
    280.4 Nonlocalized Disorder
290.0 Seventh Nerve Disorder
    290.1 Right

290.2 Left

290.3 Bilateral

300.0 Other Disorder

301.0 Tinnitus

301.1 Right

301.2 Left

301.3 Bilateral

302.0 Vertigo

310.0 Unlisted Category

320.0 Results Not Conclusive

320.1 Could Not Test

320.2 Could Not Determine

American Speech-Language-Hearing Association. "Classification of Speech-Language Pathology and Auditory Procedures and Communication Disorders," *Asha* 29 (12) (1987): 49–53.

SAMPLE LANGUAGE ARTS CURRICULUM

Below are several excerpts representing examples of the major areas of focus and objectives of key portions of a language arts curriculum for the elementary grades. Examples are provided for six skill areas including listening, speaking, oral and dramatic interpretation, oral reading, grammar, and written composition. Due to space limitations, only one representative grade level is presented for each skill area. Classroom learning activities and teaching materials are developed to support these objectives.

These examples help illustrate the communication demands placed upon children as they progress through school as well as the types of learning activities that can be incorporated into the speech-language program.

LISTENING SKILLS (KINDERGARTEN)

Major Focus

- Direction following
- Sound identification
- Stories
- Poems

Sample Objectives

- Follow oral directions for drawing pictures
- Follow directions for playing games
- Follow directions for marking worksheets
- Demonstrate body awareness of spatial words such as over, under, beside, in front, left, right, and so on
- Name a word that rhymes with a dictated word
- Arrange in the proper sequence, four or five pictures related to the story
- Answer questions using facts from the story
- Recognize the main idea in an oral presentation or story
- Name and describe the main characters in the story
- Repeat short nursery rhymes, poems, fingerplays, songs

SPEAKING SKILLS
(LEVEL 1)

Major Focus

- Story sequencing
- Sharing experiences
- Rhymes
- Poems

Sample Objectives

- Speak thoughts in complete sentences
- Supply names for concrete items and pictures
- Classification of familiar objects or pictures, (fruit—apple, orange; furniture—chair, table; clothing—dress, suit)
- Retell a story in the proper sequence
- Relate a personal experience in front of a group
- Express verbally human needs and emotions
- Describe how two objects are alike or different
- Take part in an informal exchange of ideas with others
- Present facts and ideas in an organized manner
- Recite familiar rhymes and poems

ORAL AND DRAMATIC INTERPRETATION
(LEVEL 2)

Major Focus

- Pantomime
- Role playing
- Story characters
- Human emotions

Sample Objectives

- Take part in pantomiming activities; pretend to be the animal or character
  - Animals or real people
  - Nonliving things
  - Action or series of actions
  - Emotion or series of emotions
  - Story characters
- Act out a situation in the classroom
- Participate in role playing of real-life or storybook characters

- Improvise familiar stories
- Memorize written parts
- Participate in a formal play
- Dramatize a chosen role from a favorite book or play

ORAL READING
(LEVEL 3)

Major Focus

- Expression
- Comprehension
- Clear and distinct pronunciation
- Punctuation

Sample Objectives

- Read fluently in thought units
- Use clear and distinct pronunciation when reading
- Use expression to show the mood and emotion in the story
- Reread to locate information
- Recall the sequence of the story
- Recall details of the story
- Identify the main idea of the story
- Read orally for the enjoyment of others
- Read a part in a play along with other readers

GRAMMAR SKILLS
(LEVEL 4)

Major Focus

- Punctuation
- Capitalization
- Abbreviations
- Irregular verbs
- Prepositional phrases
- Pronouns
- Usage
- Contractions
- Possessives
- Verb tense

Sample Objectives

- Write and punctuate sentence types correctly
- Use punctuation correctly in sentences
- Use capital letters
- Use correct plurals
- Identify verbs in sentences
- Identify the pronouns in sentences by underlining
- Identify the two parts of a sentence by underlining the subject and the predicate
- Identify the adjectives in sentences
- Recognize that English sentences have definite word-order patterns
- Show how changing the word-order of most English sentences will change their meaning
- Make a list of words that show ownership by adding 's to singular nouns
- Develop skill in proofreading

WRITTEN COMPOSITION
(LEVEL 5)

Major Focus

- Different points of view
- Advertisements
- Magazine articles, news stories
- Poetry; limericks
- Scripts; dialogues
- Stories—surprise endings, interesting beginnings, science fiction
- Letters
- Note taking
- Organization of ideas

Sample Objectives

- Write from the point of view of animals or other people
- Experiment with writing interesting book cards for a file as a means of pooling information about books
- Develop skill in taking notes
- Write an imaginary news story using notes
- Use information from multiple sources when writing travel ads
- Write a story about the future
- Use correct form for a friendly letter
- Combine concepts, principles and generalizations in written compositions

Developed by Jean Blosser after reviewing curricula from numerous school programs

SAMPLE FORMS USED FOR MULTIFACTORED EVALUATION AND PLANNING THE INDIVIDUALIZED EDUCATION PROGRAM

(Developed by the Akron Public School District, Akron, OH (2000)
—Brian Williams, Superintendent).

SCHOOL-AGE REQUEST FOR ASSISTANCE

Identifying Data

Name: _____   Father: _____

Date of Birth: _____   Address (if different from student): _____

Address: _____   _____

_____   Home Phone (if different from student): ___

Phone: _____   Work Phone: _____

Legal Guardian: _____   Mother: _____

Address (if different from student): _____   Address (if different from student): _____

_____   Home Phone (if different from student): ___

Phone (if different from student: _____   Work Phone: _____

Parents' Native Language (if not English): _____

Student's Native Language (if not English): _____

Student ID Number: _____

Building of Current Attendance: _____

Grade: _____   Present Teacher(s): _____

If the student or parent need assistive technology, environmental adaptation, or other such accommodations in order to attend meetings or understand the content of written and/or verbal information, please specify/explain: _____

_____

_____

_____

Reason for Request for Assistance: _____

_____

_____

_____

Educational History

Number of school districts attended: _____   Years at present school: _____

Attendance: ☐ Regular   ☐ Irregular (explain) _____

_____

Is this student age-appropriate for grade level?   ☐ Yes   ☐ No

If **No,** check all that apply   ☐ Retained (specify grade) _____
☐ Started school late
☐ Held out of school by parent
☐ Unknown

Indicate any current or past supplemental programs/services (Title 1, Preschool, Reading Recovery, etc.)

_____

_____

Attach copies of district test results (Proficiency, Competency-Based Education, etc.).

Background Information

A. Health Data

Do you suspect problems with   ☐ Vision   ☐ Hearing
Does the student   ☐ Wear glasses ☐ Use hearing aid(s)
Does the student take medication   ☐ Yes   ☐ No

If **Yes,** specify type and purpose:

_____

_____

Does the student have any health/developmental/physical problems of which you are aware? ☐ Yes
☐ No

If **Yes,** explain: _____

_____

B. Environmental Factors

Describe any specific home factors that might affect the student's performance in school:

_____

_____

_____

Areas of Educational Concern

Skill Areas: For each of the following, check areas of concern and describe the student's current levels of educational functioning in those areas as determined by current classroom-based assessments and observations. Attach additional pages as needed.

(Continued)

SCHOOL-AGE REQUEST FOR ASSISTANCE (CONTINUED)

A. Academic

- ☐ Reading
- ☐ Content Areas
- ☐ Written Language
- ☐ Math
- ☐ Other (specify): _____

1. What specific skills does the student have in the above-checked areas?

_____

_____

_____

2. What specific skills does the student not have in the above-checked areas?

_____

_____

_____

3. What instructional approach has/is being used?

_____

_____

_____

4. How much instruction does the student receive (daily/weekly) and in what setting?

_____

_____

_____

5. What has been done to address the problem?

_____

_____

_____

6. How does performance in the above-checked areas affect the student's performance in other areas of the curriculum and/or behavior?

_____

_____

_____

B. Communication

- ☐ Articulation
- ☐ Fluency
- ☐ Language Comprehension
- ☐ Social Language (Pragmatics)
- ☐ Verbal Expression
- ☐ Limited English Proficiency (English Language Limited)
- ☐ Voice
- ☐ Other (specify): _____
  _____

Describe difficulties as indicated above: _____

_____

_____

How do the difficulties affect performance in the curriculum and/or behavior?

_____

_____

_____

C. Motor

☐ Fine Motor Coordination   ☐ Visual Motor Coordination
☐ Gross Motor Coordination ☐ Other (specify) _____

Describe difficulties as indicated above: _____

_____

_____

How do the difficulties affect performance in the curriculum and/or behavior?

_____

_____

_____

D. Behavior

☐ Attention Span   ☐ Activity Level   ☐ Acting Out
☐ Withdrawal   ☐ Peer Relationships   ☐ Adult Relationships
☐ Other (specify) _____

Describe difficulties as indicated above, including the frequency, severity, and under what conditions/settings the behavior occurs: _____

_____

How do the behavioral conditions affect performances in the curriculum?

_____

_____

E. Related Areas

☐ Self-Help Skills   ☐ Study Skills   ☐ Organizational Skills
☐ Test-Taking Skills   ☐ Other (specify) _____

Describe difficulties as indicated above: _____

_____

_____

(Continued)

SCHOOL-AGE REQUEST FOR ASSISTANCE (CONTINUED)

How do the difficulties affect performance in the curriculum and/or behavior?

_____

_____

_____

F. Strengths and Interests

Describe the student's strengths and interests: _____

_____

_____

G. Parental Involvement

Date(s) parent(s) was contacted regarding the concern(s): _____

How has the parent been involved in addressing the current concern? _____

_____

_____

H. Other

Is there any other pertinent information not previously described?

_____

_____

_____

_____	_____	_____
Signatures of Person Initiating the Request for Assistance	Position or Relationship to Student	Date
_____	_____	_____
Signature of Person Receiving the Request for Assistance	Title	Telephone Number
		_____
		Date

Initial Meeting Date: _____

Outcome of Meeting: _____

_____

_____

Follow-up Meeting Date: _____

Outcome of Meeting: _____

_____

_____

Follow-up Meeting Date: _____

Outcome of Meeting: _____

_____

_____

☐ I am requesting a meeting to determine if this student may be suspected of having a disability.

_____   _____

Signature   Date

The team, which includes the parents, will review all available information and complete Form CI-211.

Note: A referral for Multifactored Evaluation (MFE) consists of the following completed forms:

1. Form CI-204, School-Age Request for Assistance;
2. Form CI-207✦, Documentation of Interventions, if appropriate; and
3. Form CI-211, Determination of Suspected Disability.

✦**Denotes optional procedure/form**

DETERMINATION OF SUSPECTED DISABILITY

Name of Child: _____   Date of Birth: ___ / ___ / ___   Age: _____

Student ID Number: _____

The following individuals met on _____ to decide if there is a suspected disability:
(Date)

_____   _____
Name and Title   Name and Title

_____   _____
Name and Title   Name and Title

_____   _____
Name and Title   Name and Title

Information used to make the decision about whether or not there is a suspected disability:
(Check information used)

☐ Request for Assistance   ☐ Observation
☐ Interview with ___Parent ___Primary Care Provider ___Child's Teacher   ☐ Screening
☐ Results of Interventions   ☐ Other (specify)
                                                           _____

Summarize the most <u>significant</u> factors used by the team to make a decision, including any other options considered and the reasons why those options were rejected: _____

_____ .

Date of Referral: _____

☐ This child is NOT suspected of having a disability and there are no further recommendations.

☐ This child is NOT suspected of having a disability; however, the following activities/interventions are recommended:

_____

_____

_____

☐ This child is suspected of having a disability. The completed Multifactored Evaluation Planning Chart (MFE-501c or MFE-501d) is attached.

_____   _____
Signature of Chairperson   Signature of Parent
[☐Agree   ☐Disagree]

☐ Although the team does not suspect a disability, I believe my child has a disability and request a multifactored evaluation.

_____
Signature of Parent(s)

If it is determined that the child is suspected of having a disability, and the parent(s) refuses permission for the multifactored evaluation (Form PS-402), the district may initiate a due process hearing.

Team members who disagree with the determination may attach a statement supporting their respective positions.

Note: A referral for Multifactored Evaluation (MFE) consists of the following completed forms:

1. Form CI-204, School-Age Request for Assistance;
2. Form CI-207✦, Documentation of Interventions, if appropriate; and
3. Form CI-211, Determination of Suspected Disability.

✦Denotes optional procedure/form

Preschool Planning Form: INITIAL MULTIFACTORED EVALUATION (MFE)

Child's Name: _____   Date of Birth: _____   Chronological Age: __

STEP 1:   In the appropriate box, document each assessment which has already occurred. Include title and/or person who conducted the assessment and the date. When applicable, include the name of the assessment tool.

STEP 2:   In the appropriate box, write the title and/or person who will conduct the evaluation(s) needed to complete the MFE.

NOTE: Information must be collected for all the areas in the left-hand column using one of the four methods listed across the top. In the area(s) of suspected deficit (indicated in bold print) which are circled, information must be collected using **all four** methods.

CIRCLE the area(s) of suspected deficit	Structured Interview	Structured Observations (2)	Standardized Norm-Referenced Tests	Criterion-Referenced/ Curriculum-Based
Background ☐ Completed				
Adaptive Behavior ☐ All needed information has been collected or completed				
Cognitive Ability ☐ All needed information has been collected or completed				
Communication ☐ All needed information has been collected or completed				
Hearing Ability ☐ All needed information has been collected or completed			Audiological Exam	
Vision Ability ☐ All needed information has been collected or completed			Vision Exam Braille	
Preacademic Skills ☐ All needed information has been collected or completed				

CIRCLE the area(s) of suspected deficit	Structured Interview	Structured Observations (2)	Standardized Norm-Referenced Tests	Criterion-Referenced/ Curriculum-Based
Gross/Fine Motor Skills ☐ All needed information has been collected or completed				
Social/Emotional Behavioral ☐ All needed information has been collected or completed				
Medical/Health ☐ All needed information has been collected or completed				

☐ The team has taken into consideration possible sources of racial/cultural bias in planning these assessments.

_____ (Signature of Evaluation Team Chairperson)Date of Plan: ____ / ____ / ____

School-Age Planning Form: INITIAL MULTIFACTORED EVALUATION (MFE)

Student's Name: _____   Date of Birth: _____   Age: _____

STEP 1:   List area(s) of suspected disability: _____

STEP 2:   In column (C), record the assessments completed within the past year by listing the assessment date and the position of the individual or agency that conducted the assessment.

STEP 3:   In the methods columns (D), indicate the position of the individual assigned to conduct the assessments listed in column (A).

(A) Assessment Areas	(B) Required to Determine Eligibility for:	(C) Completed by:	(D) Methods Interview/ Records	Observations	Direct Assessment
Physical (medical) Examination	MD, HI, VI, OH, OHI, ED, TBI, Autism				
Health and Nutrition	As needed				
General Intelligence	All, except S/L				
Academic/Preacademic Skills	All				
Educational Functioning	S/L				
Vision Abilities	All, except S/L & VI				
Eye Condition by Specialist	VI				
Braille Needs	VI				
Hearing Abilities	All except HI				
Audiological Status	HI				
Communicative Status	All				
Communication Mode	HI				
Adaptive Behavior	MD, MR (DH)				
Social and Emotional Status	MD, HI, VI, OH, OHI, SLD				
Classroom Observations	SLD		▓▓▓		▓▓▓
Informal Behavioral	ED		▓▓▓		▓▓▓
Informal Behavioral	ED		▓▓▓		
Behavior/Personality Measure	ED				
Background Information	ED				
■ Reading and Math Instruction	All				
■ Social and Cultural	MR (DH)				
■ English Proficiency	All				
Teacher Recommendations	MR (DH)				
Motor Abilities	All, except S/L				
Vocational/Occupational and Transition Needs	When needed, and as required by age 14 and age 16				
■ Aptitudes					
■ Interests					
■ Preferences					
■ Employability					
Assistive Technology Needs	As Needed				
Other:					
Other:					

☐ The team has taken into consideration possible sources of racial/cultural bias in planning these assessments.

_____   (Signature of Evaluation Team Chairperson)   Date of Plan: ____/____/____

EVALUATION FORM

Student's Name: _____   Date of Birth: ___/___/___ Age: _____

Evaluator: _____   Title: _____

Areas of Assessments:

_____

_____

_____

_____

Evaluation methods and activities:

☐ Observation(s)   ☐ Interview(s)   ☐ Trial Intervention(s)
☐ Record Review   ☐ Classroom-Based Assessment   ☐ Other
☐ Curriculum-Based Assessment   ☐ Norm-Referenced Assessment

Summary of assessment(s), including results and instructional implications:

_____

_____

_____

_____

_____

_____

_____

_____

_____

_____

Signature of Evaluator: _____   Date : ___/___/___

SUMMARY OF OBSERVATION

Student's Name: _____   Date of Birth: ____ / ____ / ____ Age: _____

(Multiple observations are required for ED evaluations. Each individual conducting an observation should complete a Summary of Observation form).

Date of Observation: ____ / ____ / ____   Setting: _____

Activity: _____

_____

Conducted by (Name and Title): _____

A. Summarize relevant behaviors:

    1. Describe behavior patterns:

    2. Describe the frequency of problem behavior(s):

    3. Describe the intensity of the problem behavior(s):

B. Describe the relationship of behavior(s) to the student's academic functioning:

C. Describe instructional implications of behavior problems:

_____   _____
Signature   Date

TEAM SUMMARY AND
INTERPRETATION OF THE MULTIFACTORED EVALUATION

Student's Name: _____ Date of Birth: ____/____/____ Age: _____

Summary of Current Performance:

Description of Educational Needs:

Implications for Instruction and Progress Monitoring:

DETERMINATION OF ELIGIBILITY

Student's Name: _____   Date of Birth: ____/____/____   Age: _____

1. Has the evaluation eliminated lack of instruction in reading or math as the determinant factor in reaching a conclusion about the presence of a disability?   ☐ Yes   ☐ No

2. Has the evaluation eliminated limited English proficiency as a determinant factor in reaching a conclusion about the presence of a disability?   ☐ Yes   ☐ No

3. Has it been determined that this student has or continues to have a disability?

   ☐ Yes (indicate disability _____   ☐ No

   _____

4. Describe how the child either meets or fails to meet the definition of the suspected disability for which the assessment was conducted.

5. Does information contained in the preceding evaluation summary confirm that the disability condition has an adverse affect upon the educational performance?   ☐ Yes   ☐ No

   The following individuals participated in reaching the determination about this child's or student's eligibility for special education and related services (Signatures required for all team members for SLD, ED, PS, and IBA/MFE):

NAME	TITLE	DATE	AGREE	DISAGREE*	SIGNATURE
	Parent				
	Teacher				

*Team member/individual must file a statement of disagreement.

INVITATION TO INITIAL
INDIVIDUALIZED EDUCATION PROGRAM (IEP) MEETING

Name of Child: _____   Date of Birth: ___/___/___

Dear Parent:

At the time you gave consent for a multifactored evaluation, you were informed that you would be an equal participant in the meeting(s) to determine your child's educational program.

This letter serves as an invitation to a meeting for the following purposes:

☐ **1.** To discuss the results of the multifactored evaluation, share other information the school may have about your child, and provide an opportunity for you to contribute additional information.

☐ **2.** To determine your child's educational needs, and develop goals and objectives to meet your child's needs.

☐ **3.** If your child is eligible for special education services, we will, together with you, determine if special education services are necessary. If special education services are necessary, we will write an IEP and determine where those services should be delivered to meet your child's needs.

☐ **4.** If your child is preschool age, we will discuss transition from early childhood to school-age programs.

☐ **5.** If your child is 14 (or younger, if appropriate), we will discuss transition from high school to post-high school activities.

The meeting is scheduled for _____ at _____ at

  (Date)   (Time)

_____ .

  (Location)

Other people in attendace may include

_____   _____

(Name and Title)   (Name and Title)

_____   _____

(Name and Title)   (Name and Title)

_____   _____

(Name and Title)   (Name and Title)

If we will be discussing <u>transition activities</u>, we will invite a representative(s) from the following agency(ies).

_____   _____

(Agency)   (Agency)

Your attendance and participation is especially encouraged, as it is critical to have your input. Please plan to attend this meeting. You may bring others who you feel can assist in this important planning

(Continued)

INVITATION TO INITIAL
INDIVIDUALIZED EDUCATION PROGRAM (IEP) MEETING (CONTINUED)

for your child. If you do not attend, you will receive a copy of the IEP within 30 days after the meeting with a request for your approval and signature.

If you have any questions, or need additional information, please contact

_____   _____
Name   Telephone Number

PLEASE RETURN THE ATTACHED PAGE (FORM CI-209)

☐ **Services Plan**

Individualized Education Program (IEP)

Name _____ Date of Birth ___/___/___ Grade Level _____ ☐ Male ☐ Female

Student Identification Number _____

Child/Student Address _____

Parent/Guardian _____

Parent Address _____ Home Phone _____ Work Phone _____

Effective Dates from _____ to _____ Meeting Date _____ ☐ Initial IEP ☐ Periodic Review

District of Residence _____ District of Service _____

Step 1   **Discuss Vision:** *Future Planning.*

Step 2   **Discuss Present Levels of Performance.**

(Continued)

COMMUNITY PARTICIPATION LONG-TERM OUTCOME: _____

Current Year Activities and Services	Responsible Person/Provider	Initiation/Duration (Specify Date)	Goals/Objectives that Support Activities/Services

Vocational Evaluation ☐ Needed ☐ Not Needed   Date Completed _____

Functional/Daily Living Evaluation ☐ Needed ☐ Not Needed   Date Completed _____

Student's Needs	Annual Goals	Objectives
Step 3 **Identify Specialized Needs for this IEP**	**Step 4** **Identify Measurable Goals, Objectives, and Assessment Procedures**	

| Step 4 (continued) Assessment of Student Progress | | | | | Step 5 Identify Needed Services | Initiation/ Duration | Step 6 Determine Least Restrictive Environment (LRE) |
Procedures	Who	Criteria	Schedule	Progress			

(Continued)

Discuss and Document a Statement of Needed Transition Services

| Name of Student _____ | Date _____ | Person(s) Responsible for Coordinating Transition Services _____ |

Write a statement of transition service needs that focus on the student's courses of study during his or her secondary school experiences (beginning at age 14 or younger, if appropriate).

- Long-term Outcomes—What is the vision for the student exiting education?
- Activities and Services—What needs to be accomplished in one year to support the student in meeting long-term outcomes?
- Activities and services must include community experience.
- If activities and services are instructional based, they must be reflected in goals/objectives of IEP.
- The courses of study during the student's secondary school experiences must support the student's long-term goals.

| FOR 16 YEARS AND OLDER | | COMPLETED AFTER IEP DEVELOPMENT |

EMPLOYMENT AND POSTSECONDARY LONG-TERM OUTCOME: _____

Current Year Activities and Services	Responsible Person/Provider	Initiation/Duration (Specify Date)	Goals/Objectives that Support Activities/Services

POSTSCHOOL/ADULT LIVING LONG-TERM OUTCOME: _____

Current Year Activities and Services	Responsible Person/Provider	Initiation/Duration (Specify Date)	Goals/Objectives that Support Activities/Services

338

STATEWIDE AND DISTRICTWIDE TESTING

Student Name: _____ Student's Grade: _____ Student ID: _____

School Year: _____ IEP Meeting Date: _____

STATEWIDE TESTING

Areas of Assessment	Grade Level of Test to be Administered	Required		Will Take Test without IEP Accommodations	Exempted		Will Participate in Alternate Assessment
		Will Take Test without IEP Accommodations	Will Take Test with IEP Accommodations		Will take test with Allowable IEP Accommodations	Will take test with IEP Extended Accommodations	Alternate Assessment
		B	C	J	K	L	N
Reading							
Writing							
Math							
Science							
Citizenship							
Work Keys							
ITAC							

DISTRICTWIDE TESTING

Grade Level of Test to be Administered	Will Take Test without Accommodations	Will Take Test with Accommodations	Will Participate in Alternate Assessment

ACCOMMODATIONS (FOR CODES J, K, AND L)

Areas	STATEWIDE			DISTRICTWIDE	
	List Accommodations to Statewide Testing	Reasons for Exemption or Alternate Assessment (Check Box)	List Accommodations to Local Testing	How Student will be Assessed in Alternate Assessment	
Reading		☐ Substantial modifications in curriculum ☐ Accommodations exceed allowable criteria			
Writing		☐ Substantial modifications in curriculum ☐ Accommodations exceed allowable criteria			
Math		☐ Substantial modifications in curriculum ☐ Accommodations exceed allowable criteria			
Science		☐ Substantial modifications in curriculum ☐ Accommodations exceed allowable criteria			
Citizenship		☐ Substantial modifications in curriculum ☐ Accommodations exceed allowable criteria			
Work Keys					
ITAC					

CC: Testing Coordinator
      EMIS Coordinator

BUILDING-LEVEL PROBLEM ANALYSIS AND INTERVENTION PLAN

Student: _____   Grade: _____   Date: _____

Teacher: _____   Collaborators: _____

_____

_____

_____

STEP 1. BEHAVIORAL DESCRIPTION OF THE PROBLEM:
(specific and observable behavior)

_____

_____

_____

STEP 2. BEHAVIORAL STATEMENT OF DESIRED GOAL OR OBJECTIVE:
(objective written in precise terms)

_____

_____

_____

STEP 3. BRAINSTORM POSSIBLE INTERVENTIONS:
(list without evaluating)

_____

_____

_____

STEP 4. CLARIFY AND EVALUATE POSSIBLE INTERVENTIONS:
(outline interventions)

_____

_____

_____

STEP 5. DEVELOP AN INTERVENTION PLAN:
(attach intervention plan)

STEP 6. EVALUATE EFFECTIVENESS OF INTERVENTION PLAN:
(dates, modifications, measures of effectiveness)

_____

_____

_____

PROGRESS MONITORING

DEFINITION: **Progress monitoring is a systematic procedure for the frequent and repeated collection and analysis of student performance data.**

WHAT ARE THE BENEFITS OF PROGRESS MONITORING?

FOR STUDENTS: ■ **Monitoring provides a clear idea of expectations for performance.**

■ **Continuous feedback on performance enhances motivation.**

■ **Student outcomes improve.**

FOR TEACHERS: ■ **Monitoring provides timely feedback on the effectiveness of an intervention.**

■ **Data collection provides an objective data base for decision-making.**

■ **Continuous feedback improves instructional planning.**

■ **Progress monitoring is an important tool for problem-solving.**

WHY SHOULD I MONITOR PROGRESS?

No way to predict that interventions will be successful.

Increased emphasis on the demonstration of outcomes.

Student outcomes improve.

Allows us to make decisions based on the pattern of performance.

RELATIONSHIP OF THE DEGREE OF LONG-TERM HEARING LOSS TO PSYCHOSOCIAL IMPACT AND EDUCATIONAL NEEDS

DEGREE OF HEARING LOSS BASED ON MODIFIED PURE TONE AVERAGE (500–4000 HZ)	POSSIBLE EFFECT OF HEARING LOSS ON THE UNDERSTANDING OF LANGUAGE & SPEECH	POSSIBLE PSYCHOSOCIAL IMPACT OF HEARING LOSS	POTENTIAL EDUCATIONAL NEEDS AND PROGRAMS
Normal Hearing −10–+15 dB HL	Children have better hearing sensitivity than the accepted normal range for adults. A child with hearing sensitivity in the −10 to +15 dB range will detect the complete speech signal even at soft conversation levels. However, good hearing, does not guarantee good ability to discriminate speech in the presence of background noise.		
Minimal (borderline) 16–25 dB HL	May have difficulty hearing faint or distant speech. At 15 dB student can miss up to 10% of speech signal when teacher is at a distance greater than 3 feet and when the classroom is noisy, especially in the elementary grades when verbal instruction predominates.	May be unaware of subtle conversational cues which could cause child to be viewed as inappropriate or awkward. May miss portions of fast-paced peer interactions which could begin to have an impact on socialization and self concept. May have immature behavior. Child may be more fatigued than classmates due to listening effort needed.	May benefit from mild gain/low MPO hearing aid or personal FM system dependent on loss configuration. Would benefit from soundfield amplification if classroom is noisy and/or reverberant. Favorable seating. May need attention to vocabulary or speech, especially with recurrent otitis media history. Appropriate medical management necessary for conductive losses. Teacher requires in-service on impact of hearing loss on language development and learning.

Degree			
Mild 26–40 dB HL	At 30 dB can miss 25–40% of speech signal. The degree of difficulty experienced in school will depend upon the noise level in classroom, distance from teacher and the configuration of the hearing loss. Without amplification the child with 35–40 dB loss may miss at least 50% of class discussions, especially when voices are faint or speaker is not in line of vision. Will miss consonants, especially when a high frequency hearing loss is present.	Barriers beginning to build with negative impact on self esteem as child is accused of "hearing when he or she wants to," "daydreaming," or "not paying attention." Child begins to lose ability for selective hearing, and has increasing difficulty suppressing background noise which makes the learning environment stressful. Child is more fatigued than classmates due to listening effort needed.	Will benefit from a hearing aid and use of a personal FM or classroom. Needs favorable seating and lighting. Refer to special education for language evaluation and for educational follow-up. Needs auditory skill building. May need attention to vocabulary and language development, articulation or speechreading and/or special support in reading. May need help with self esteem. Teacher in-service required.
Moderate 41–55 dB HL	Understands conversational speech at a distance of 3–5 feet (face-to-face) only if structure and vocabulary controlled. Without amplification the amount of speech signal missed can be 50% to 75% with 40 dB loss and 80% to 100% with 50 dB loss. Is likely to have delayed or defective syntax, limited vocabulary, imperfect speech production, and an atonal voice quality.	Often with this degree of hearing loss, communication is significantly affected, and socialization with peers with normal hearing becomes increasingly difficult. With full time use of hearing aids/FM systems child may be judged as a less competent learner. There is an increasing impact on self-esteem.	Refer to special education for language evaluation and for educational follow-up. Amplification is essential (hearing aids and FM system). Special education support may be needed, especially for primary children. Attention to oral language development, reading and written language. Auditory skill development and speech therapy usually needed. Teacher in-service required.
Moderate to Severe 56–70 dB HL	Without amplification, conversation must be very loud to be understood. A 55 dB loss can cause child to miss up to 100% of speech information. Will have marked difficulty in school situations requiring verbal communication in both one-to-one and group situations. Delayed language, syntax, reduced speech intelligibility and atonal voice quality likely.	Full time use of hearing aids/FM systems may result in child being judged by both peers and adults as a less competent learner, resulting in poorer self concept, social maturity and contributing to a sense of rejection. In-service to address these attitudes may be helpful.	Full time use of amplification is essential. Will need resource teacher or special class depending on magnitude of language delay. May require special help in all language academic skills, language based subjects, vocabulary, grammar, pragmatics as well as reading and writing. Probably needs assistance to expand experiential language base. In-service of mainstream teachers required.

(Continued)

DEGREE OF HEARING LOSS BASED ON MODIFIED PURE TONE AVERAGE (500–4000 HZ)	POSSIBLE EFFECT OF HEARING LOSS ON THE UNDERSTANDING OF LANGUAGE & SPEECH	POSSIBLE PSYCHOSOCIAL IMPACT OF HEARING LOSS	POTENTIAL EDUCATIONAL NEEDS AND PROGRAMS
Severe 71–90 dB HL	Without amplification may hear loud voices about one foot from ear. When amplified optimally, children with hearing ability of 90 dB or better should he able to identify environmental sounds and detect all the sounds of speech. If loss is of prelingual onset, oral language and speech may not develop spontaneously or will be severely delayed. If hearing loss is of recent onset speech is likely to deteriorate with quality becoming atonal.	Child may prefer other children with hearing impairments as friends and playmates. This may further isolate the child from the mainstream, however, these peer relationships may foster improved self concept and a sense of cultural identity.	May need full-time special aural/oral program with emphasis on all auditory language skills, speechreading, concept development and speech. As loss approaches 80–90 dB, may benefit from a Total Communication approach, especially in the early language learning years. Individual hearing aid/personal FM system essential. Need to monitor effectiveness of communication modality. Participation in regular classes as much as beneficial to student. In-service of mainstream teachers essential.
Profound 91 dB HL or more	Aware of vibrations more than tonal pattern. Many rely on vision rather than hearing as primary avenue for communication and learning. Detection of speech sounds dependent upon loss configuration and use of amplification. Speech and language will not develop spontaneously and is likely to deteriorate rapidly if hearing loss is of recent onset.	Depending on auditory/oral competence, peer use of sign language, parental attitude, etc., child may or may not increasingly prefer association with the deaf culture.	May need special program for deaf children with emphasis on all language skills and academic areas. Program needs specialized supervision and comprehensive support services. Early use of amplification likely to help if part of an intensive training program. May be cochlear implant or vibrotactile aid candidate. Requires continual appraisal of needs in regard to communication and learning mode. Part-time in regular classes as much as beneficial to student.

Type of Loss	Possible Impact on the Understanding of Language and Speech	Possible Psychosocial Impact	Potential Educational Needs and Programs
Unilateral One normal hearing ear and one ear with at least a permanent mild hearing loss	May have difficulty hearing faint or distant speech. Usually has difficulty localizing sounds and voices. Unilateral listener will have greater difficulty understanding speech when environment is noisy and/or reverberant. Difficulty detecting or understanding soft speech from side of bad ear, especially in a group discussion.	Child may be accused of selective hearing due to discrepancies in speech understanding in quiet versus noise. Child will be more fatigued in classroom setting due to greater effort needed to listen. May appear inattentive or frustrated. Behavior problems sometimes evident.	May benefit from personal FM or soundfield FM system in classroom. CROS hearing aid may be of benefit in quiet settings. Needs favorable seating and lighting. Student is at risk for educational difficulties. Educational monitoring warranted with support services provided as soon as difficulties appear. Teacher in-service is beneficial.

Note: All children with hearing loss require periodic audiologic evaluation, rigorous monitoring of amplification, and regular monitoring of communication skills. All children with hearing loss (especially conductive) need appropriate medical attention in conjunction with educational programming.

References

Olsen, W. O., Hawkins, D. B., VanTassell, D. J. (1987). Representatives of the Longterm Spectrum of Speech. *Ear & Hearing*, Supplement 8, pp. 100–108.

Mueller, H. G. & Killion, M. C. (1990). An easy method for calculating the articulation index. *The Hearing Journal*, 43, 9, pp. 14–22.

Hasenstab, M. S. (1987). *Language Learning and Otitis Media*, College Hill Press, Boston, MA.

Developed by Karen L. Anderson, Ed.S & Noel D. Matkin, Ph.D (1991).

Adapted from: Bernero, R. J. & Bothwell, H. (1966). Relationship of Hearing Impairment to Educational Needs. Illinois Department of Public Health & Office of Superintendent of Public Instruction.

Peer Review by Members of the Educational Audiology Association, Winter 1991.

*Reprinted with permission of authors and *Seminars in Hearing*.

REFERENCES

Adams, P. R. and Marano, M. A. (1995). Current estimates from the national health interview survey, 1994. *Vital Health Statistics,* 10, 193. Washington, DC: National Center for Health Scientists.

Adler, S. (1973). Data Gathering: The reliability and validity of test data obtained from culturally different children. *Journal of Learning Disabilities* 6: 429–34.

Ainsworth, S. (December 1965). The speech clinician in public schools: participant or separatist? *Asha* 7: 495–503.

Akron Public School District. (2000). Individualized education program forms. Akron, OH.

Alpiner, J., Ogden, J. A., and Wiggens, J. (December 1970). The utilization of supportive personnel in speech correction in the public schools: A pilot project. *Asha* 12, 599–604.

American Speech-Language-Hearing Association (1983). Ad Hoc Committee on Extension of Audiological Services in the Schools. Audiology services in the schools position statement. *Asha* 25 (5): 53–60.

American Speech-Language-Hearing Association. (2000). Ad Hoc Committee on Reading and Writing Language Disorders. Roles and responsibilities of speech-language pathologists related to reading and writing in children and youth. Rockville, MD: American Speech-Language-Hearing Association.

———. (1999a). Frequently asked questions about speech-language pathology assistants. ASHA website.

———. (1999b). Guidelines for the roles and responsibilities of the school-based speech-language-pathologist. Ad Hoc Committee on the Roles and Responsibilities of the School-Based Speech-Language Pathologist. Rockville, MD.

———. (1999c). National outcomes measurement system for speech-language pathology and audiology (NOMS). Rockville, MD: American Speech-Language-Hearing Association.

———. (1997). Guidelines for Audiologic Screening. Panel on Audiologic Assessment. Rockville, MD.

———. (1996). Guidelines for the training, credentialing, use, and supervision of speech-language pathology assistants. *Asha* 38 (Supplement 16), 21–34.

———. (1994a). Admission/discharge criteria in speech-language pathology. *ASHA Desk Reference* (Vol. 3, pp. 158–158b).

———. (1994b). Code of ethics. *Asha* 34 (March Supplement 9): 1–2.

———. (1993). Committee on Language, Speech, and Hearing Services in the Schools. Guidelines for caseload size for speech-language services in the schools. *Asha* 35 (10), 33–39.

———. (1985). Committee on the Status of Racial Minorities.

———. (1992). Task Force on Clinical Standards. *Preferred Practice Patterns for the Professions of Speech-Language Pathology and Audiology.* Draft for Review. Rockville, MD: American Speech-Language-Hearing Association.

———. (1991a). Council on Professional Standards. Proposed change in scope of ESB accreditation (Revised). *Asha* 33 (11), 63.

———. (1991b). Educational Standards Board. Supervision of student clinicians. *Asha* 33 (6/7), 53.

———. (1990). Guidelines for screening for hearing impairment and middle ear disorders. *Asha* 32 (Supplement 2): 17–24.

———. (1989). Issues in determining eligibility for language intervention. *Asha* 31, 113–18.

———. (1988). Committee on Supportive Personnel. Utilization and employment of speech-language pathology supportive personnel with underserved populations. *Asha* 30 (11), 55–56.

———. (1993). National Joint Committee for the Communicative Needs of Persons with Severe Disabilities.

———. (1985). Committee on Audiologic Evaluation. Guidelines for identification audiometry. *Asha* 27 (5), 49–52.

———. (1984). Committee on Language, Speech, and Hearing Services in the Schools. Guidelines for caseload size for speech-language services in the schools. *Asha* 26 (4), 53–58.

Anderson, K. L. (1991). Hearing conservation in the public schools revisited. In C. Flexer (Ed.). Current audiological issues in the educational management of children with hearing loss. *Seminars in Hearing,* 12 (4), 340–64.

Baker-Hawkins, S. and Easterbrooks, S. (Eds.). (1994). Deaf and hard of hearing students: Educational service guidelines. Alexandria, VA: National Association of State Directors Of Special Education.

Bankson, N. W., and Bernthal, J. E. (1990). *Quick Screen of Phonology.* San Antonio, Texas: Special Press, Inc.

Barrett, M. D., and Welsh, J. W. (1975). Predictive articulation screening. *Language, Speech, and Hearing Services in Schools,* 6, 91–95.

Beitchman, J. H., Nair, R., Clegg, M., and Patel, P. G. (May 1986). Prevalence of speech and language disorders in 5-year old kindergarten children in the Ottawa-Carleton region. *Journal of Speech and Hearing Disorders,* 51, 98–110.

Bender, R. E. (1960). *The Conquest of Deafness.* Cleveland, Ohio: The Press of Western Reserve University.

Berg, F. S. (1987). *Facilitating Classroom Listening: A Handbook for Teachers of Normal and Hard of Hearing Students.* Boston: College-Hill Press.

Bergman, M. (1964). Screening the hearing of preschool children. *Maico Audiological Library Series, III,* Report 4, Maico Electronics, Inc.

Bess, F. H. (1988). *Hearing Impairment in Children.* Parkton, MD: York Press.

Bess, F. H., Dodd-Murphy, J., and Parker, R. (1998). Children with minimal sensorineural hearing Loss: Prevalence, educational performance, and functional status. *Ear and Hearing,* 339–354.

Blachman, B. (1998). Early intervention and phonological awareness. A cautionary tale. In B. Blachman (Ed.). *Foundations of reading acquisition and dyslexia, implications for early intervention.* Mahwah, NJ: Erlbaum.

Blackstone, S. W. (1995). For consumers: Supporting parents and family members. *Augmentative Communication News,* 8 (6), 4–5.

Blosser, J. and DePompei, R. (1994). *Pediatric traumatic brain injury: Proactive intervention.* San Diego, CA: Singular Publishing Group.

Blosser, J. and Kratcoski, A. (1997). PACS: A framework for determining appropriate service delivery options. *Language, Speech, and Hearing Services in Schools,* 28, 99–107.

Blosser, J. and Park, L. (1996). "Kids are Consumers Too" Satisfaction Survey. Annual Convention. Rockville, MD: American Speech-Language-Hearing Association.

Blosser, J., Subich, L., and Ehren, T. (1999). ASHA Functional communication measures: Reliability and validity in the school age population. A final report submitted to the American Speech-Language-Hearing Foundation.

Bluestone, C. D. and Klein, J. D. (1996). Otitis media, atelectasis, and eustachian tube disfunction. In C. D. Bluestone, S. E. Stool, and M. A. Kenna (Eds.). *Pediatric Otaloaryngology* (3rd ed. Vol. 1, pp. 338–582). Philadelphia: Saunders.

Byrne-Saricks, M. C. (June/July 1989). School services and communication disorders. *Asha* 31 (6/7): 79–80.

Caccamo, J. M. (1973). Accountability—A matter of ethics? *Asha* 15: 411–12.

Cappadona, J. (2000). Where we work—Nassau BOCES: Services for schools in the new millennium. *ASHA Leader, 5,* 1.

Catts, H. and Kamhi, A. (Eds.). (1999). *Language and reading disabilities.* Boston, MA: Allyn & Bacon.

Chamberlain, P., and Landurand, P. (1990). Practical considerations—In the assessment of bilingual students. In E. V. Hamayan and J. S. Damico (Eds.) *Limiting bias in the assessment of bilingual students.* Austin, TX: Pro-Ed.

Chomsky, N. (1957). *Syntactic structures.* The Hague: Mouton.

Clark, G. M., Carlson, B. C., Fisher, S., Cook, J. D., and D'Alonzo, B. J. (1991). "Career development for students with disabilities in elementary schools." A position statement of the Division on Career Development. *Career Development for Exceptional Individuals, 14,* 109–120.

Clark, J. G. (1980). Central auditory dysfunction in school children: Compilation suggestions. *Language, Speech, and Hearing Services in Schools.*

Clausen, R., Corley-Keith, M., Gould, N. C., and Lebowitz, S. *Preparation for a due process hearing.* Montgomery County Schools, Rockville, Maryland. Presentation.

The Communication Aid Manufacturers Association (CAMA), 518–26 Davis St. Ste. 211–212, Evanston, IL. 60204-1039; 800-441-CAMA.

Costello, M. R. and Curtis, R. (1989). The Early Years: History of the Michigan Speech, Language and Hearing Association. MSHA *Journal* 23: 20.

Coventry, W. F. and Burstiner, I. (1977). *Management: A Basic Handbook.* Englewood Cliffs, NJ: Prentice-Hall, Inc.

Crais, E. R. (1991). Moving From 'Parent Involvement' to Family-Centered Services. *American Journal of Speech-Language Pathology* 1 (1) (1991): 5–8.

Creaghead, N., Estomin, E., Freilinger, J. J., & Peters-Johnson, C. (1992). Focus on School Issues: Classroom Integration and Collaborative Consultation as Service

Delivery Models. Teleconference, Rockville, MD: American Speech-Language-Hearing Association.

Damico, J. (1987). Addressing language concerns in the schools: The SLP as consultant. *Journal of Childhood Communication Disorders,* 11 (1), 139–179.

Damico, J. S., and Nye, C. (1990). Collaborative issues in multicultural populations. In W. A. Secord and E. H. Wiig (Eds.). *Best practices in school speech-language pathology. collaborative programs in the schools: Concepts, models, and procedures.* San Antonio, TX: The Psychological Corporation.

DeFur, S. H. and Patton, J. R. (1999). *Transition and school-based services.* Austin, TX: PRO-ED.

Donnelly, C. A. (1984). Changing the role of the speech-language pathologist in the public schools. Presentation at the American Speech-Language-Hearing Association Convention, San Francisco, CA.

Downs, M., Mencher, G., Dahle, A., Gerber, S., Stein, L., Cherow, E., and Rubin, M. (1982). Joint Committee on Infant Hearing: Position Statement. *Asha, 24,* 1017–18.

Dublinske, S. (May 1986) Collective bargaining: What can it do for you? *Asha,* 28: 31–34.

Dublinske, S., Minor, B., Hofmeister, L., and Taliaferro, S. (1988). School issues: Effective integration of speech-language services into the regular classroom. Asha Teleconference Seminar. Rockville, MD: The American Speech-Language-Hearing Association.

Dunn, H. M. (June 1949). A speech and hearing program for children in a rural area. *Journal of Speech and Hearing Disorders.* 166–70.

Dustrude, S. R. (May 1990) Thoughts of a speech-language pathologist: An inside perspective. *Computer Users in Speech and Hearing* 6 (1): 46–49.

Eger, D. L. (1997). Outcomes measurement in the schools. In C. M. Fratteli (Ed.). *Measuring Outcomes in Speech-Language Pathology.* New York: Thieme.

Eger, D., Adamczyk, D., Baker, A., Ekin, M. A., Hartman, K., Klein, D., Levy, M. Matta, C., Miller, R., Nalitz, N., Proto, J., Tempalski, D., Veraldi, J., Vukas, C., and Wood., M. (1990). Planned courses: Speech and language program. Exceptional Children's Program, Allegheny Intermediate Unit, Pittsburgh, PA.

Ehren, T. (1999). Developing a professional growth plan for speech-language pathologists. In-service meeting for Broward County School District, Ft. Lauderdale, FL.

Finn, M. S. and Gardner, J. B. (1984). Teacher interview: A better speech-language screening technique. Area Education Agency AEA XI, Ankeny, Iowa and Des Moines Public Schools. The American Speech, Language, Hearing Association Convention. San Francisco, CA.

Flexer, C. (1999). *Facilitating hearing and listening in young children* (2nd ed.). San Diego: Singular Publishing Group, Inc.

Flexer, C. (1992). Management of hearing in an educational setting. In J. G. Alpiner and P. A. McCarthy, *Rehabilitation Audiology: Children and Adults* (2nd ed.). Baltimore, MD: Williams & Wilkins, Inc.

Flexer, C. (1991). Access to communication environments through associative listening devices. *Hearsay: The Journal of the Ohio Speech and Hearing Association,* 6 (1), 9–14.

Flexer, C. (1989) Neglected issues in educational audiology. *Journal of the Aural Rehabilitation Association* 22, 61–66.

Flexer, C., Wray, D., and Ireland, J. (1984). Preferential seating is not enough: Issues in classroom management of hearing-impaired students. *Language, Speech and Hearing Services in Schools, 20,* 11–21.

Flower, R. M. (1984). *Delivery of Speech-Language and Audiology Services.* Baltimore, MD: Williams and Wilkins.

Frattali, C. M. (1998). *Measuring outcome in speech-language pathology.* New York: Thieme.

Frattali, C. M. (1991). From quality assurance to total quality management. *American Journal of Audiology* 1 (1), 41–47.

Frattali, C. M. Quality Assurance Today: Learning the Basics. Adapted from Fratelli, C. "Are We Reaching Our Goals?": Developing Outcome Measures. In P. Larkins (Ed.). *In Search of Quality Assurance: What Lies Ahead?* Rockville, MD: American Speech-Language-Hearing Association.

Gillette, Y. and Robinson, J. (1992). The individualized family service plan: A systematic approach. From The CATCH Guide to planning services with families: Coordinated transition from the hospital to the community and home.

Goldstein, D. and Ehren, T. (1999). Guidelines for supervising speech-language pathology assistants. Broward County School District, Ft. Lauderdale, FL.

Haines, H. H. (1965). Trends in public school therapy. *Asha, 7,* 166–170.

Hales, R. M. and Carlson, L. B. (1992). Issues and trends in special education. Federal Resource Center of Special Education. University of Kentucky.

Halpern, A. S., Herr, C. M., Wolf, N. K., Doren, B., Johnson, M. D., and Lawson, J. D. (1997). *NEXT S.T.E.P.: Student Transition and Educational Planning.* Austin, TX: PRO-ED.

Hanson, M. J., Lynch, E. W., and Wayman, K. I. (1990). Honoring the cultural diversity of families when gathering data. *Topics in Early Childhood Special Education, 10* (1), 112–131.

Harris, G. (1985). Considerations in assessing English language performance in Native American Children. *Topics in Language Disorders.*

Healey, W. C. (April 1973). Notes from the associate secretary for school affairs, task force report on data collection and information systems. *Language, Speech and Hearing Services in Schools,* 4 (2): 57–65.

Hepworth, D., Rooney, R., & Larson, J. (1997). *Direct social work practice: Theory and Skills* (5th ed.). Pacific Grove, CA: Brooks/Cole Publishing.

Hess, R. (1976). Guidelines for a cooperating clinician in working with a student clinician in the schools. *Ohio Journal of Speech and Hearing, 11,* 83–89.

Holzhauser-Peters, L. and Husemann, D. A. (1988). *Alternative service delivery models for more efficient and effective treatment programs.* Alexandria, VA: The Clinical Connection.

Homer, E. M. (1997). Making time in the schools: A program of caseload management. American Speech-Language Hearing Convention.

Huffman, N. (1992). Educational reform: New challenges. *Asha, 34,* 41–44.

Huffman, N. (1995). Education reform: New challenges and messages for speech-language pathologists and audiologists in educational practice. *HEARSAY: The Journal of the Ohio Speech and Hearing Association, 10(1),* 6–12.

Hull, F. M. (1964). National speech and hearing survey interim report. Project NO. 50978. Washington, DC: Department of Health, Education, Bureau of Education for the Handicapped.

Idol, L., Paolucci-Whitcomb, P., and Nevin, A. (1986). *Collaborative consultation.* Rockville, MD: Aspen.

Individuals with Disabilities Education Act of 1990, 20 U.S.C. 1400 *et. seq.*

Individuals with Disabilities Education Act Amendments of 1997, 20, U.S.C. 1400 *et. seq.*

Irwin, R. B. (1959). Speech therapy in the public schools: State legislation and certification. *Journal of Speech and Hearing Disorders,* 24: 127.

Jackson, P. (1986) Akron public schools speech-language priority rating and eligibility service scale. *HEARSAY: The Journal of the Ohio Speech and Hearing Association,* 55–58.

Johnson, A. (1997). ASHA Functional communication measures: Reliability and validity in medical speech-language pathology. A final report submitted to the American Speech-Language-Hearing Foundation.

Kreb, R. (1991). *Third Party Payment for Funding Special Education and Related Services.* Horsham, PA: LRP Publications.

Kulpa, J. I., Blackstone, S., Clarke, C. C., Collingnon, M. M., Griffin, E. B., Hutchins, B. F., Jernigan, L. R.,

Mellott, K. E., Rao, P. R., Fattali, C. M., and Seymour, C. M. (1991) "Chronic communicable diseases and risk management in the schools." *Language, Speech, and Hearing Services in the Schools* 22, 345–52.

Kuster, J. (2001). *Net Connections for communication sciences and disorders.* An Internet guide by Judith Magginis Kuster. <http://www.mnsu.edu/dept/comdis/kuster2>

Lastohkein, T., Glay-Moon, C., and Blosser, J. (1992) "Improving Collaborative Efforts Through the QI Process." *HEARSAY, The Journal of The Ohio Speech and Hearing Association* 7 (1): 19–22.

Lawrence, C., Katz, K., and Linville, J. (1991). Ages of phonological processes suppression: a clinical assessment tool. Poster session presented at The American Speech-Language-Hearing Association Annual Convention. Atlanta, GA.

Leavitt, R. J. (April 1987). Promoting the use of rehabilitation technology. *Asha* 29 (4): 28–31.

Leconte, P. M. (1999). Vocational evaluation. In S. H. deFur and J. R. Patton (Eds.). *Transition and School-Based Services: Interdisciplinary Perspective for Enhancing the Transition Process.* Austin, TX: Pro-Ed.

Leith, W. R. (1984). Handbook of clinical methods in communication disorders. Austin TX: Pro-Ed.

Lesner, S. A. (1991). A practical update in amplification for speech-language pathologists. Ohio Speech and Hearing Convention. Akron, OH.

Levinson, E. M. and Murphy, J. P. (1999). School psychology. In S. H. deFur and J. R. Patton (Eds.). *Transition and School-Based Services: Interdisciplinary Perspectives for Enhancing the Transition Process.* Austin, TX: Pro-Ed.

Listen Foundation. (1991). Five options for teaching deaf and hearing-impaired children. *The Listener.* Englewood, CO: The Listen Foundation, Inc.

Markward, M. and Kurtz, P. D. (1999). School social work. In S. H. deFur and J. R. Patton (Eds.). *Transition and School-Based Services: Interdisciplinary Perspectives for Enhancing the Transition Process.* Austin, TX: Pro-ED.

Marvin, C. A. (1990). Problems in school-based speech-language consultation and collaboration services: Defining the terms and improving the process. In W. A. Secord and E. H. Wiig (Eds.). Best practices in school speech-language pathology collaborative programs in the schools: Concepts, models and procedures. San Antonio, TX: The Psychological Corporation.

Matkin, N. (1991). Educational Audiology Association. Membership application brochure.

Miller, L. (1989). Classroom-based language intervention. *Language, Speech and Hearing Services in Schools,* 27, 122–131.

Montgomery, J. (2000). The role of the school-based speech-language-pathologist vis-à-vis IDEA'97. <http://www.professional.asha.org>

Moore, G. P. and Kester, D. (March 1953). Historical notes on speech correction in the preassociation era." *Journal of Speech and Hearing Disorders, 18,* 48–53.

Moursund, J. (1990). *The process of counseling and therapy.* (2nd ed.). Englewood Cliffs, NJ: Prentice-Hall, Inc.

National Education Goals Panel. (1996). *The National Education Goals Report.* Washington, DC.

National Information Center for Children and Youth with Disabilities (NICHCY). (1993). Transition Summary. Transition services in the IEP. Vol. 3, No. 1, 1–28.

National Institute on Deafness and other Communication Disorders. (1995). Research in human communication. (Annual Report). Bethesda, MD.

National Institutes of Health. (1993). *Early identification of hearing impairment in infants and young children: Consensus development conference.* Bethesda, MD: NIH.

Neidecker, E. A. (1976). Supervision in the school clinician practicum situation: Roles and responsibilities. *Ohio Journal of Speech and Hearing, 10* (Spring 1976).

Nelson, N. (1993). Childhood language disorders in context: Infancy through adolescence. New York: Macmillan.

Nelson, N. W. (1989). Curriculum-based language assessment and instruction. *Language, Speech, and Hearing Services in Schools, 21,* 170–184.

Niskar, A. S., Kieszak, S. M., Holmes, A., Esteban, E., Rubin, C., and Brody, D. J. (1998). Prevalence of hearing loss among children 6 to 19 years: The third National Health and Nutrition Examination Survey. *Journal of the American Medical Association (JAMA), 279,* 1071–1075.

Norris, J. A. and Damico, J. S. (1990). Whole language in theory and practice: Implications for language intervention. *Language, Speech, and Hearing Services in Schools, 2,* 212–20.

Northern, J. L. and Downs, M. P. (1991). *Hearing in Children* (4th ed.). Baltimore: Williams & Wilkins Company.

O'Brien, M. (1991). Third party billing for school services: The school's perspective. *Asha, 33,* 43–45.

O'Toole, T. J. (1971). Accountability and the clinician in the schools. *Speech and Hearing Service in Schools* 3: 24–25.

Ohio Coalition for Equity and Adequacy of School Funding. (1998) Columbus, OH.

Ohio Department of Education, Division of Special Education, Statewide Language Task Force. (1991).

Ohio handbook for the identification, evaluation, and placement of children with language problems. Columbus, OH: Ohio Department of Education.

Ohio Department of Health Hearing Advisory Committee. (1990). *Policies for hearing conservation programs for children: Requirements and recommendations.* Columbus, OH: Ohio Department of Health.

Orelove, F. P. and Sobsey, D. (1996). *Educating children with multiple disabilities: A transdisciplinary approach* (3rd ed.). Baltimore: Brookes.

Osberger, M., Moeller, M., Eccarius, M., Robbins, A., and Johnson, D. (1986). Expressive language skills. In M. Osberger (Ed.). Language and learning skills in hearing impaired students. *ASHA Monographs,* 23, 54–65.

Paden, E. P. (1970). *A History of the American Speech and Hearing Association 1925–1958.* Washington DC: American Speech and Hearing Association.

Patton, J. R. and Dunn, C. (1998). *Transition from school to young adulthood: Basic concepts and recommended practices.* Austin, TX: PRO-ED.

Paul-Brown, D. (1995). Clinical record keeping in audiology and speech-language pathology. Rockville, MD: The American Speech-Language-Hearing Association.

Paul-Brown, D. (1991). *Communication Problems of Adolescents: Identification, Impact, Intervention.* Presentation to The New York Branch of the Orton Dyslexia Society Annual Conference

Pediatric Otolaryngology (3rd ed. Vol. 1, pp. 338–582). Philadelphia: Saunders.

Pershey, M. G. (1998). Collaboration models and projected outcomes for school-based language therapy: Sampling the buffet. *HEARSAY, The Journal of The Ohio Speech and Hearing Association, 12, 1,* 32–38. Columbus, OH.

Peters-Johnson, C. (1990). Medicaid and third-party reimbursement for schools. *Language, Speech, and Hearing Services in the Schools* 21 (2), 121.

Peterson, H. A. and Marquardt, T. P. (1990). *Appraisal and Diagnosis of Speech and Language Disorders.* Englewood Cliffs, NJ: Prentice-Hall, Inc.

Phillips, P. (1975). *Speech and Hearing Problems in the Classroom.* Lincoln, Nebraska: Cliff Notes, Inc.

Power-deFur, L. (October 1999). Medicaid billing in public schools: Is this health care or education? Special Interest Division 11: Administration and Supervision. Rockville, MD: American Speech-Language-Hearing Association.

Prentke-Romich. (1989). *How to Obtain Funding for Augmentative Communication Devices.* Wooster, OH: Prentke-Romich Company.

Public Agenda Online. (1999). Overview: The issue at a glance. <http://www.publicagenda.org>

Quigley, S. P. and Kretschmer, R. E. (1982). *The education of deaf children.* Baltimore, MD: University Park Press.

Rebore, R. W. Sr (1984). *A Handbook for School Board Members.* Englewood Cliffs, NJ: Prentice Hall, Inc.

Reed, V. A. and Miles, M. C. (1989). *Adolescent Language Disorders: A Video Inservice for Educators.* Eau Claire, WI: Thinking Publications.

Reinhartsen, D., Edmondson, R., and Pierce, D. (1995). Technology for Infants and Toddlers Made Easy. North Carolina Department of Human Resources, Division of Developmental Disabilities/Mental Retardation/Substance Abuse and the North Carolina Department of Environment, Health and Natural Resources, Division of Maternal and Child Health.

Reynolds, M. C. and Rosen, S. W. (May 1976). Special Education: Past, Present, and Future. *The Educational Forum, 40,* 551–62.

Ribbler, N. (1999). Sample professional growth plan for a speech-language pathologist in Broward County School District, Ft. Lauderdale, FL.

Ross, M. and Giolas, T. G. (Eds.). (1978). *Auditory Management of Hearing-Impaired Children.* Baltimore, MD: University Park Press.

Ross, M., Brackett, D., and Maxon, A. (1982). *Hard of hearing children in regular schools.* Englewood Cliffs, NJ: Prentice Hall, Inc.

Rothstein, R. (1998). Where's the money going? Economic Policy Institute. The American School Board Journal.

Rules for the Education of Handicapped Children, (1982). Worthingon: Ohio Department of Education, Division of Special Education.

Savage, R. (1994). Identification, classification, and placement issues for students with traumatic brain injury. In J. Blosser and R. DePompei (Eds.). *Journal of Head Trauma Rehabilitation: School Reentry Following Head Injury, 6* (1), 1–9.

Scarvel, L. D. (1997). Standardizing Criteria for Evaluating Physical Facilities and Organizational Patterns of Speech, Language and Hearing Programs. *The Journal of the Pennsylvania Speech and Hearing Association* 10, 17–19.

Schoolfield, L. (1937). *Better speech and better reading.* Magnolia, MA: The Expression Company.

Shepherd, J. and Inge, K. J. (1999). Occupational and physical therapy. In S. H. deFur and J. R. Patton (Eds.). *Transition and School-Based Services: Interdisciplinary Perspectives for Enhancing the Transition Process.* Austin, TX: Pro-Ed.

Shibley, R. (1998). Ohio Newsline. Nationally, paperwork is number 1 obstacle for special education teachers. The Ohio Federation Council for Exceptional Children. Issue 3, pg. 4. Cleveland, OH.

Silverman, F. H. (1989). *Communication for the Speechless.* Englewood Cliffs, NJ: Prentice Hall, Inc.

Simon, C. S. (1987). Out of the broom closet and into the classroom: The emerging SLP. *Journal of Childhood Communication Disorders, 2(1),* 41–46.

Spady, W. G. (1994). *Outcome-Based Education: Critical Issues and Answers.* Arlington, VA: The American Association of School Administrators.

Steer, M. D. (July 1961). Public school speech and hearing services. A special report prepared with support of the United States Office of Education and Purdue University. *Journal of Speech and Hearing Disorder, Monograph Supplement 8:* Washington, DC: U.S. Office of Education Cooperative Research Project No. 649 (8191).

Sudler, W. H. and Flexer, C. (October 1986). Low cost assistive listening device. *Language, Speech and Hearing Services in the Schools, 17,* 342–43.

Swift, W. B. (April 1972). How to begin speech correction in the public schools. *Language, Speech and Hearing Services in the Schools, 3,* 51–56.

Terrell, B. Y. and Hale, J. E. (1992). Serving a multicultural population: Different learning styles. *American Journal of Speech-Language Pathology, 1 (2),* 5–8.

U.S. Congress. (1997). Individuals with Disabilities Education Act of 1997. (IDEA97; Public Law 105-17). *Federal Register.*

U.S. Congress. (1991). National Literacy Act of 1991 (Public Law 102-73). *Federal Register.*

U.S. Department of Education. (1998). To assure the free appropriate public education of all Americans: Twentieth annual report to Congress on the implementation of the Individuals with Disabilities Act (Pub No 1998-716-372/93547). Washington, DC: U.S. Government Printing Office.

U.S. Department of Education. America Reads Challenge. (1997). Read "right" now. Washington, DC: Author.

U.S. Department of Education. (1991). *Thirteenth Annual Report to Congress on the Implementation of The Individuals with Disabilities Education Act.* Washington, DC: U.S. Department of Education, Office of Special Education Programs.

U.S. Department of Labor. (1979). *Dictionary of Occupational Titles.* Washington, DC, United States Government Printing Office.

Van Riper, C. and Erikson, R. L. (1973). *Predictive Screening Test of Articulation,* 3rd ed. Kalamazoo: Continuing Education Office, Western Michigan University.

Vanderheiden, G. C. and Lloyd, L. L. (1986). Communication systems and their components. In S. W. Blackstone and D. M. Bruskin (Eds.). *Augmentative Communication: An Introduction,* 49–161. Rockville, MD: The American Speech-Language-Hearing Association.

Vanderheiden, G. C. and Yoder, D. E. (1986) Overview. In S. W. Blackstone and D. M. Bruskin (Eds.). *Augmentative Communication: An Introduction,* 1–28. Rockville, MD: The American Speech-Language-Hearing Association.

Wehman, P. (1992). Life beyond the classroom: Transition strategies for young people with disabilities. Baltimore, MD: Paul H. Brooks Publishing Co.

Weinberger, H. (Ed.). (1990). The BGSU University supervisor. Bowling Green, OH: Office of Field Experiences, College of Education and Allied Professions, Bowling Green State University.

Weiner, F. and Wacker, R. (1982). The development of phonology in unintelligible speakers. In N. Lass (Ed.). *Speech Advances in Basic Research and Practice 8,* 51–125. New York: Academic Press.

Westman, M. J. and Broen, P. A. (1989). Preschool Screening for Predictive Articulation Errors. *Language, Speech, and Hearing Services in the Schools, 20,* 139–48.

Wiig, E. & Secord, W. (1991). Best practices in school speech-language pathology. San Antonio, TX: The Psychological Corporation.

Wing, D. M. (January 1975) A data recording form for case management and accountability. *Language, Speech and Hearing Services in Schools* 6: 38–40.

Work, R. S. (1989) "Statewide eligibility criteria for programs for the speech and language impaired of florida." *Tejas* XV: 33–34.

World Health Organization. (1980). International classification of impairments, disabilities, and handicaps. Geneva, Switzerland: Author.

Yorkston, K. M. and Karlan, G. (1986). Assessment procedures. In S. W. Blackstone and D. M. Bruskin (Eds.), *Augmentative Communication: An Introduction,* 163–96. Rockville, MD: The American Speech-Language-Hearing Association.

SUBJECT INDEX

RUMBLE, YOUNG MAN, RUMBLE

RUMBLE, YOUNG MAN, RUMBLE

BENJAMIN CAVELL

F
CAVE

ALFRED A. KNOPF ✦ NEW YORK 2003

This Is a Borzoi Book Published by Alfred A. Knopf
Copyright © 2003 by Benjamin Cavell

All rights reserved under International and Pan-American
Copyright Conventions
Published in the United States by Alfred A. Knopf, a
division of Random House, Inc., New York, and simultaneously in Canada
by Random House of Canada Limited, Toronto. Distributed by
Random House, Inc., New York.
www.aaknopf.com

Knopf, Borzoi Books, and the colophon are registered
trademarks of Random House, Inc.

Library of Congress Cataloging-in-Publication Data
Cavell, Benjamin.
Rumble, young man, rumble / Benjamin Cavell.— 1st ed.
p.   cm.
ISBN 0-375-41464-9 (alk. paper)
1. Young men—Fiction.   I. Title.

PS3603.A9 R8 2003
813'.6—dc21   2002027525

Manufactured in the United States of America
First Edition

TO MY MOTHER AND FATHER

THE HANDS CAN'T HIT WHAT THE EYES CAN'T SEE.
FLOAT LIKE A BUTTERFLY, STING LIKE A BEE.
RUMBLE, YOUNG MAN, RUMBLE.

—Bundini

CONTENTS

RUMBLE, YOUNG MAN, RUMBLE

BALLS, BALLS, BALLS

On Thursday, a man comes into the store and asks me how to kill his wife. I know, because it's my business to know, that what he really wants to ask is how to kill his wife and not get caught.

The man wears a short-sleeved button-down shirt and dark blue Dockers. His face is cratered with acne scars. It looks like the surface of the moon. I know without being told that this man works at one of the tech firms that have sprung up in the last year or so all along the road from Albany. He has never lifted a weight in his life. He has probably never been in a fight. He has never even been paintballing. But for some reason I feel sorry for this poor, bony fool and so I ask him whether he has a gas furnace.

I explain how to drill a hole in the main line that will allow a tiny stream of gas to trickle into his basement. The emission is so gradual that his wife is unlikely to notice. This is less detectable than disabling the pilot light on a gas stove. Also, it's more controllable than blocking the return-air vents and filling the house with carbon monoxide. Then I tell him that he'll need a spark.

The spark can come from anything. The static electricity

of shoes scuffing a rug, the momentary discharge from the flipping of a light switch, the red power light on a clock radio that usually clicks on when the alarm sounds, a lightbulb that has been filled with gasoline and then screwed back into the socket—each can become a trigger that will *turn out all the lights*, if he knows what I mean. He does. He buys the Taskmaster Tool Kit (Deluxe Set), $179.99 on sale.

In the afternoon, I tell a nineteen-year-old in a fatigue jacket how to make napalm from gasoline and frozen orange juice concentrate (just mix equal parts—diet cola and gasoline works also) and then he buys a superthin Maxi-Grip C-series folding knife ($124.99)—which can be concealed in a boot or even inside a shirt collar for easy access—and a telescoping graphite police baton ($64.95). I tell him two stories about my time in the SEALs and show him my tattoo of Freddie the Frogman and then sell him *The Mercenary's Guide to Urban Survival* ($19.99, paperback), and he leaves smiling and even salutes me, almost dropping his new baton.

The tattoo is temporary (I got a whole box of them two years ago at a novelty shop in Jersey City) and I've never been in the Navy. I've never even been farther than Philadelphia. And I can't swim.

My name is Logan Bryant. I sell sporting goods.

Actually, I sell sporting goods, hardware, athletic equipment, patio furniture, barbecue grills and hobby literature.

But don't get me wrong: I'm not just some wanna-be. Truth is, I *could* have been a SEAL if I'd ever bothered to learn to swim. I hold at least a green belt in several fighting disciplines and am nearly a black belt in Thai kickboxing (I just haven't had time to take the test). I am the uncontested star of what is generally acknowledged to be the fourth-best paintball team in the tristate area. (We were scheduled to compete for the national title on ESPN2 but were scratched at the last second. Politics.) I have a full collection of green and brown face paint in various shades. I was All-Conference at middle linebacker my junior year of high school and would have been All-State or maybe even Honorable Mention All-America the next year if I hadn't quit. I used to have subscriptions to *Soldier of Fortune* and *Guns and Ammo* until Barry told me that no one reads those anymore. Also, I am confident in my willingness to take the life of another human being.

And I can almost bench-press three eighty-five.

Barry arrives as Lou and I are totaling Thursday's receipts. Lou nods to him and Barry swaggers around a standing rack of catcher's mitts and ducks under the counter. Barry is wearing a lime-green New York Jets warm-up jacket.

"The average American," I am telling Lou, "has an IQ around seventy-three. At that level of intellect, even basic functioning requires considerable effort. Decisions that you or I would consider simple border on impossible for Joe Citizen. That's why people are so easily swayed by celebrity pitchmen and Oprah Winfrey and demonstrations of the new-and-improved Spic and Span. That's why a presidential candidate can give the same speech over and over—they're all talking to five-year-olds. People are just like children."

"But all people *were* children at one point," Lou says.

"So?"

"So, if they're children now, what were they then?"

I sigh. "I'm trying to illustrate a point."

"And what is that?"

"What is what?"

"The *point,* guy, the *point.*"

"My point is that people, for the most part, have no understanding of the realities of the world. That's why it's so easy for guys like you and me to get ahead."

Lou finishes with his receipts and lays them down on the counter in a neat stack. "Isn't that the same point you made on Monday?"

"No," I say, exasperated. "My point on Monday was that college degrees are meaningless and that the only useful intelligence is street smarts. And that guys like you and me should really be running this country—and *would* be if we had little pieces of paper that said we'd gone to Princeton. Also, my point on Monday was based on the figure they released over the weekend, which put the average national IQ around seventy-six. In light of the most recent data, the conclusions must be even more extreme."

"And who," Lou says, "is compiling this data?"

I stare at him. "What do you mean? It's a study."

"By who?" He smiles. "Who's 'they'?"

Before I can answer, Barry says, "Do you doubt what he's saying, Louie?"

Lou shrugs. "I just don't know if people are so dumb."

"Don't *know*," Barry says. "Look around you, man. We have the corrupt, liberal media. We have unchecked and unquestioned federal power. We have suppression of the First *and* Second Amendments, babies being murdered, kids' shows that promote homosexuality, twenty-four-hour music videos, political correctness, celebrity magazines that promote homosexuality, celebrity talk shows, school shootings, celebrity profiles, celebrity political campaigns, celebrity fund-raisers for homosexual causes. This country is in the midst of a moral, racial, political, economic, social, sexual, military, environmental, educational, moral, fiscal, ethical, moral, class-based, moral crisis. We have forgotten our morality. We need a leader with *character*, who can provide moral stewardship and protect our kids from nudity and foul language and violence in the media and from entertainment with a homosexual agenda and who will institute a foreign policy to keep the ragheads in check *and* who has the compassion necessary to phase out the welfare system that lets *fifty million* unwed, teenage black mothers live lazily in the veritable lap of luxury by sucking on the overtaxed teat of real, hardworking Americans. Instead, we get these goddamn midwestern smooth talkers, chosen—by *fifty-three percent* of voters according to the most recent statistics—on the basis of *height*, for Chrissake. And you don't know if people are dumb?"

I watch Lou triumphantly.

"That's quite a speech," he says.

"Damn right," Barry says. "I always have one ready for you goddamn bleeding hearts."

Lou frowns. "Are you sure there are fifty million black girls on welfare?"

"Sure I'm sure," Barry tells him.

I'm tired of losing," Barry says.

"At paintball?" I say.

"That's right."

"We don't lose too often."

"Often enough."

We're at our gym, which is called Size, and Barry and I are taking turns on the leg press. He is wearing a tan leather weight belt to support his lower back. I pull the pin out of the weight stack—it was at two hundred, the weight Barry uses—and slide it into the hole marked four twenty-five.

There are only a few sluts in the weight room, stretching on the mats in the corner or else working on the lat pull-down, all of them dressed in spandex and string-strapped tank tops. I wait until a few of them are done with their various sets and then I lie back on the red-padded machine and set my feet shoulder width on the dimpled metal plate and push hard against it. The rack I am on slides away from the unmoving metal plate, and next to me four hundred twenty-five pounds of Bodysmith Nautilus weights creak upward in a quivering pile.

I can't see anything but the white plaster of the ceiling, but I know the sluts must be looking. Even if they hadn't already noticed me, the sound would have gotten their attention.

The ideal weight-lifting sound is never very loud. If you scream, you look like you're trying too hard. The sound should combine the moan of sex with a muted angry roar. It should grow louder with each repetition, ending at about the same volume as a normal speaking voice.

When I am finished with the set, I sit up with my legs hanging off the edge of the machine and blot my face with a towel, looking out the side of my eye at one of the wall-size mirrors, inspecting the veins on my arms and the bulges of my chest and shoulders under the T-shirt.

I stand and Barry lies down for his next set.

"I've decided to bring in an expert," he says.

"What kind of expert?"

"You know—an operator, a specialist, a mechanic."

"Like a mercenary?"

He glances around us to see if anyone heard and motions for me to lean toward him, and when I do, says, "Like a mercenary."

I keep my breathing normal. "Where's he from?"

Barry smiles, our faces still close together, and says, "Israel, I think."

"Why Israel?"

"Because they're experienced."

I groan. "But they don't even *lift*. He probably has skinny little arms."

Barry stares at me.

"Also," I say, "what does some *yid* have to teach me about being hard?"

"He might know more about it than you think. And don't say 'yid.' "

"Sorry, but this all comes as quite a shock."

"He'll be here for our morning session on Saturday."
He waves for me to move away from him and starts his set.

I n the locker room, after we shower, Barry and I examine each other's bodies and give constructive criticism. I know this sounds bad, but I just want to assure everyone that I'm not a fag. In fact, I would hate fags except that I read somewhere that hating fags meant you were a fag yourself. So I don't hate them. I'm just not one. Really.

M y apartment looks onto a grassless soccer field and the abandoned hulk of a paper mill and then onto the bright gray surface of Route 90, stretched out between banks of rust-colored trees, separated from the soccer field by a chain-link fence.

I turn on the television and slouch, sore-limbed, on the sofa. I drink a ready-mixed vanilla Met-Rx. The light from the television flickers across my face as I prepare the hypodermic and line up the bottles of pills—Dianabol, Nolvadex, Maxibolin, creatine phosphate. After I swallow the pills, I give myself the injection of B-12 and, so that doesn't keep me up all night, follow it with two Seconal capsules the color of velvet-red cherries. I take four chalk-white zinc pills to keep the steroids from putting zits on my back and then I lie back and watch the bright gray screen.

The champion has teased hair and a sequined dress. She sings "I'm Still Here." She is seven years old. She would like to thank God and her parents. She smiles all the time. The judges give her three and a half stars.

The challenger is an eleven-year-old boy with blond hair that flops over the sides of his head. He smiles wider than the girl. He sings "Yankee Doodle Dandy," marching energetically in place. Suddenly, I have a vision of this boy in fifteen years, bruised, crying, track marks all along his arms. He is curled in a ball on the floor grabbing at the ankles of a V-bodied stud in leather pants. The big stud is saying, "It's over, Julian. It's . . . over."

The judges give the challenger two and three-quarters stars.

The Seconals take hold and I am drifting and my chin sags to touch my chest. My eyelids droop closed and then pop open and droop closed again and do this over and over until finally they do not open anymore and I am asleep and the television is saying, "Kill, kill, kill."

On Friday morning a blond slut in a purple tank top comes into the store and asks me about recumbent stationary bicycles. I am wearing a dark blue T-shirt with the Navy SEAL crest over the heart and UNITED STATES NAVY SEAL TEAMS across the back in white. The sleeves hug my biceps. My jeans are dark and boot-cut (I never wear a taper). My boots are tan Timberlands ($59.99 with the staff discount).

The slut stares at me hungrily. I lift up my T-shirt, using the bottom to wipe some imaginary grime from underneath my eye, showing her the cobblestone abs and the striations of the obliques.

"Are you an athlete?" she asks.

"I'm captain of the store paintball team."

"Are you any good?"

"Bill Cookston said I was almost the best he ever saw. He said I could make any team I wanted, including Shockwave."

"What's that?"

"You've never heard of Shockwave? They're only the winningest team in the *history* of the World Cup of paintball."

"So, were you guys ever in that tournament on ESPN?" she says.

I snort. "ESPN."

"I thought those guys were the best."

"That's what a lot of people think," I say. "But for the serious MilSim competitor, that stuff is a sellout. It dilutes the purity of the sport."

"What's MilSim?"

I look at her for a few seconds and then say, "Military Simulation. What do you think we're talking about?"

"I thought it was called war games."

I can feel the muscles tighten in my shoulders. "It's not a game."

"Sorry."

"Don't worry about it," I say, teeth clenched.

To calm myself, I put my hand on the seat of the Ergometer 9000 with optional heart-rate monitor and reading rack ($1,499.95).

"The recumbent feature," I say carefully, "is particularly important if there will be any men riding the unit. Studies have shown that the upright models tend to promote impotence."

"How do they do that?"

"Excuse me?"

"Promote impotence. The upright bicycles. How do they do it?"

"Well . . . I believe it has something to do with"—I look around for Lou, but I don't see him anywhere—"with the ah . . . the heat of the testicle walls."

Stevie is the only other salesman on the floor. He is showing a Merry Men compound bow ($334.99) to a fat-body in jungle camouflage complete with bush hat. I catch Stevie's eye and he says something to the fat-body and walks toward me. The fat-body lays down the bow and begins fingering various arrowheads and stroking his thick mustache.

"Hello," Stevie says when he reaches us.

"Hello," the slut says. She is looking at Stevie with the same expression she had when I showed her my stomach.

Stevie is taller than I am, but thin, and I wonder whether I am misreading her reaction.

"I was just explaining how upright bicycles cause impotence by overheating the testicle walls," I say.

"Well," Stevie says, smiling at me, "of course, that's part of it. Also, the pressure restricts blood flow and damages the soft tissue."

He walks the slut toward the displays of upright bicycles.

When erect, my cock is nine and a half inches long and as thick as some men's wrists. A year ago, Stevie started working at the store and I heard from some slut we both know that he was packing almost eleven. Since then I have been seriously considering the experimental penile-enlargement surgery, which has been performed (I understand) with great success by two doctors in Sweden.

On the way into Champagne Dreams, the bar we go to on Friday nights, Barry points out two men in suits standing on the corner and tells me that they could be from the secret police.

I say, "This country doesn't have any secret police." I frown. "At least, I've never heard of any."

Barry shakes his head. "Why do you think they call them *secret*?"

Inside, the place glows blue and orange from neon signs that hang outside the windows. The room is full of sluts dressed to show their belly buttons and the narrow strip of skin between their inflated breasts.

"I could never fuck a girl with a tit job," Lou says.

"I don't care if she's had a tit job," I say, "as long as she *looks* like she's had one. And not one of these cut-rate three-grand hack jobs where you can still see the scar. I'm talking about seven thousand *per*."

Ken, who is the fifth member of our paintball team and the only one who doesn't work at the store, is sitting in a horseshoe-shaped corner booth with two brunette sluts. We all slide into the booth, the sluts crowding closer to Ken to make room.

The slut sitting next to Barry looks at the gold that glitters on each of his fingers (including the thumb) and at his platinum necklace, which she probably thinks is silver, and asks him what he does for a living.

"I own a store called Balls, Balls, Balls," Barry says.

"On the highway? 'Everything for the New American Sportsman,' or something like that?"

"That's the one."

"And what about the rest of you?" the other slut says.

"They work for me," Barry says. "Except for Ken. But he used to."

"So you're the boss," she says.

Later, Barry and I will take turns fucking these sluts. We'll tie them up. We'll beat them with phone cords and Spiritbreaker riding crops (two for $79.50). But now I just smile at them and then I go to the bar.

Waiting for the drinks, I talk to Samson Taylor, who is the largest man I know. He is slumped, sullen, close to the surface of the bar. In the dimness the features of his face are nearly indistinguishable. He is a gray-haired, mahogany mountain.

"How many years you play, again?" I ask him.

"Five," he says, his eyes closed.

"All in Minnesota?"

"Yeah."

"So, why'd you stop so early?"

He sighs. "Can we not talk about this right now?"

"Sure, sure. Whatever you want. I heard it was drugs."

"You shouldn't believe everything you hear."

"What do you mean?"

He shrugs.

"Barry's bringing in a professional," I say, "to help with our training. He gets here in the morning. I'm worried that Jew fuck is trying to phase me out of the team. I practically *built* that team for him. You think they'd be fourth-best without me? The fuck they would. None of those bitches has my skills."

He puts one of his enormous hands on my forearm and I almost jerk away. I stare at the hand, imagining that I can smell the blackness rising from it.

"You're my friend, right?" he asks.

"Of course."

"Then leave me alone a while."

"Okay. Leave you alone. No problem. Done and *done*."

He removes his hand from my arm and I take a deep breath.

"I knew you'd understand," he says. "You're the only one who understands."

The bartender brings my drinks and pours two more shots for Samson, who does not open his eyes but smiles slightly when he hears the shots set down in front of him. A tear dribbles down his cheek.

I walk back to the booth, thinking that Samson Taylor is not as tough as I thought.

I am nervous that my cock shrinks too much when it's limp. I read once that black guys don't actually have larger dicks, it's just that they grow less, so they walk around bigger.

Sometimes I even wonder whether I am really as good as I think, whether all the sluts who have screamed my name and begged for more, more, more weren't in it for the sex but were trying to attach themselves to my rising star. I have heard that, sooner or later, all great men have that worry.

One slut I used to know—I think her name was Laura—told me when I broke up with her that I was selfish in bed.

I said, "I tried to give you everything I have. You're just not deep enough."

I drive Ken and Stevie to practice on Saturday morning in my black Pathfinder, which I got for *well* under the list price from some Panamanians Barry knows.

I have the tuner set to National Public Radio.

The host of the show says, "We're talking America's foreign policy woes. Do you have the solution? Our lines are open."

Sitting in the passenger seat, Ken says, "How can you take this crap?"

I say, "I need to have the information."

"This isn't information, it's opinion."

I wave him off. "It's not my fault if you don't care about being educated."

"But they're all so self-satisfied."

"It's a small price to pay."

He shakes his head. "Carl Kassel can kiss Ken's crevice."

" 'Crack,' " Stevie says from the backseat.

"What?"

"Use 'crack.' It's funnier."

"There's nothing funny about using crack."

"I mean instead of 'crevice.' "

Ken turns around in his seat to look at him. "Just say no, guy."

The practice site is a replica of a few blocks from Beirut circa 1985, contained inside an immense warehouse that is owned by a paintball-organizing company called Marked for Dead. When we arrive, all of us dressed in gray-and-white urban-camouflage jumpsuits, Barry is there already, standing next to a full-scale model of a bombed schoolhouse. He is with Lou and a man I don't recognize. My heart is thumping fast. My face has begun to sweat.

When we reach them, Barry introduces us to the new man, whose name is Jack.

"Jack what?" Ken says.

"Just Jack," Barry tells him.

"Like Madonna," Stevie says.

Jack smiles. "That's right."

He is my height and twenty pounds lighter, which is considerably larger than I imagined. Even so, I doubt he can bench-press three-fifteen. But he *is* thick through the shoulders and awfully cut, the veins in his arms raised like seams. I get a view of him in profile and, I have to admit, he doesn't look too kikey. His nose is short and broad. His head is shaved almost to the scalp. His skin is as dark as mine. I wonder where he does his tanning.

He is wearing a light blue short-sleeved flannel shirt and beige pants, which are made from a horrible, coarse-looking material but which, as far as I can see, do not taper. His shoes are low-top boots that are probably not *half* as expensive as my Timberlands (if I had paid full price), although they might be more durable.

"How old are you?" I ask him.

"Thirty."

"Mmm," I say, "I would have guessed older. But still, thirty might be a little old for this business. Killing, as I'm sure you know, is young men's work."

"I'll be all right."

"Your English is pretty good."

He looks at me for a moment. "I'm from Pittsburgh."

"Barry said you were from Israel."

He shrugs. "I worked there for a while."

"What did you do before that?"

"I was in the Navy."

"Doing what?" Stevie asks.

Jack shrugs again. "Let's just say I wasn't a sailor."

My face is suddenly hot. I sit down on the charred remains of a swing set and lean my head down, pretending to retie my boots, hoping that no one will notice.

Jack makes us run laps around the inside of the warehouse to warm up. He keeps us running for forty minutes. When we stop, I open my duffel bag. Sweat stings my eyes. I take out my goggles, which are made by V-Shock. I put on the goggles and then take out the face mask (also by V-Shock). Jack looks at the mask.

"What are you putting on a mask for?" he says. "This is paint*ball*, not paint*pussy*. Not paint*ovary*. I see why you guys never win."

I open my mouth, but I can't make a sound, so I begin setting up my weapon, which is a Hicap 180-round front-loader with Trimount sight rail and TF90 reflex sight, all from Gods of War. I walk to the high-pressure air pump behind the jagged ruins of a small apartment building and fill the gun's tank (I *never* use carbon dioxide for propulsion).

When I come back, Jack is checking the sight of a pistol that looks like a Beretta automatic.

"Who makes that?" I say. "Spyder? Hardboilers? Gods of War? Bloodsports?"

"No," he says.

"Who then? It looks so real."

He glances up at me. "It *is* real."

Somebody once told me that the average man experiences his greatest rate of hair loss at age twenty-three, so for the last five years (since my twenty-first birthday) I have been using Rogaine (Maximum Strength formula) twice a day, every day. I haven't detected any sign of fallout.

· · ·

Sitting on the sofa Saturday night after practice, too tired to move, waiting for the Seconals to kick in, I hear one of the square-jawed network anchormen say that the average American now has an IQ of seventy-one. He starts a story about the stock market and then interrupts himself for breaking news: the national IQ has dropped below sixty. This has resulted in record sell-offs. While he is telling me this, the IQ drops to fifty-three, then to forty-seven. As I succumb to the Seconals, the number continues to plummet. By the time I am completely surrounded by blackness, it is approaching twenty.

For Sunday's practice, we are simulating night fighting. All the windows are covered with blackout blankets. The ceiling of the warehouse is a glowing map of stars with a perfectly rounded moon in the center. The bomb-cratered buildings of our Beirut are lit dimly with recessed floor lights and dull floodlights that line the edges of the course. We sit on broken seesaws in the playground beside the schoolhouse, waiting for our eyes to adjust to the gloom.

"He's not such hot shit," I am whispering to Lou. "It's not like he was in Vietnam or anything. All he's done is ran a lot and swam a lot, and jumped out of some planes. Big deal. I've sky-dived; you've sky-dived."

"I don't know," Lou says. "He seems to know what he's doing."

"He *can't* be better than I am."

We practice house-to-house assaults. Door kicking, Jack calls it. Cardboard silhouettes pop up to confront us as we enter some of the ruined houses and we pepper the targets with small yellow blotches. Occasionally we shoot each other.

We break after finishing each block. During the second-to-last break, all of us lying on the floor of a gutted, roofless mosque, Jack sits next to me and looks at the false sky.

"You have anything you want to say to me, Logan?"

I feel the muscles behind my testicles contract, but I keep my voice as normal as I can and say, "I've been wondering how much combat experience you've had."

"Ah," he says.

"Because I personally don't like someone passing themselves off as some kind of expert when they don't have the *credentials*. Playing soldier in California doesn't do much for me. I mean, being able to swim don't make you a dolphin."

"Mmm," Jack says, nodding. He reaches into the front pocket of his tan windbreaker and comes out with a crumpled pack of Pall Mall unfiltereds.

I smile at him, little chills of relief running along my spine. "You know, everything I've read says that commandos shouldn't smoke. Especially in the dark. Ruins the night vision."

He ignores me, lighting one of the cigarettes and sucking on it until the tip glows orange.

"Don't feel bad that you didn't know," I say, dizzy from the chills. "You've probably never been on long patrol."

He takes the cigarette out of his mouth and looks at me and then presses the burning end to the back of his hand and holds it there as we listen to the quiet sizzling. His expression does not change.

"Jesus Christ," Stevie says.

I feel the circular exterior wall of the mosque begin spinning around us. The stars twinkle like strobe lights. Gray smoke floats from under the edges of the cigarette. Ken and Barry have their hands held against their eyes.

Jack stares at me all the time, not blinking, grinding the flaming tip into his hand. My chills have disappeared. My mouth is hanging open. And then I feel nothing. I cannot move. All I can do is watch the gleaming coal of the cigarette reflected in Jack's eyes.

• • •

can't remember anything else until we are sitting in our booth at Champagne Dreams. Jack is there, laughing with Lou and Stevie. They are talking about Bosnia. I lean my mouth close to Ken's ear. "*Lots* of guys can put cigarettes out on their hands," I whisper.

"Not lots," Ken whispers back.

"I must've seen it in a hundred movies."

"That's *movies*, guy. Can *you* do it?"

"I think so," I say.

Ken shakes his head and turns away from me. I walk to the bar, dazed.

Samson Taylor is in his usual seat, a line of empty shot glasses in front of him. I sit down next to him.

"I thought about what you said," he tells me.

"Yes," I say.

"About the expert. I don't think it's a real challenge to you. I mean, you know Sugar Ray Robinson was a better fighter than the guys who trained him."

"What are you talking about?"

"Sometimes the guy with the knowledge isn't the guy with the skills."

I look at the sluts around the room and wonder how many people know what happened with the cigarette.

"You know," I say to Samson Taylor, "you really are a silly nigger."

"What?" He is blinking, trying to focus his eyes.

"You," I say. "Are. A. Silly. Nigger."

"I don't understand."

"What's to understand?"

"You're my friend."

"Bullshit. I'm not friends with silly-nigger winos. No wonder your kids won't see you. I wouldn't either."

There are tears running down his cheeks. "No," he says. "No, no, no, no."

"What do you mean, no?"

"You're my friend. My friend."

"Wrong, nigger. I'm better than you." I look around the
bar. "I'm better than all these stinking people. I'm the kind
of man who knows how to get ahead. You're nobody. That's
why somebody else gets to fuck your wife every night."
He groans.
"Do you wonder about it?" I say. "You must. You must
wonder if she likes it, if she makes different noises with him
than she did with you. Maybe that's why she left—you
couldn't make her scream."

His groan turns into a growl and then into a roar, and his
tree-trunk arm comes around, much faster than I was expecting, and knocks me off the stool and onto the floor. He stands
over me, his bulk blocking out everything else. He picks up
the stool to smash on my head and I brace for it and then
there is someone on his back, who I think might be Stevie,
and there is someone else hanging from one of his arms.
Then there is confusion and bodies flying through the air
above my head and then there is a moment of calm and I see
that Samson has thrown off everybody and lifted the stool
again and I can only see one other person, who is standing
behind Samson and to the side and has one arm extended
with a handgun on the end of it. The gun is pointed at Samson's temple, but he does not notice. We are frozen like that.

Then Samson screams again and hurls the stool against a
wall and runs out of the bar. I can hear him roaring in the
street. I sit up.

Jack is standing above me, his arm still extended, the pistol held steadily in his hand, sighting down the barrel just
like the textbooks teach.

"He could have killed me," I say.
He nods.
"Why didn't you put him down?" I say.
"I don't know."
"Well, I guess you *better* fucking know. This is my *life*."
He lowers his arm and shakes his head. "I *wanted* to fire,"
he says. "I was all ready." He shakes his head again. "Hunt-

ing scuds, we always tried to avoid everybody. Never had to shoot. Not in Somalia, either."

I hear sirens in the distance.

Jack kneels beside me. His mouth is inches from my face. "I never killed anybody," he whispers. "But I *could*. I'm sure I could."

ALL THE NIGHTS
OF THE WORLD

In the car, snowflakes floating against the windshield and then melting in the defrost and streaking the glass like tears, Chris tells me how nervous she is. I make the turn. My hands are cold against the steering wheel. "Why should you be nervous?" I say.

"This is *my* audition," she says.

I glance over. She is huddled inside her coat. She has my jacket wrapped around her legs and her hat pulled down low over her ears. The only part of her I see is her nose, peeking from under the mass of clothing, windburn red and tiny and perfect. She is sitting on her hands.

"Is that what you think?" I say. I turn back to the road.

We drive in silence for a while.

Chris says, "Is he going to like me?"

"I told you before," I say.

"Tell me again," she says and I do.

As I am making the turn onto the street that runs in front of the restaurant, Chris says, "Am I going to like him?"

I laugh. "Everybody likes him," I say. "He's a star."

We pull into the parking lot. I ease into a space near the

entrance. I turn off the engine. Then we sit, not moving, the car clicking, and before we open the doors I tell Chris how much I love her and she nuzzles my shoulder.

My father is never late.

He is already at the table when we enter the room. Several of the waiters have recognized him. They are gathered around him excitedly. He is telling a joke. When my father finishes the joke, the waiters laugh too loudly. He half-smiles and picks up his glass of water and drains it. The glass disappears in his fist.

The room is red-carpeted and dark-walled and is filled with men who have never torn off another man's ear. The men are soft and pink-faced. They sit separated from their dates by cream-colored tablecloths. The dates are young models with skeletal fingers and long legs or middle-aged wives with faces like marble floors.

The maître d' leads us to the table. When he sees us, my father stands and steps past the group of waiters. He throws his arms around me and claps me on the back. I am drowning in Old Spice and the familiar smell from his shirt. I am shocked, as I always am, by the size of him. He steps away from me and looks at Chris.

"You must be Christina," he says. He leans down very far to kiss her delicately on the cheek.

The waiters are nervous with my father standing. They disperse quickly.

Without all the coats wrapped around her, Chris seems very small. The men in the room notice her, as they always do. I watch my father notice them noticing.

I pull out Chris's chair for her and we sit.

The menus are leather-bound. They do not list prices.

"What *is* this place?" I say.

"First class," my father says. "It's first class."

Chris reaches into her purse and brings out a black jewelry box. She hands it to my father. "Happy birthday," she says.

He opens the box and peers inside.

"It's a tie clasp," I say.

He begins to nod and then catches himself. He picks up the tie clasp. In his hand it looks like a toothpick.

"Chris made it," I say.

He smiles at her. "It's wonderful," he says.

Chris smiles back at him.

A waiter slides in to take our drink orders. When he's gone, I say, "How was the flight?"

My father shrugs. "Made it in before the storm."

"I suppose we should have come down," I say.

"Please," he says. "I had to fly so much when I was playing, I could practically *pilot* one of those things."

The waiter returns with the drinks.

"Should we order?" I say.

"We're waiting for Don," my father tells me.

"Will you tell one of your stories?" Chris asks him.

"What do you want to hear?"

"I'm not sure. I don't know much about sports."

"Me neither," he says and they laugh. He begins to tell her about Bobby Layne jumping into the pool at the Hyatt in Philadelphia from his window on the third floor, but he stops and looks at the front of the room. When I look, Don Erskine is standing beside the maître d'.

The maître d' walks toward the table. Don Erskine lumbers after him. He is almost as tall as my father and not quite as thick through the shoulders. In front of him he carries a hard-fat gut like a swollen hot-water bottle.

We introduce Don to Chris. He shakes her hand and glances at me. He sits across from me and says, "I hate the winters in this city."

"Move," my father says.

"Play nice. It's your birthday."

The waiter comes back with a gray-haired man in a white dinner jacket. This is the owner. I know it before he tells us. The collar of his shirt is open. The skin of his chest is the same unnatural tan color as his face.

The owner puts his hand on my father's shoulder and says, "I just want you all to know what an honor it is to have you dining with us this evening."

"Glad to be here," my father tells him.

"Does anyone need recommendations? We have some five-pound lobsters. Just got them this morning. Watched them get unloaded myself. Also, I hope you will do me the courtesy of being my guests."

"That would be fine," my father says. "Thank you."

"After your meal, perhaps we could take a picture together for the wall."

"Why not?"

"I'd like to bring my son over to meet you. If he's going to run this place, he's got to learn how to treat our special guests."

"We'll help you break him in."

We order the food. The waiter and the owner disappear.

Chris says, "You never finished your story."

Don Erskine says, "What story?"

"Bobby Layne at the Hyatt," my father tells him.

"That's a good one."

"I'm always telling stories," my father says. "I want somebody to tell me a story for a change. I want Chris to tell me the story of her life."

"That's not so easy," she says.

"It's easier than you think. There are only tiny parts of it that anyone wants to hear."

"Where should I begin?"

"Tell what you do for a living."

"He hasn't told you?"

"He doesn't tell me much."

"I'm a dancer."

"Ballet?"

"I'm with a jazz company."

"I don't know anything about jazz dancing," my father says.

The waiter brings the salads.

When Chris is in the ladies' room, Don Erskine says, "A shiksa?"

"I'm not exactly Jackie Mason," I tell him.

He nods. "But you're not Pat Boone, either."

"He never liked the Catholic girls," my father says.

"Jesus Christ, Pop," I say, "you haven't been inside a church in twenty years."

"First of all, you're too young to remember what I did twenty years ago. Second, not going to church doesn't make me not a Catholic. Sure as hell doesn't make me a *WASP.*"

He eats a bite of his steak.

"You going to marry this girl?" Don Erskine says.

"It's a little early for that. She only just met the old man."

"So what?"

"So he'll charm her for me. Then I won't have to marry her."

"Careful. Your old man might not be as glamorous as you think." Don smiles. "Anyway, answer me seriously."

"Seriously, I don't know."

"What's to know?"

"What if I don't love her?"

"Don't marry her."

"I mean, what if it turns out I don't?"

"It never *turns out.* Either you do or you don't. When you're under the covers in the dark, either you're the only two people on earth or you aren't."

"That's not much."

"That's all there is."

"That's all you need," my father says. His face is a picture of solemnity.

We look at him for a moment. Then I say, "How lyrical of you."

He can't hold it. His lips force their way up at the sides and he smiles and then he laughs with his head thrown back.

"Jesus," Don Erskine says. "I'm just trying to give your son a little fatherly advice."

My father's eyes are shining. He says, "If the earth moves then she's the one? That's not advice, that's pillow talk. The only romantic advice you need is give her an enema before you fuck her in the ass. That and abs. Girls like abs. Don't let yourself go the way Don has."

"Fuck you, you prick. It's part of the aging process."

"I weigh thirty pounds less today than I did the day I quit playing."

"Different metabolisms," Don mutters.

My father pours himself more wine. He looks at me. "I assume you inherited your father's cock. That'll keep a woman better than any ring."

"Comes a time when a woman needs you to settle down," Don says.

"If you're poking her in the kidneys every night, she'll deal with the uncertainties."

"So why'd you get married?"

My father looks at him. "I don't have bastard kids."

Don shakes his head. "Never take romantic counsel from a man who can't invite his ex-wife to his fiftieth birthday."

When the owner brings his son over, my father tells them about the night he broke Mike Webster's nose. The owner's son is tall, nearly my height. The top of his head would be even with my father's chin. He has blow-dried hair and caps on his teeth. He smiles as often as possible.

My father tells about reaching under Webster's face mask and grabbing and tearing and how he felt the bone give and how the blood poured as though someone had turned on a faucet. He tells about the sound that Webster made and how he clawed at my father's hand and pulled the index finger out of its socket and bent it back so far that it touched the back of the hand. My father shows them the crooked finger.

The owner and his son are very happy. My father tells them about thumbing Gene Upshaw in the Adam's apple and how Upshaw went down on his hands and knees and vomited. The other men from the Raiders' line were insane with rage. They tried to get even on every play. Finally Art Shell stomped my father in the groin near the end of the third quarter and he pissed blood for a week.

I examine Chris's face while my father speaks. I expect her to be excited or disgusted. She only looks sad.

"You know," the owner says, "my son was a halfback in college."

"Mine, too," my father says.

"Where?" the son asks and I tell him.

My father says, "Nobody your age knows how to play ball."

"There are a few," Don Erskine says.

"Maybe," my father allows. "Who's that boy they have now—the one with hands the size of pie plates?"

"I don't think you can say 'boy,' " I tell him.

"You can't say anything these days."

The waiter brings coffee and the dessert cart. After he leaves, my father says, "I'm twenty-five years old in every story I tell."

"We're famous for playing a little boys' game," Don tells him.

"You're not really *famous*."

Don smiles. "No, I suppose not."

"I'm not complaining, you understand. It keeps me fed. They put my name on the letterhead and give me an office and a partner's salary, and all I have to do is sit around and tell war stories. I haven't really worked in fifteen years."

"Wonderful," Chris says.

I clear my throat. "We need to think about going. It's only supposed to get worse out there."

"All right," my father says. "I still have to give the jock sniffer his picture. Don'll drive me to the hotel."

We stand. Chris kisses my father and Don Erskine.

In the coatroom, I say, "Every time I see the way he affects people, I feel like I'm going to be a failure."

Chris turns around and looks at me. "That's the dumbest thing you've ever said."

Before I can ask what she means, the girl is back with our coats and then my father has come up behind us and put an arm around each of us and is walking us to the parking lot. I decide to ask her on the way home, but by the time we are in the car I have forgotten what it is I was going to ask.

C hris is so cold when we get back to my apartment that she is unable to speak. Her teeth chatter wildly. She strips off her clothes and throws herself onto my bed. She wraps the blankets close around her.

I undress more slowly and fold my clothes and then fold hers and lay them all at the foot of the bed. I turn on the stereo with the volume low. I light an orange candle that smells like ginger tea.

Chris is still shivering when I climb in next to her. She has bedclothes clutched against her chin. I slide down under the covers and blow warm breath on her body. I take each of her feet between my hands and rub it hard until the sole loses its iciness. Then Chris turns on her side and I emerge from under the bedding, dripping sweat. I wrap myself around her and breathe hot against the back of her neck.

She stops shaking. Her breathing slows. I go back under the sheets and kiss my way down her back. She squirms slightly each time I press my lips against her. When I reach her underwear, I kiss along the waistband and then gently turn her over onto her back. I kiss the front of her panties and the soft outlines of what is underneath. She moans.

When I come up again, we are both breathing deeply. She pushes her mouth against mine very hard.

"I think you impressed my father," I say in a voice I don't recognize.

"It wasn't him I was trying to impress."

We push our mouths together again and then we lie together. Light from the candle flickers over us. Snow falls past my window in bloated flakes. Below, the street bustles silently.

We lie like that a long time.

KILLING TIME

Ray sits with his eyes half closed and does not look at the girls. The girls look the way they always look. They sit across the room all in a row on the banquette, whispering to each other, giggling, staring at our table. We order a second round and Milt Bailey says, "Maybe I should go show those three a little piece of Philadelphia."

Davey Manzelli says, "A very little piece," and we laugh. Dave's face looks like a boiled dinner.

"Fuck you, Garlic," Milt Bailey says.

"Up your ass, you jungle-bunny fairy."

Frank Patterson, the bodyguard, sits beside Ray and does not watch the girls, either. He is wearing a white suit. He leans far back in his chair. The only parts of him that move are his eyes.

"What time is it?" Davey asks.

"Eleven-thirty," Milt tells him.

"You sparring in the morning, Ray-Ray?"

Ray shrugs without looking up. "Ask Sunshine."

"Well?" Davey says.

"Well, what?" I say.

"Are you sparring in the morning or not?"

"Fuck should I know? It's up to Doc. I'm not the trainer."

"Well, Doc ain't here. I think maybe we ought to call it a night."

"Hey, Dave," I say, "I already have a mother. And a wife."

"Hey, fuck you, Mike. I'm just trying to be the voice of reason. These niggers would stay out all fucking night. Can't even hardly tell time."

"Why are you in such a rush?" I ask him. "The new *Playgirl* just come out?"

Ray smiles for the first time. "Hey, Dave," he says, "did you suck cock before Dannemora or did the spade sodomites make you into a bitch and one day you discovered you liked it?"

Dave smiles slightly. "It was Folsom, and who you calling a spade?"

Ray brightens further. "You mean the pot and the kettle? Well, get one thing straight: I ain't no spade, Daddy. I'm a high-yellow, gold-colored African prince with a cock that hangs to my knees."

Dave says, "Doesn't it get in the way when you *drop* to your knees?" and we laugh and Ray reaches across the table and musses Dave's hair and Dave slaps his hand away.

"**Y**ou're Ray Martin," the girl says.

"That's right," he tells her.

"We think you're the sexiest. Except for Oscar De La Hoya."

Ray nods. "Fuck Oscar De La Hoya."

The girl smiles nervously.

"Who's your friend?" one of the other girls says.

"That's Mike Larkin."

"Are you a fighter too?" she asks.

"Not anymore," I tell her.

The third girl is brunette and prettier than the others. She wears a black wrap skirt that clings to her hips. She smells like a peach. "Don't you worry about your face?" she says.

Ray laughs. "It's not much to begin with."

"Doesn't it hurt when you get hit?" one of the others asks. "Whenever I hit my head—getting out of a car, or whatever—I always want to cry."

"Not Ray," I tell her. "Ray didn't even cry when the doctor slapped him on the ass. They thought he was stillborn."

Ray's smile fades, but does not disappear. He says, "Mike is so tough he doesn't even have to throw punches. He just *scares* them to death."

"Would it hurt if I hit you?" asks one of the girls who is not the pretty girl.

"Depends," Ray says. He looks only at the pretty one.

She smiles. "On what?"

"On what you hit me with."

"What about with my fist?"

"Try it on Mike first."

Her eyes are wide. "Can I?"

"He doesn't mind."

When Ray takes the two girls into the men's room with him, I am alone with the pretty one and I ask her why she didn't go.

"I'm no groupie," she says.

"Of course not."

"What's that for?"

"Sorry. Sometimes this gets me down."

"This happens often?"

"Fight week is nasty," I tell her.

"So why are you here?"

"Because I'm his friend."

We are silent for a while. I sip my drink.

She says, "Have you known him a long time?"

"Ten years."

"How did you meet?"

"We used to fight sometimes in the amateurs."

"Who won?"

"We split pretty even."

"What about now?"

"What do you mean?"

"Could you beat him now?"

Across the room, Ray has reappeared, smiling hard, one of the girls on each arm. When she sees them, the pretty girl shakes her head.

"I'm glad you didn't go with them," I tell her.

On the street, mist makes the lights stretch out long. Frank Patterson sits beside me while I drive. The Navigator rides high in front like a motorboat.

"You guys won't say anything to Doc?" Ray says.

We are silent.

"Come on," he says. "The whole worry is the legs, right? Well, I was sitting the whole time. I made them do all the work. All I had to do was stay hard. I didn't even move the hips."

I listen to the breathing sound our tires make against the wet pavement.

"Fuck this," Ray says. "Who's the fucking champ here, anyway?"

"You are," Davey says.

"So I must be doing something right. If clean living won titles, Mike would be champ. Hey, Frank, you're on my side, aren't you?"

Frank shifts in his seat.

"Well, then fuck you too," Ray screams. "You want to shut me up, you big fuck? I don't care that you're Man-Mountain Dean. You think you can whup me?"

"No, Ray," Frank mumbles.

"What's that?"

"No," he says. "I can't."

. . .

We lie in the twin beds with the lights out, staring at the ceiling, unable to sleep. We listen to the cars passing and to the sounds from the sidewalk outside the casino. Ray says, "These beds make me feel like we're at camp."

"You never went to camp," I say. "Besides, they don't sleep two to a room there. They sleep in cabins with lines of beds. Like a barracks."

"All right. College, then."

"You never went to college, either."

"Fuck you, man."

After a while I say, "You want to play cards?"

"I don't have the energy. I wish we could just sleep."

"I miss my wife," I say.

"Mikey," he says some time later.

"Yeah."

"I don't know if I can take it."

"Just two more days," I tell him.

Ray walks into the gym from the lobby wearing track pants and a white T-shirt with a gold lion's head in the center. He sits on a folding chair at the gray plastic table next to the ring and Davey comes over and sits across from him. They do not speak. Ray puts his right hand on the table, palm down, and Davey lifts it gently and begins wrapping it in a light-brown cloth bandage.

"We on colored-people time this morning?" Doc says from across the room.

Ray shakes his head. "Too early for bullshit, Doc."

"Sorry. I thought we were training for a fight."

"Nobody else has to spar the day before."

"What if, for a little while, I was the trainer and you were the fighter?"

Ray shrugs.

When Ray is finished having his hands wrapped, I put in

my mouthpiece and strap on the headgear and check my cup. I slide on the pillowy sparring gloves and mount the portable metal steps and duck through the ropes and into the ring. The chinstrap from the headgear is chafing and I try to adjust it by rubbing it with my shoulder. Davey helps Ray into his gloves and then Ray climbs into the ring and stands in front of me.

"Light," Doc tells us. "Light."

"Careful of the face," Ray says through his mouthpiece. "Press conference tonight."

We circle. Ray hops easily from foot to foot. I stalk, crouched low, forcing him into the corner, narrowing his angles of escape, cutting off the ring. I throw a short combination to his body, pulling the punches so that they thud harmlessly against his belly and his pulled-in forearms. He counters by hammering a left hook behind my ear. He bobs once and then throws an uppercut into my ribs. He slips my next few punches. He works his way out of the corner with jab-jab-hook. I hook him as he weaves past me and he counters with a right hand over the top that lands on the bridge of my nose and makes white flashbulbs explode in my head. I shake the haze away and I can see again and now the flashbulbs are like furry white bees that dart around the edges of my vision. I bully Ray into a corner again and he brings his right leg even with his left and squares his shoulders and pounds uppercuts just above my belt. I pound him back. I lean my head against his shoulder and weave with him. I watch the muscles in his chest to know when he's punching. He works his way out this time with a seven-punch combination to my head. The punches are so fast that the sound of them runs together. As he dances away, I throw a big, looping hook at him that misses terribly. He winks at me.

Doc lets us go for fifteen minutes before he rings the bell.

• • •

The first two Mexicans come in and stand by the entrance, working hard to look tough. After a few seconds, Bennie Suarez sweeps in behind them. And then comes Pachanga, flanked by one of his brothers and a kid with a mean-looking puckered pink scar running along his jaw. Pachanga is wide-shouldered and shorter than Bennie Suarez. Bennie is thin and careful in his movements. He spots us and oozes toward the table. Pachanga follows. The four Mexicans move with Pachanga.

"Good evening, Raymond," Bennie says.

Pachanga looks only at Ray. Pachanga's brother and the first two Mexicans glower at each of us in turn. Davey glowers back. The kid with the scar looks only at Frank Patterson. Frank seems about to fall asleep.

"You been working on your accent there, *vato*?" Ray says to Bennie Suarez.

"I am making an effort at assimilation," he says.

Ray snorts. "Wearing a mink shirt?"

Bennie shrugs. "I forgive myself a few little eccentricities."

"You just buy one of those word-a-day calendars?" I say.

"There's nothing wrong with sounding educated."

"Maybe you ought to teach your boy a little something," I say. "How long's he been here and he still can't speak the language? People are starting to think he's retarded."

Bennie half-smiles. "He knows what he needs to know."

"Doesn't take too much education for 'No mas,' " Ray says.

There is grumbling from the Mexicans. Pachanga raises his hand.

"I haven't quit yet," he says quietly.

"He hasn't *queeeet*," Davey says.

Pachanga does not look at him.

"Maybe," Ray says. "But you're at middleweight now, *cabrón*. I ain't no hundred-thirty-five-pound spic."

"You going to say that to the cameras?" Bennie asks.

Ray smiles. "You using an interpreter?"

"Of course."

"Too bad. Throws off my timing."

"All apologies."

A blue-jacketed hotel security guard comes through the double doors and says, "Five minutes."

Bennie says, "Time to get mean."

Ray says, "You tell your boy, he pulls any shit today and I'll ruin him for you."

The Mexicans head for the exit from which they will enter when the reporters are seated. When they are almost to the side door, Pachanga stops and turns around. "You piss blood tomorrow, *mayate*," he says.

Ray blows him a kiss.

"He *peeees* blood," I say.

We are already on the stage when the reporters are let in. Milt Bailey and Bennie Suarez are standing behind us with the promoters and the head of the commission, in front of the white sheet dotted with Budweiser crests that hangs at the back of the platform. When the reporters are seated, Pachanga enters behind Cleveland Henderson, his trainer. They are followed closely by Pachanga's brother and the kid with the scar. Cleveland Henderson sits next to Doc at the center of the table. Pachanga flops into the chair beside him, calm and brown and tough. Ray leans forward and grins at Pachanga. Pachanga pretends not to notice. He keeps staring straight ahead.

The reporters begin asking questions.

"How do you feel?" they say.

Pachanga mumbles into the microphone. The interpreter says, "I am an Aztec warrior. I have heart. I fight no matter how I feel."

"How's the eye?" they say.

"I am an Aztec warrior. I feel no pain."

"The bell hasn't rung yet," Ray says and everyone laughs.

"How long will the fight go?" they ask Pachanga.

"If he faces me like a man and does not run, the fight will be very short. If he runs like a rabbit, we will be there longer."

"I have no question that I will win," the interpreter says. "I am an Aztec warrior."

When it's Ray's turn, he says, "I've been in with Hopkins. I've been in with Jones. Who's *he* been in with?"

Ray says, "I'm not an idiot. I'm not going to bang with him. But I'm not planning on doing much running. He's used to guys standing in front of him. I don't do that. I can't see him being able to find me."

Ray says, "As far as that rabbit business, ask him about it after the sixth when he can't breathe and I'm still bouncing. I don't like watching these clumsy guys fight. It's not artistic. Makes me feel like a thug."

Ray says, "Sure, he has a chance—there's always a *chance*. But if you're asking me where to put your money, I'd have to think that's easy." He smiles. "When you're at a bullfight, you don't bet on the bull."

They are weighed on a black balance scale. The head of the commission slides the weights along the beam and calls out the numbers. The cameras chatter and flash. Pachanga wears sunglasses. Ray smiles and flexes his biceps.

Afterward, they pose together for the photographers. They face each other, hands up, trying to look bored.

The morning of the fight, we eat pancakes and eggs in our suite. We watch television. We do not answer the phone. Ray drinks as much water as he can handle. We play rummy and don't keep score.

At noon Ray eats two bananas and two hard-boiled eggs.

When he's finished with the second egg, he says, "You pissed at me?"

"Don't break your concentration," I say.

"You want me to apologize 'cause I'm better than you?"

I am silent.

"You don't have nothing you want to say?" he says. "I can look in your eyes and see what you're thinking. Why don't you grow some balls and tell me?"

"Careful, Ray."

"Careful of what? If you was my friend you'd tell me what you thought. But you get *paid* to be my friend, so you have to shut up and take what I give you. I throw my punch a little faster than you throw yours and it lands a little harder and that means you spend your life with your tongue in my ass. What do you think of that?"

"I think fight week is a tough week."

"Yeah, it's *my* tough week."

"Fine," I say.

It is hot in the locker room under the arena. Ray dances between us over the cement floor and throws combinations in the air. Sweat pours off him. He is dressed in gray sweatpants and his ring shoes. The noise of the crowd breaks in above our heads. The walls shake with the force.

When Ray stops shadowboxing, he stands shuffling his feet, unable to keep still. Davey sits on a high stool in front of him and massages the sweat into his chest and shoulders.

"I'm ready," Ray says.

"Goddamn right," Milt Bailey tells him.

"Bring that motherfucker," Ray says, his voice rising.

"He don't even belong in the same ring with you. He's never been in with anybody serious."

"He hits like a bitch."

"He can't break popcorn."

"I'm gonna take that motherfucker *out*."

"It's your ring, baby. It's *your* ring."

Milt is almost screaming now. Ray, his eyes wild from the tension, pulls himself away from Davey and begins flying around the room again and throwing bombs with both hands.

Milt screams at him as he throws. "There ain't nobody else, baby. They can't *see* you. He'll be lucky to make it through the first."

One of the security guards appears in the doorway. Thunder from the crowd pours in behind him. He shouts over the roar, "You boys ready to exchange trainers? They want to wrap Pachanga."

Doc is sitting on one of the benches in front of the banks of lockers. He glances up and nods.

"I'll go," I tell him.

He nods again.

The security guard motions into the hallway. Cleveland Henderson glides past him. Cleveland Henderson is small and caramel-colored. His fists are the size of grapefruits.

"Doc," he says. "Ray."

"Cleve," Doc says.

Ray sits on the high stool in front of Dave Manzelli. I walk toward the door.

"Your boy looks a little edgy," Cleveland Henderson tells me as I pass him.

"You know how he gets," I say.

The security guard leads me down the hallway. We pass lines of event staff and cameramen with laminated cards hanging from chains around their necks. We pass ring-card girls in sequined bikinis craning their necks for a glimpse of the crowd.

The Mexicans are gathered outside the dressing room, near the entrance to the tunnel. The kid with the scar slouches elaborately against one of the walls and looks fierce.

Inside the room, Pachanga sits on a padded table, staring at the floor. His brother sits next to him on a wooden chair. The inspector from the commission is the only other person in the room. In the corner, an immense radio blasts Tito Puente. Pachanga's brother nods at me and does not speak. He begins wrapping Pachanga's hands with white gauze.

Pachanga does not move. When the hands are wrapped, I inspect them. I check the knuckles for lumps. The inspector takes the gloves out of his bag and sets them on the table. The brother puts the gloves on Pachanga and laces them and covers the laces with tape. I examine the gloves and the covered laces. I pull a fat marker from my pocket and write "M. Larkin" over the tape on each wrist.

As I leave, the brother nods again and still does not speak. Pachanga is still staring at the floor.

Ray is standing in the center of the room when I get back. He is stripped down to his shorts. The sweat on his body gleams. Davey is on his knees in front of him, retying the laces of the ring shoes.

"How'd he look?" Ray asks me.

"Scared," I tell him. He nods.

Cleveland Henderson chuckles.

Ray jerks his head at me. I cross the room and lean in close to him.

"Thanks, Mikey," he says.

I look at him.

He lays a gloved hand on my shoulder.

Dave finishes with the shoes. Ray takes his hand from my shoulder and then he is weaving again. He uses the back of his forearm to wipe the sweat from his eyes.

"How we gonna do it?" he shouts at Milt Bailey.

"Limb from limb!" Milt Bailey shouts back.

"All night long!" Milt Bailey shouts.

Cleveland Henderson watches them peacefully, half-smiling.

The rest of us stand back and let Ray get himself ready.

EVOLUTION

PART ONE: SEX

On our first date, Heather Gordon orders the Maryland crab cakes with red-pepper polenta and when I walk her home she asks me to take her to bed. On our second date, she has portabello and endive salad followed by veal tenderloin with poblano chiles and we make love on the swing set of an empty playground. On our third date, she tells me she is going to marry me.

For our one-month anniversary, Heather lights candles all around my bedroom and strips me naked and walks me to the bathtub, which is filled with warm water and rose petals. After three months, she takes me to Paris for the weekend. When we have been dating for six months, she asks me to kill her father.

. . .

"The first thing we have to do," Kelly says when I tell him, "is cross over."

"Cross over," I say.

"Cross over the line between the good people and the bad people."

"There's a line?"

"Sure," he says. "Actually, there are several. We'll cross them in stages. We'll work slowly. We'll keep upping the ante."

"Did you get this from a book?"

He shakes his head. "No books. This is about personal experience. We must walk the path."

"The path."

"The path to emotional detachment."

"Are you making this up?"

He shakes his head again. "It's in all the latest literature."

I stare at him. "I thought you said no books."

He frowns. "From now *on*," he says.

We are sitting on the sofa in our apartment watching Kelly's high-definition television, which is shaped like a fish tank. The picture is so sharp that it reveals the individual pores in human faces.

Kelly says, "Everything's going cerebral these days. If we want to resist that trend, we have to master the physical world. If we want to be masters of the physical world, we have to know about life and death."

"Kel," I say, "are you sure you want to do this?"

He looks at me in silence for a while. Then he says, "This is what we've been waiting for."

The room is cavernous and blue-carpeted and honey-combed with tiny cubicles. The analysts sit in the cubicles between eighty and a hundred hours each week. The traders come in at eight-thirty and leave at five.

A green digital stock ticker rushes along the edges of the ceiling.

Kelly and I are sitting in brown leather armchairs outside a glass-walled conference room. Inside the conference room is a long cherry table with a podium at one end.

A kid about our age wearing Ferragamo lace-ups strolls past the analysts and pours himself a cup of coffee from the cart next to us.

Kelly says, "You have to come all the way over here every time you want coffee?"

The kid shrugs. "Can't put it on the trading floor. Someone would crash into it."

"You a trader?" Kelly says.

"Apprentice. You the boys from Merrill?"

Kelly shakes his head.

"We work for a start-up," I say.

The kid frowns. "But you're wearing suits."

"We're in new investment."

"You're here to pitch us?"

"Something like that," Kelly says.

The kid nods. "You guys have one of those cute tech names where you change the first couple letters of an existing word? Like Verizon. Or Cinergy."

"We're called eVolution," I tell him.

"Small ee, big vee?"

"That's right."

He smiles. "So what does it do?"

"The small ee, big vee?"

"The *company*."

I look around the room at analysts hunched over keyboards and at traders in shirtsleeves shouting into telephones. "I really don't know," I tell him.

• • •

You can open a car door without a slimjim by bending a hanger into a squared hook and inserting it between the window and the weather stripping and using it to catch the lock rod. Sometimes you can open the door by using a key from the same manufacturer.

It is possible to hot-wire the car from the inside, but to do this you need to remove the ignition mechanism and complete the circuit manually. This risks severe electric shock. It also damages the car.

It is better to pop the hood and run a wire from the positive side of the battery to the positive side of the coil wire. The coil wire is red. Use a pair of pliers to hold the starter solenoid to the positive battery cable. This fires the engine. To unlock the wheel, insert a screwdriver into the steering column and use it to push the locking pin away from the wheel.

Kelly says, before you can kill you have to know what it is like to die.

Before you can know what it is like to die, he says, you have to know what it is to live.

"Do you know the life span of the common housefly?" he asks me.

"One day."

"One day," he says. "Twenty-four hours in which to pack all his loving and hating and living and dying."

I say, "I don't think a housefly does much loving and hating."

I change the channel on the high-definition television. The news is running a feature on school shootings.

Kelly sighs. "You're missing the point."

I shrug. "His life isn't short if he doesn't know it's short."

Kelly frowns and wrinkles his forehead and then says, "He only gets one sunrise and one sunset."

"And you only get a few thousand."

"Hopefully more than a *few*."

"Even so," I say.

Kelly nods. "Even so."

We are in a taxi. The driver wears a green knit hat and loafers with no socks. He has a stick of incense burning on the dashboard, which makes the air smell and taste like hot soap. I am sitting in the middle, between Kelly and my boss. My boss wears a linen suit. His tan is perfectly even.

Looking out the window at skyscrapers like enormous gray wafers, I say, "I don't understand my job."

My boss says, "What's to understand?"

"Shouldn't we bring a programmer with us?"

"Didn't I explain this to you last week?"

My scalp itches. I say, "It's just that I've been thinking some more about it and I figure it couldn't hurt to have an expert along."

My boss sighs. I look at Kelly. He is shaking his head. My boss says, "Our investors didn't grow up covered with zits."

"Excuse me?" I say.

"These people made their money the old-fashioned way—they inherited it. And they'll *never* give it away to some fruitcake in clear-framed glasses who wears his jeans two sizes too small. The key is charm, not knowledge. You were born for this."

Kelly is smiling at me. I ignore him. "But what if they ask me"—I lean close to my boss and whisper—"*technical* questions?"

"Do they ever?"

"They *could*."

He rolls his eyes. "Make something *up*. We're *salesmen*, for Chrissake."

"What are we selling? We don't make anything."

He looks at me. "We make *money*, kid. I sell experience. Kelly sells cool. You sell cheekbones and green eyes and leading-rusher-in-Ivy-League-history."

"Second-leading."

"My mistake," he says.

"It's just," I say, "that I don't know anything about computers."

He shakes his head. "This isn't about *computers*. Do you think Rockefeller knew anything about oil? Do you think Carnegie knew anything about steel? All you have to know is what people want and how to tell them they want it from you."

"But what if you don't know what people want?"

He shrugs. "Then you have to know how to tell them what they want."

When you die violently, your bowels let go. It's called involuntary-sphincter-release response and it means that you spew all the foul waste from inside you, more than you ever imagined possible.

Kelly says the next step after crossing over is the planning phase.

Really, he says, the two steps are simultaneous.

I am sitting in our living room, listening to the steam heat, and Kelly is telling me that evolution means the extinction of the weak.

"Every human and animal characteristic is the result of random genetic mutation."

"Yes," I say.

"Think of the creatures who lived before certain features developed. Think of the ones whose mutations failed to increase their fitness."

I close my eyes and picture ancient sea creatures with

squat bodies and tails like embryonic alligators', bobbing on
the tide, near powerless with their shrunken fins, watching
one of their fellows crawl out of the surf and onto the beach.
He will go on to populate the world. The rest will be prey
for prehistoric sharks or else will have descendants who will
be less and less suited to the sea and will eventually drown
as infants or occasionally flop their way onto the sand. I wonder whether these creatures know that they are the footnotes
of history while their friend on the beach is the ancestor of
an entire planet. I think of all the animals not selected for
a place on the ark. I think of the thieves crucified next to
Jesus.

"Eyelids," Kelly says.

I open my eyes. "What?"

"Eyelids are the result of random genetic mutation."

"Yes," I say.

"You have to be able to imagine how it felt before eyelids.
If you looked at the sky during the day, your retinas would
burn. You'd have to walk with your face pressed into the
ground, dirt in your mouth all the time. You'd have to sleep
with your eyes open."

"Yes," I say.

Kelly nods. "You need to be able to imagine the time
before tear ducts."

Heather's father leaves his office between six-
eighteen and six-fifty-one, Monday through Friday.
On Saturday and Sunday he works noon to five. It takes him
between four and seven minutes to make his way down to
the garage, depending on the elevators. He drives a black
Lexus sedan.

There ought to be two men in bland suits who drive
Heather's father to and from work and sit all day behind
Plexiglas in the hallway outside his office and shadow him
wherever he goes.

This would make for more of an operation.

In that case, we might use a pipe bomb. We might use an incendiary device underneath the backseat. We might use a sniper. If the bodyguards blocked sight lines to the subject whenever they were out in the open (as they should), we might use the sniper to take out the bodyguards and use a chase man to go after the subject if he broke and ran. Of course, it is better to snipe in two-man teams. And neither of us knows how to use a rifle.

I am pressing my face into Heather's neck and smelling her perfume and her shampoo and the soap she uses, which is goat's milk and honey and costs twenty dollars a bar. Even through all of that, I can still catch the scent of her skin.

Heather is wearing a pair of my boxer shorts and a T-shirt from the gym I go to, which is called Advance.

We are watching 2001 on my DVD player.

I stop nuzzling Heather's neck and sit back into the sofa with my legs extended in front of me. Heather rests her head on my chest. The light from the television twinkles all around us.

"It's less than two thousand years since the fall of the Roman Empire."

"Is that right?" Heather says.

"That's right," I say. "Less than two thousand years after chariot races, we have airplanes and space shuttles and movie-theater popcorn."

"Amazing."

She shifts the position of her body and nestles into my chest.

I say, "We weren't even the same *species* until about twenty thousand years ago. Before that we were Cro-Magnons."

"Fascinating," Heather murmurs. Her breathing is becoming deep and slow.

"Until recently, we were carrying clubs and living in caves."

She is silent.

I watch the television. Keir Dullea has just shut down the supercomputer. This is immediately before the part I don't understand, in which he imagines himself sitting in a room that looks like the smoking room from the world's fanciest mental hospital and then sees himself as an old man and a fetus.

I say, "Kelly and I are making preparations."

Heather stirs for a moment and then relaxes back onto me. "Mmm," she says sleepily. "Preparations for what?"

"Never mind," I say. "It's all right if you don't want to talk about it."

Kelly says, "You're the bastard who gave measles to the Yanomami." He is talking to the waiter, whom he has just accused of sneezing over his Parmesan-and-onion tartlet. "These people lived in isolation for hundreds of years and then you goddamn sociobiologists and you save-the-rain-forest fairies came in and gave them a measles vaccine, except that there *were* no measles in the rain forest until you brought them. And when the vaccine made some of the people sick, you refused them treatment on the grounds that you wanted to study a society completely free from outside influence."

The waiter is trying to figure out whether Kelly is making fun of him. The men sitting next to Kelly are laughing. One of them says, "This guy is a card. A goddamn *card*."

The other one nods and says, "The genuine article."

Kelly says, "Do you have any *idea* how many germs live in the mucus inside your nose?"

We are in a restaurant called Neoterra in which each of the tables has a different shape than the others and none of them is round. Our table is shaped like a lima bean or like a slug writhing to death under a blanket of salt.

The men we are eating with all wear suspenders and Kenneth Cole glasses and have their sideburns trimmed every other day. There are five of these men. They are venture capitalists. I cannot remember any of their names, so I have assigned names to them at random. When I cannot remember the name that I have assigned, I say the first name I can think of. They do not seem to notice.

One of the men next to Kelly is saying, "The plain ones are always the most suggestible. The pretty ones tend to be too uppity and the ugly ones are too wary. The plain ones are up for what*ever.*"

Kelly says, "How do you know who's pretty and who's ugly?"

The man says, "You *look.*"

"But how do you assign categories? Certain features make you feel physical attraction, but these features are different from culture to culture and even, sometimes, from person to person. It is a selection-based instinct to want to combine your genes with the genes of someone physically attractive, in order that you will have attractive offspring whose appearance will make them more likely to have reproductive success. Of course, you have a chicken-and-egg problem there. Also, that does not account for differences of opinion."

The man stares at him.

Kelly says, "Do you ever try to imagine the time before dilating pupils?"

When I open my eyes, the man to my right is speaking earnestly to my boss. He is asking to see the business plan.

My boss shifts in his chair.

"You do *have* a business plan," the man says.

My boss clears his throat. "Of course we have a plan," he says. "But we're not planning to be captains of industry. This isn't industry. We're not planning to be the world's leading distributor of butt plugs. We're sure as *hell* not planning to build the world's best shuffleboard Web site so that some Daddy Warbucks can stroll up and pat us on the head and pay us twenty-five million to split twenty-four ways, so we can buy a town house and a Benz and some pussy and live goddamn upper-middle-class. Upper-middle-class means *dick*. Fuck the suburbs. Fuck commuting. Fuck neighbors. Our plan here is to be rich enough not to *have* neighbors. To be able to stand in front of your house and turn around in a circle and own everything you see. Not season tickets, not even courtside. I'm talking about owning your own team. No Internet millionaires here. Fuck that, too. I'm talking about Internet *billionaires*. What we're offering you is the opportunity to be part of that."

The man to my left, whom I have decided (I think) to refer to as Gill, looks at me and says, "So, you played halfback at Princeton?"

"Not Princeton," I tell him.

"Of course not," he says. "How tall are you? Six feet?"

"Why not?"

"You weigh around two hundred?"

"One-ninety."

He smiles. "What's your forty time?"

"My forty time."

He nods.

"I don't know these days."

He frowns.

"I'm not really an athlete anymore," I explain.

"Hmm," Gill says.

We drink in silence for a while. Suddenly Gill looks at me. I lean back toward him.

Gill says, "What's your body-fat percentage?"

. . .

We are standing at the urinals in the bathroom at Neoterra and Kelly is saying, "The difference between assault and aggravated assault is mostly about the severity of the injuries."

I say, "How bad does it have to be to be aggravated?"

"It's subjective."

We zip up. The urinals flush automatically when we walk away.

We hold our hands under the faucets, waiting for the sink to recognize that we are not just dust particles blowing in front of the electric eye.

Kelly says, "Last night I was reading about the human botfly."

"I thought you said no books."

He nods. "I think we're going to have to forget that rule."

"I already did," I tell him.

The water begins to spray from our faucets.

He glances at me. "When?"

"From the beginning."

"Why didn't you tell me?"

I shrug. "I don't care much about it. As long as we don't say no movies."

"Of course not," he says. "That would ruin everything."

"The human botfly," I remind him.

"Right, right. Anyway, when it bites you, it raises a bump like a mosquito bite. Except that the fly has burrowed its way into your arm and the bump is covering it. It incubates for a while until it gets hungry and then it begins to consume you. You can feel it eating its way up your arm."

We take our hands from under the faucet and the water stops. We stand with our hands under the nozzles of the hand dryers.

Kelly says, "There are tiny parasitic worms that can live

in drinking water. Once they're inside you, they gather in sores on your legs. The only way to get rid of them is to immerse them in water and allow them to flow out of the hole they'll open in your skin."

They are laughing when they leave the club and weaving as they walk. Both of them wear white baseball caps emblazoned with the letters of their fraternity.

Kelly says, "Are you ready for this?"

I nod.

"Deep breaths," he says. "Try to swallow."

I nod again.

The frat boys do not notice us until they are only a few feet away. Then they stop.

Kelly is wearing a long black overcoat and leather gloves with lead studs sewn into the knuckles on the inside. He says, "You boys sure you're all right to drive? You look a little under the weather."

The frat boys are silent.

Kelly says, "Is this your car?"

"Yeah," one of them says.

"This a Corvette?"

The frat boy snorts. "Try Lamborghini."

"Ah."

He narrows his eyes. "You fuck with the alarm or something?"

Kelly smiles. "Now why would you think that?"

"Should be going off with you sitting on the hood."

"Well," Kelly says, "we're not as heavy as we look. The camera adds ten pounds." He laughs.

The frat boy says, "If you get off the car by yourselves, we'll give you a running start." He spreads his hands, palms up. He is thick through the chest and shoulders. His friend is taller than he is and wide.

Kelly slides off the car onto his feet. The frat boy smiles and turns his head to glance at his friend and when he turns back Kelly throws a straight right hand into the middle of his face. The gloved fist makes a dull-hollow slapping sound when it lands, followed immediately by the crunch of the nose breaking, and the frat boy's head disappears in red mist and then he has fallen to his knees. His friend is staring, openmouthed, and does not notice me standing up off the hood. He is reaching for Kelly when I kick him in the groin as hard as I can. He crumples next to the other one. And then we are on top of them.

I take the big one, who is curled into a ball with his hands cupped between his legs. He is dry-heaving. White lines of saliva hang from his chin. I kick him a few times in his kidneys and he rolls onto his back and I stomp his forearm with the heel of my boot and I am pretty sure I feel bones breaking. He screams. I kick him in the stomach and listen to him gasp as the air rushes out of him. Now he has no breath to scream and he is gagging. I drop onto his chest and, as I do this, I bring my elbow straight down into his mouth and feel the teeth give. He brings his arms up to cover his face and I punch the broken forearm. He screams again. When he moves the forearm, I drive my fists into him over and over. The skin splits along his eyebrows and forehead and cheekbones and blood seeps through the cracks like lava. Sweat is rolling down my face, plastering my hair to my forehead. I feel like crying.

Kelly says, "Enough."

I stand up and look at the big frat boy at my feet. His wrist is bent at a terrible angle. His mouth looks like a tomato with ripped skin. There are teeth sticking through his upper lip.

I look at Kelly, who is also standing. "Wallets?" I say, my chest heaving.

Kelly shakes his head. "This is assault, not robbery."

"Two birds, one stone?"

He chews his bottom lip and considers this. "Fuck it," he says. He reaches inside his frat boy's jacket and pulls out his wallet. The frat boy groans. Kelly kicks him in the ribs.

"We taking the car?" I say.

"No," Kelly says. He looks at the frat boy below him. "Don't take it too hard, fellas," he says. "We've just grown past you. You're the giraffes whose necks never stretched." He pulls off his gloves. "You're the elephants with short noses."

"I think we're ready for the next level," Kelly says.

I glance at him. The streetlights we pass turn his face ghostly white and run the shadow of the windshield wipers along his profile. I massage the fingers of my left hand against the knuckles of my right, which are scraped bloody and have already begun to swell.

"What's the next level?" I say.

Kelly turns his head slightly so that the wiper shadow now flows over his face asymmetrically, making a jagged line on his nose. He is smiling enough for me to see the tips of his teeth.

"It's time to shoot somebody," he says.

Heather is wearing a red dress with no back. The dress is longer on one side than the other. On the short side, it rises almost above her hip.

The skin on Heather's thighs is the color of butterscotch.

We are standing under an enormous crystal chandelier that hangs over a crimson staircase. Everywhere I look, there are men in tuxedoes. Heather has the fingers of her left hand laced through the fingers of my right.

The poster next to the theater door shows two immense eyes and, above that, the word "Gatsby" in white letters.

Heather is talking to Cynthia Lowell-Wellington and

Vanessa Mather Coppedge Bryson, who are jammed up against us by the crush of people. Cynthia's boyfriend, who is taller than I am and has a dimpled chin, looms on my left, just behind Cynthia. I am fairly certain that he was on the crew team at Brown, but it is possible that he was on the lacrosse team at Penn. He shakes my hand at every opportunity.

For dinner, Heather had the New Orleans–style catfish with chipotle dipping sauce.

She is saying, "If you're going to use a bronzing agent of *any* kind, you *have* to couple it with a good moisturizer."

Cynthia says, "Should I be looking for one with sunblock in it?"

"I suppose it couldn't hurt. But really, you should be keeping yourself out of the sun completely. That's what the bronzer is for."

Vanessa leans toward Heather and says, "So, do you put it *every*where?"

Heather nods. "No white should show."

I say, "Can you picture the time before melanin?"

Heather raises herself on the balls of her feet and kisses the side of my mouth.

The mob surges all around us, moving with tiny shuffling steps.

We are sitting in a private box on the left side above the orchestra. The house lights are down and the women onstage are singing to each other and staring into the audience. According to the program, they are singing in English, but it is impossible to understand them and my attention is focused on the seat backs of the row in front of us where a thin digital screen shows a scrolling transcription of the lyrics.

Heather is sucking my thumb.

Next to me, Cynthia's boyfriend, Clay Harrison Adams, whispers, "When's your IPO?"

I say, "We're not trying to be the world's leading distributor of butt plugs."

He says, "Oh."

The stage is darker now and the women are gone. They have been replaced by a dancing mob and bright-colored balloons. In the background a tiny green light is flashing.

Suddenly I have the urge to climb on top of my seat and throw my head back and scream. I have this urge every time I go to the theater. I believe it is a similar instinct to the one I have to turn on the engine of my car when the mechanic has his hand inside it. Or the impulse I feel on subway platforms to push the man next to me in front of the oncoming train. Or when I imagine swerving my car into a group of pedestrians and feeling the dull cracks of their heads against my windshield and gazing at the wet smears of their blood. Or when I think of diving through the plate glass of the Rainbow Room at Rockefeller Center and plunging, back arched, head up, gleaming shards of glass falling all around me, into the middle of the herd of ice-skaters circling sixty-seven stories below.

Clay says, "Johnson and Johnson?"

"What?" I say, turning to him.

"The butt plugs. Leading distributor."

I sigh. "I don't *know*, guy."

"Oh," he says.

I think about throwing him over our balcony and watching him drop, arms and legs windmilling, into the front row.

With all these impulses, there is the idea stage, then the imagination stage, then the spine-tingle, adrenaline-shot, testicle-clench moment when you *know* that you are actually going to do whatever it is.

But you never do.

• • •

During intermission Heather and I get on one of the mirror-walled elevators and ride it until we are alone. She pushes the Run-Stop button. A voice comes over the intercom asking if everything is all right. Heather begins unbuttoning my shirt. The voice from the intercom says that if the elevator does not begin moving in the next five minutes it will call the fire department. Heather licks my chest. I put my arms around her. The voice tells us not to panic.

Heather pulls away from me and takes two steps backward, smiling slightly, and presses herself against the brass handrail. As she leans onto the handrail, her dress drifts up and I can see the thin black string of her panties. I move close to her and she kisses me hard and runs her hand along the back of my neck and along my shoulder and down my arm and then she takes my hand and puts it gently between her legs. Her underwear is already moist. I grab hold of it and pull so that the narrow strip rubs against her. She gasps. I slide my hand under the wet fabric and touch the soft, slick skin and then I ease my middle finger inside her. She tips her head back and moans. I suck on the skin of her neck. Her perfume has a bitter taste.

She says, "Oh my God."

I kneel down in front of her and grip the backs of her thighs and pull her close to me, resting my head just below her ribs.

She strokes my hair. "How much do you want me?" she whispers.

I groan against her stomach.

Back in my seat, I can smell Heather on my fingers and I can taste her when I lick my lips.

In front of us, dozens of miniature chandeliers hang on long cords from the ceiling. In the hallways behind us, the lights flash off and on and an usher closes the door to our box. The cords begin to retract and the chandeliers float toward the high ceiling.

Heather whispers, "What's wrong with you lately?"

"What do you mean?"

"You've been even more distant than usual."

I say, "I've been walking the path to emotional detachment."

She frowns. "This is Kelly's idea?"

I nod. "We're working in stages."

She opens her mouth to say something else, but the two women are singing again. They are slumped in lawn chairs. They wear straw hats and white dresses. They draw out a single note so long that I have to take a deep breath in sympathy. The urge to scream washes over me again.

The words click by in white block letters on the digital screen in front of me. IT'S HOT, says the screen. IT'S HOT.

PART TWO: VIOLENCE

The man by the door is wearing a beige turtleneck and a leather jacket. He leans us against the wall and frisks us quickly.

Kelly says, "Won't you at least buy me dinner first?"

The man sighs. "Haven't heard that one yet this week."

Dexter is sitting in the far corner on a hydraulic chair that looks like a life raft. The man cutting his hair wears a long white shirt that says MECCA across the chest. The room smells of cocoa butter. The floor is covered with hair.

The man beside Dexter is almost as thick as he is and has

a big jagged scar along his jaw. He wears a cream-colored suit and a silk shirt.

The only other man in the barbershop lounges on a leather sofa in the corner opposite Dexter. His entire body seems frozen, including his eyes, which are locked on mine.

Dexter raises his head and looks at me in the mirror. "Looking good, baby," he says.

I smile. "You remember Kelly?"

He shrugs. "Why not?"

"Good to see you again," Kelly says.

Dexter grunts. He jerks his head toward the window. "That your new whip?"

"Yeah."

"Whip?" Kelly whispers.

"Car," I tell him.

Dexter whistles. "Fuckin' ay. You niggers must be *flush*."

"We can't complain," I say.

"I thought you were supposed to call me before you went public."

"We will."

He frowns. "So how come you niggers are rolling Bill Gates–style all of a sudden?"

I look around at the bodyguards. "You think you have enough security?"

"Can't be too careful."

"I don't remember anyone ever taking a shot at Butkus."

Dexter grins. "He wasn't a Nubian king."

"All right, I don't remember anyone taking a shot at Willie Lanier."

"That was a different era. It's all haters out there these days. Can't stand to see a brother living the dream."

"Is *that* what you're doing?"

Dexter's barber opens a drawer in the counter in front of him and changes the guard on his clippers.

Dexter says, "You watch me in the Pro Bowl?"

I nod.

He says, "They've never seen anything like me."

The barber removes the guard from his clippers and carefully shapes Dexter's sideburns. He unsnaps Dexter's maroon smock and passes the razor over the back of his neck. He pours alcohol onto a cotton ball and runs it around Dexter's hairline. He douses him with talcum powder.

Dexter says, "That's enough. Don't give me any of that Afro-Sheen shit."

The barber nods.

Dexter shrugs out of his smock and stands. He is an inch or two taller than I am. He is wearing a white knit tank top. His body is like a clenched fist.

"Shame the way you're letting yourself go," I say.

Dexter snorts. He takes a fat wad of bills from his pocket, peels one off the top, and hands it to the barber.

The man in the corner is moving now. He is on his feet and coming toward us. I can't remember seeing him stand up.

Dexter says, "This is Wilton."

"Wilton?" I say.

Dexter smiles. "Him a yardie, y'know."

"What?" Kelly says.

"He's Jamaican," I say.

Wilton looks at Dexter. "That accent's a little Harry Belafonte."

Dexter says, "So are you."

Wilton is wearing gray wool slacks and a black ribbed turtleneck sweater.

Dexter says, "These are the boys I told you about."

Wilton nods. He does not move to shake our hands.

I say, "Dexter tells me you used to work for Mike Tyson."

He shrugs.

"You know what we're working on?"

He shrugs again.

"We're trying to reach the next stage in our development."

Wilton stares at me.

Kelly says, "For most mammals, grooming is a sign of affection. That's why I cut my own hair."

Wilton is saying, "You'd be amazed how long it takes some guys to die."
I say, "Doesn't it depend on where they get hit?"
"Not always."
We are at an outdoor shooting range, lying on our stomachs beside green T-shaped shooting benches, facing white-and-black silhouette targets set up in front of a stone wall. I am leaning on my elbows on the concrete apron, sighting down the barrel of a rifle that looks like it is made out of Legos.
I say, "I wish these things still looked like they used to."
"Why?"
"It would make me feel more real."
Wilton says, "Draw down center body mass on everybody. No head shots."
"What about bulletproof vests?"
"That's just movie shit."
"*Someone* must wear them."
"Sure. But they'll still be incapacitated if they take one in the chest, provided you have enough stopping power. Even with body armor, a heavy load can break ribs and collapse lungs."
I squint through the aperture and place my crosshairs on the center of the target.
"Raise your aim four inches at two hundred yards, ten inches at three hundred."
"Why?" I turn my head to look at him.
"Gravity," he says.
"What do I do past three hundred?"
"You miss."
I nod.

Wilton says, "How you know Dexter?"

"We went to high school together."

"You play ball with him?"

"Sure."

He frowns. "I thought he was from Cleveland."

"So?"

"So, you don't look too Cleveland to me."

I shrug, gently so as not to lose my target picture. "Near Cleveland."

"Shaker Heights?"

"Something like that."

He smiles. "Always knew that motherfucker was wanna-be hard."

"Don't need to be from the ghetto to be hard."

"It helps." He looks at Kelly, who is on his stomach fifty feet to my right, sighting down the barrel of his Lego rifle. "What about the ofay?"

"Why is he an ofay and I'm not?"

He shrugs. "Ain't just about skin color."

"Mmm," I say. "We lived together in college."

Wilton nods. "He's a fuckin' fruit loop."

Sometimes, particularly when you can anticipate the precise location of your target, it is preferable to snipe at a near-flat trajectory. For countersniping, because you cannot predict your target's whereabouts and because the target will likely be concealing himself from anyone on the ground, it is vital to occupy the highest position possible.

In close quarters, the pistol is ideal because of its conceal-ability and ease of use. However, its effectiveness drops sharply as range increases. It is very difficult to be accurate with a pistol at distances greater than fifty feet. Past a hundred, it is almost impossible.

· · ·

My boss is riding in the cart in front of us with a man from Goldman who has skin like tapioca. We all wear green sweaters and brown-and-white spikes. Kelly is driving our cart, bouncing over ruts in the dirt path. The air tastes like the dirt thrown up by the other cart. Kelly is saying, "Why doesn't he have an accent?"

"He told me he lost it."

"He talks like a goddamn Yalie."

"He's self-educated."

Kelly snorts. "You *must* know what that means."

"What?"

"Anytime a Nubian says he's self-educated, ten to one he was reading with his ass to the wall."

"Prison?"

He nods. "Probably has one of those correspondence diplomas."

"That's not fair."

He glances at me. "You two have been getting awful close lately."

"He's been *teaching* me."

"I hope you're not losing perspective."

"Perspective on what?" I say.

"Just make sure you keep in mind what it is we're doing."

The cart in front of us stops dustily. Kelly pulls in behind it. We sit off to the side on a wooden bench while the man from Goldman sets himself over the tee.

Kelly says, "In gorilla societies, each adult male has his own position in the hierarchy. You don't look directly at anyone higher than you. Eye contact indicates provocation for all primates. No one looks at the alpha male, unless they are ready to challenge for his position. If you look him in the eye before you're ready for him, he will tear your limbs off."

· · ·

I am sitting in the backseat, between Heather and her father. We are on the way to the opening of an art gallery called Cave Paintings. Heather is gazing out the window.

Her father is my size with big hands. He has a thin white scar under his right eye. I am trying not to look at him.

He is saying, "Sometimes we would wait all night and not see anyone. Some nights we would all see movement on the road and we would blow the claymores and launch flares and pour fire into the tree line and when we walked down, we wouldn't find anything except the craters we'd made."

I say, "How'd they get away?"

"Who?"

"Whoever was on the road."

He looks at me. "There *wasn't* anybody on the road. We imagined it."

"You all imagined the same thing?"

"The visions are contagious. One guy points at what he sees and you make yourself see it, too."

"So, after a while, why didn't you stop believing something was there?"

"Because sometimes something *was* there."

"What were those nights like?"

He shakes his head. "You don't want to hear about *those* nights."

"Sure I do."

He says, "Later on, I was with Recon and we did less search-and-destroy, but we still had visions."

"Does it give you nightmares?"

"Nightmares?"

"Because you hated it so much."

He frowns. "Did I say that?"

"I just assumed. I thought everybody hated it."

He says, "It was the happiest time of my life."

• • •

We are sitting in a rented van at the curb across the street from Heather's father's office building and Kelly says, "What about knives?"

Wilton looks at him. "This ain't *West Side Story*."

"It's just that I thought we were supposed to learn these things in stages."

"You niggers want to learn knives, you can do it on your own time."

Wilton is shielding his eyes from the sun and staring up at the building, which looks like a giant milk carton. He says, "Next time we're doing reconnaissance, you ought to bring a jacket."

Kelly says, "Why not just keep the heat on?"

Wilton says, "Three guys sitting by the curb all day in a car with the motor running might as well hang out a sign that says STAKEOUT."

"Why are we here at all? We already know his schedule."

"*You* already know it. I want to see it for myself."

"You don't trust us?"

Wilton shakes his head. "You can't learn this stuff from books."

"And you've learned it through experience."

"That's right."

"So when we have the experience we'll be as good as you."

Wilton shifts his eyes to look at Kelly. He says, "You can't have a late start."

Armor-piercing or KTW rounds can puncture steel doors and pass through bulletproof vests. Their drawback is that they make neat, surgical wounds.

Full-metal-jacketed rounds also have a better penetration value than standard loads, but they are less streamlined than the armor piercers and cause more tissue damage.

Hollowpoints carry low penetration values but expand on impact. This is also true for dum-dums.

You can create a hollowpoint effect by cutting cross-shaped grooves into the tips of your cartridges. On impact, the round will flatten out along the grooves, disintegrating muscle and bone. (Note: Handmade loads may tend to jam an automatic.)

I am kneeling by an open window on the ninth floor of the Ritz, looking past the Public Garden at Beacon Street, and Wilton says, "Blue suit with the grocery bag."

"Got it," says Kelly.

"Why him?" I say.

"I don't know," Wilton says. "Easily identifiable."

Kelly says, "It doesn't pay to stand out."

They are on their feet next to me, binoculars held to their faces. I open and close my hands against the rifle and blink my eyes and watch through the scope as the man scratches his neck, magnified ten times.

"I don't know if I can," I say.

Wilton sighs. "This is what you said you wanted."

"I know. I just wasn't expecting him to be so *alive*."

Kelly says, "I'll do it."

"Wait your turn," Wilton says.

The man stops walking and checks his watch.

I say, "Won't they be able to tell where the shots came from?"

"Who's 'they'?"

"I don't know. Somebody."

"Unlikely. The flash isn't too apparent in daylight."

"What about the sound?"

"It'll echo off the buildings. It'll seem to come from everywhere."

"What if somebody sees us?"

"The chances of that increase with every second you don't take the shot."

The man is whistling now. I steady the crosshairs on the top button of his suit jacket. I close my eyes and imagine the way his face will look when the bullet hits him and the noises he'll make and the way his body will come apart. I wonder whether he will drop the groceries. I open my eyes.

Wilton says, "Deep breaths. Squeeze, don't pull."

The man smiles suddenly and switches his grocery bag to the other arm. A young girl with blond hair runs into the sight picture. The man bends down and scoops her up with his free hand and spins her around in a circle. She kisses him on the cheek.

I draw back from the scope and lay the rifle on the windowsill and stand up. I shake my head. "Not in front of his daughter."

Kelly looks at me. "The fuck you care?"

"She'll never recover."

"Nobody recovers from anything. Your experiences shape who you are. You have a chance to be the defining influence in this girl's life."

I don't say anything.

"If you're so worried about it," he says, "maybe we should do her too."

"No," I say. "I won't do that."

He groans. "Have Wilton do it."

"The girl can't die."

"She can and she will. The only question is when."

"Not today."

"What difference does it make? Today, tomorrow, eighty years from now. She won't be in a position to care."

"But in eighty years, when she feels it coming, she'll be able to look at all the things she did. Now she could only think of what she didn't do."

"So what if this girl has an unpleasant last few minutes in which she imagines the life she didn't live? It'll probably be better when she imagines it than it would have been to live it. It'll be better than remembering all the things she could never quite do. Besides, it's only a few minutes at the end. And if you hit her right, she won't even have that. Like flipping off a light switch."

Wilton turns to look at him. "I don't wash anybody for free."

"We'll pay you," Kelly says.

On the street below us, the man has put the girl down and is holding her hand. Holding the girl's other hand is a pretty blond woman in a blue cardigan.

Wilton turns back to the window. The family is moving away from us. They round the corner onto Charles Street.

I say, "They'll go home tonight like they do every night and they'll never know that they just lived through the most important moments of their lives. They don't even know we exist."

Kelly says, "Goldfish have thirty-second memories. Everything that happened more than thirty seconds ago is erased to make room for the new things. That means that at the very end, when they look back, they've been dying their whole lives."

Wilton grunts. When Kelly shoots him, his body clenches and he half turns from the waist, head rigid, pupils crammed to the sides of his eyes, trying to look at Kelly behind him. Then he sags against the glass, blood spraying from the big exit wound in his chest. The sound of the handgun is much softer than I am expecting. It is the dry crack of a twig snapping over and over.

"Sorry about that," Kelly tells me.

"You're crazy," I say quietly.

He smiles. "I doubt it. It's just that I've developed a more complete understanding of our situation."

"Do you understand that Dexter's other boys will be looking for us now? Along with God-knows-who-else."

He shrugs. "I hope you see why it was necessary."

I stare at him.

He stands very close to Wilton, who is gurgling. "It's

all perfectly natural. Today we're selecting for people who draw their guns on time." He smiles. "We're selecting against surly tarbabies who don't know how to watch their mouths."

We are sitting on long sofas in the dark-maple locker room at the Harvard Club and my boss is saying, "If poor people were as smart as rich people, they'd be rich by now."

The man next to him is soft everywhere and colors his hair red-brown. He netted eleven million dollars last year. He chuckles.

My boss says, "Every generation of a family has a chance to hit it big. If they keep missing, after a while you have to assume that something's wrong with the genes."

The carpet is blood-colored. The walls of the locker room are covered with lacquered plaques that show vertical columns of men's names. Kelly and I have our legs stuck out in front of us and crossed at the ankles. We are wearing white Izod shirts and gray shorts. We have long-handled rackets laid across our laps.

The television that hangs from the ceiling of the locker room shows a pretty blond woman with straight teeth and a gray-haired man, also with straight teeth, sitting at a curved desk in front of Corinthian columns and windows that show false sky. At the bottom of the screen, stock prices churn by in a blue strip.

Kelly whispers, "Ancient chieftains developed efficient methods of agriculture so that they could throw banquets to show their power."

"What?" I say.

"It wasn't to better provide for their people. For that, the old methods were sufficient."

I stare at him.

"Technology develops not to advance the species but to consolidate the power of individuals."

"Listen," I say, "I don't have any idea what you're talking about."

"I'm talking about the death of emotion and the sublimation of desire."

"I thought the death of emotion was what we wanted. I thought you said we were walking the path to emotional detachment."

He nods. "Yes. I've come to reexamine our position. At the beginning I thought we were working to evolve into things capable of murder. I thought we were trying to divorce mind from body. I thought we were trying to resist going cerebral." He sighs. "I realized recently that our problem is that we had already *gone* cerebral. We had already separated mind and body. We've been denying our instincts. For human beings to be able to kill, they don't need to evolve, they need to regress. All these computer-geek faggots live in the world of the cerebral and they've probably never been in a fight. They can't fight, they can't fuck, they have no physical *presence*. You and I have been trying to regain our instinctive behaviors. We're trying to get back to basics."

"But my instinct was to feel sorry for those frat boys and for the guy I was supposed to shoot."

"You're making the mistake of classifying compassion as a human emotion. Really, your natural instincts are to do what's best for yourself and to eliminate anything that challenges your success. You do for you, I do for me, everyone does for themselves, shake it all up and the cream rises to the top. It's mathematics."

"How can you tell me what my instincts are?"

"Because human behavior has been completely dissected. The genome is mapped. There are no more secrets."

My boss is smoothing a terry-cloth headband over his hairline. He looks at the man next to him, who is still chuckling. My boss says, "Take the Gettys, for example."

The pretty blond anchorwoman looks into the camera and

says something, but I can't hear it because the sound on the television has been muted. Her words appear in a black closed-caption box below her. The black box says, "Now, the day's headlines."

I ignore the first two stories, both of which include videotape of rolling tanks. When the third story begins, a graphic appears over the anchorwoman's shoulder featuring a painting of the Ritz-Carlton Hotel splattered with enormous puddles of blood. Written over this painting in white block letters are the words "Ritz Murder."

Kelly says, "Normally they don't make so much fuss over a shine killing."

My boss says, "Location, location, location."

The man sitting with him says, "Such a waste."

Kelly says, "We don't know if it's a waste. It's not like this was some kid on the honor roll. Maybe this was just a big, mean dog who ran into a bigger, meaner dog. These things happen."

The man turns to look at him.

"Do you know any of the men on the walls?" I say quickly.

"Sure," he says. "Most of them."

"That must be hard."

He turns away from Kelly to look at me. "What must be hard?"

"To lose so many friends."

"Lose?"

"In the war."

He shakes his head. "The war dead are in the lobby, kid. These are the trustees."

"Oh," I say.

Kelly leans close to me and whispers, "Human beings have come to treat death differently than other animals do. When lions get too old, they lose their place in the pride and are forced to wander, scavenging for food, unable to hunt, until eventually they die of starvation or disease or they become immobilized by starvation or disease and are then eaten alive by hyenas. When sharks are injured, other sharks come from miles around and tear them to pieces. Human beings are the only species that tries to prolong life artificially after the subject has outlived his usefulness. We are the only creatures that mourn our dead."

"Elephants," I say.

"Elephants?"

"Elephants mourn their dead."

"That's impossible," he tells me.

We are standing in Dexter's living room, surrounded by Persian rugs and sliding glass doors and a glass-topped coffee table dusted with cocaine residue. The residue is smeared into white streaks. On the floor beside the table are three long-stemmed champagne glasses and a metal ice bucket.

On the other side of the glass doors are the floodlit patio and the swimming pool and the hot tub, both of which have underwater lights, and past all that are evergreen-covered hills that loom black in the darkness.

Dexter is in the hot tub with one of the girls. The other girl, naked and brown and smooth and gleaming, is standing on the edge of the pool and swaying in time to faint music. They are all laughing. I can't tell where the music is coming from.

Kelly motions toward the glass doors. He is dressed entirely in black. His face is covered in greasepaint.

"What if they hear?" I whisper.

"They won't," he whispers back. "And, even so, if they look back at the house they'll be looking from the light into the dark."

"It's not really *dark* in here."

"Dark enough."

I slide one of the doors open. It hisses on its runner. I freeze. Dexter and the girls keep laughing. I slip through the opening and onto the slate of the patio. Kelly follows me. We move slowly, crouched low, careful to keep our footfalls silent.

The dancing girl sees us first. She stops swaying and opens her mouth. Kelly shows her his gun. She does not speak.

I kneel down behind Dexter and press the barrel of my automatic into the back of his neck. His body shudders and tenses. The girl next to him gasps. She has long hair and skin the color of coffee ice cream.

I say, "Where are the roughnecks?"

"We're the only ones here," Dexter says. His voice is very steady.

"Bullshit," Kelly says.

"I swear to God."

Kelly says, "If you're lying, I'm going to slice your eyeballs open with a razor."

"I'm not lying."

"After that, I'm going to pour gasoline into your eye sockets and pull off your fingernails one by one. Then I'm going to tie your hand to the side of this pool and mash it with a cinder block. Then I'm going to take a pair of garden shears and cut your tongue in half while it's still in your mouth."

The girl in the hot tub starts to cry.

Kelly turns to her. "Is he lying?"

She shakes her head.

Kelly says, "If he is, I'm going to do the same thing to you."

She sobs more loudly. She keeps shaking her head.

Kelly looks at me. "I believe it."

I stand and walk around in front of Dexter. "It's me," I say.

He squints at my face. "Jesus Christ," he says. "You almost made me piss myself."

Kelly says, "Don't think I didn't mean what I said."

Dexter says, "What do you want?"

"We need to talk," I tell him.

Dexter is sitting on the black leather sofa in his living room and wearing a white robe that pulls very tight across his shoulders. I am seated facing him on a ceramic barstool that I dragged in from the kitchen. Kelly is on the other side of the room, leaning on a mantelpiece. The girls are upstairs in the windowless walk-in closet in Dexter's bedroom. We slid a heavy bureau in front of the closet door. We balanced a mirror between the bureau and the door. Kelly told the girls that if we heard the mirror break he was going to come upstairs and pull out their teeth with pliers and shove straightened coat hangers into their ear canals to rupture the drums.

"Where'd the hitters go?" I ask Dexter.

He says, "Wilton's disappeared. They're trying to find him."

"They have any ideas?"

He shrugs. "Not that I know of."

I glance at Kelly. He shakes his head.

"I don't believe you," I say to Dexter.

"I can't help that."

Kelly says, "The next time you lie, I'm going to shoot you in the hip. Won't be too many more Pro Bowls after that."

"Tell us," I say.

Dexter says, "They think maybe you two clipped him."

"You try to talk them out of that?"

"I tried. They weren't sure anyway."

"They have a theory?"

"They think Wilton's that thing at the Ritz."

"I thought that guy couldn't be identified."

He looks at me carefully. "Yeah, somebody put some caps

in his face. Blew out his teeth and everything. Also, they took his wallet and cut off the tips of his fingers."

"So what makes them think it's Wilton?"

"It's just a guess right now. That's why you're still walking."

"How long before it's not just a guess?"

"Who knows? Depends what they find."

"Any chance you can get them off of us?"

He shakes his head. "They're looking for payback. I can't call them off."

"What are they doing now?"

"They're checking you out."

"Any prediction about what their conclusion will be?"

"Again," he says, "it depends."

"On what?"

He stares at me. "On what you've done."

"What's your instinct?"

"These guys are pros. They'll put this together in their sleep. They'll take just enough time to be certain." He takes a breath. "Then, Kelly goes for sure. I tried to tell them that *you* couldn't have been involved. They'll spend a little while thinking about that."

"And then?"

"And then I figure you go too."

"Unless?"

He shrugs. "Unless you're gone to somewhere they can't find you."

"Or they aren't good enough," Kelly says.

"They're good enough," Dexter tells him.

"Wilton wasn't."

We are silent for a while.

Dexter says, "I'll try to warn you."

"Why would you do that?" Kelly says.

Dexter jerks his head at me. "He's my friend. It isn't fair for him to get burned just because of the company he keeps."

"You're so sure it was me?"

"Sure enough."

Kelly smiles. "Then how do you know I won't do you too?"

"Because I'm your early-warning system."

"How can you warn us when you don't know where they are?"

"They still check in." He frowns. "That reminds me—how'd you get past the alarm?"

Kelly's smile widens. "I think you may need a new one," he says.

Heather comes out of the dressing room wearing blue jeans made from some kind of stretch material. She lifts the bottom of her sweater, showing a narrow strip of belly. The jeans ride low on her hips.

"What do you think?" she says.

"Great," I say.

"That's what you always say."

"I always mean it."

She examines herself in a long mirror on the wall.

"I like them," she says. "You can wear them with a blouse. You can wear them with a halter."

"You're sexy," I tell her.

She turns her head toward me and smiles. "You're sweet."

The walls of the store are lined with light brown shelves. Most of the shelves hold scented candles and kitchenware and lamps with rice-paper shades. The shelves in back hold thirty-dollar T-shirts.

Heather walks to the narrow doorframe of the dressing room and leans her head inside. She pulls her head out and says, "Still empty."

She takes my hand and leads me into a pine-smelling corridor lined with stalls. The door of one of the stalls is hanging open and Heather pulls me inside. She closes the door behind us and throws the bolt. Her jacket is lying on the gray bench in the corner. Her shoes are on the floor under the bench. Each wall, including the back of the door, is completely covered by a mirror. The mirrors reflect each other's reflections. We are surrounded by infinite versions of ourselves that extend as far as we can see in every direction. We can see ourselves from every angle.

Heather runs her tongue along the edge of my ear. She puts her palm between my legs. I feel myself stirring against the zipper of my pants. I grip her shoulders and gently push her away. She frowns at me.

I say, "I'm sorry if my behavior has been strange lately."

"I hadn't noticed."

"I've been under a lot of pressure."

"Work?"

"Not really. I've been dealing with some personal issues."

She presses me down onto the gray bench and sits across my knees with her arms around my neck. "Like what?" she says.

"Oh, I don't know. I've been working on my development."

"As a person?"

"Sort of."

She strokes my hair. "I want to get married."

"I know. You told me after our third date."

"I mean I want to get married soon. I want to take care of you. I want you to take care of me."

"I don't have *anything*," I tell her. "At least let's wait and see what happens with the company."

"I don't like waiting. Besides, my father is practically *made* of money."

"I don't want your father to take care of us."

"No," she says, "neither do I."

•   •   •

Kelly's sketch has wide eyes and too much nose. Mine is a cross between Errol Flynn without the mustache and Paul Bunyan without the beard. The sketches are superimposed side by side on the blue-sky background behind the pretty blond anchorwoman with the stock ticker flowing beneath her.

We are sitting on the sofa in our living room.

Kelly says, "I don't like her as much on the HDTV. She wears too much makeup."

"Everyone wears makeup on television."

"She has bumps on her face. She looks like a pickle."

The anchor is talking to a brunette with thin lips who is standing in front of the Ritz in the rain, looking concerned. The anchor also looks concerned.

I say, "Aren't you a little bit worried?"

"About the sketches? You can't tell it's us unless you know what you're looking for. Even then, they're kind of a stretch. They made me look like Groucho, for Chrissake."

"Maybe we ought to lay low. Get out of the apartment. *Some*thing."

"Forget it. Those pictures could be almost anybody. The cops aren't gonna find us with these descriptions unless they're already onto us."

"And what about Dexter's boys?"

"The Jamaicans?"

"How do you know they're Jamaicans?"

He shrugs. "Wilton was."

"Fine, then," I say. "What about the Jamaicans?"

He sighs. "The important thing is for us to stay on-mission."

"On-mission?"

"Heather's old man."

"Are you serious?"

"We have to finish what we started."

The back of my neck is hot. "I'm not sure about that."

"You don't have to be sure. I'm telling you it's going to be done."

"I think I may have made some kind of mistake."

"Trust me," Kelly says. "This is best for everybody. This is what you said you wanted."

"I think I've changed my mind."

Kelly nods.

The sketches are gone. The anchorwoman is smiling now.

Kelly stands up from the couch and walks to the door.

"Where are you going?" I say.

He opens the door and walks into the hallway. I listen to the door click shut behind him. I turn back to the television.

When the phone rings an hour later, I pick it up immediately. "Kel?" I say.

There is no answer.

"Where are you?" I say.

I hear the ticking of the open line.

I say, "Just come back and we can talk about it."

I hold the receiver against my ear and listen to buzzing static and then Dexter's voice says, "They're coming."

PART THREE: CLIMAX

"**Y**ou don't look good," my boss says.

"I had to get a hotel room last night."

He half-smiles. "You have a fight with your boyfriend?"

"We're having some work done," I say.

We are looking out the big window of the Credit Suisse

luxury box at the Fleet Center, squinting at tiny players on a tiny floor hundreds of feet below us. It is almost impossible to tell what they are doing. When we want to see the game, we watch wide-screen televisions in the corners of the room.

My boss says, "I was trying to reach you. I called the cell phone."

"It didn't get reception in the hotel."

"You need to be available to me twenty-four hours. Where's Princess Grace?"

"He's not here?"

My boss shakes his head. "If you two want a job where you don't have to come in on Sundays, go work at the post office."

"I *am* in," I say.

A young trader is screaming at one of the televisions. His friends sit in front of the television in leather armchairs, Frisbeeing paper plates at the screen.

My boss says, "Any of these guys would kill for your job."

The skin on my face feels very tight. "So would I."

I imagine throwing my boss through the tinted window and watching him plummet into the middle of the court. I can see the stain of him spreading on the bleached wood.

My boss says, "Let's see some of that."

I pull my gun from inside my coat and touch the barrel to his eyebrow. "Open your mouth," I say.

"What?"

I hit him in the forehead with the side of the gun. He steps back. Blood trickles down his face.

"Get on your knees," I say.

He does.

"Open your mouth."

The traders have stopped making noise. I know that people around the room are looking at us. No one moves. My boss opens his mouth.

"Wider," I say.

I shove my gun deep into his mouth. It clatters against his teeth.

I say, "You're going to have to learn how to treat people."
He nods. He is shivering.
I say loudly, "You're a ridiculous man. You don't even understand your job. I don't know who put you in charge. I'm younger than you, I'm better than you. I don't even need this gun. I could kill you with my *hands*."
A dark patch has appeared on my boss's light gray trousers. There are tears running down his face.
I say, "You don't have the balls for this kind of work."
I take my gun out of his mouth.
Everyone stares at me uncertainly. A few of the traders applaud.
"Thank you," I say.
My boss is slumped on the floor, moaning. I smile at the room. I put my gun away and give one last wave and then walk quickly to the door.
I say, "If I see this door open while I'm still in the hallway, I'm going to come back and choose two of you at random and shoot you in the balls."
When the elevator opens, it is full of security guards. They have their guns drawn.
I say, "There's some maniac in there with a gun. He has baggies of nitroglycerin taped all over his body. He said he would detonate if he heard anyone trying to come in. If you shoot him, the whole place might go up. Can you imagine what that would be like? You'd spend days sifting through body parts. You'd have to make piles of limbs. Can you imagine an enormous pile of severed arms?"
One of the security guards says, "Get behind us."
They push past me and fan out around the entrance to the luxury box. One of them puts a finger to his lips and leans his ear against the door.
I step inside their elevator and press Lobby.
Standing on the sidewalk next to the Fleet Center, listening to the sirens approaching, I take out my cell phone and call Heather.

I say, "How soon can you be at South Station?"

"Is this a joke?" she says.

"It's not a joke. I'm leaving. Will you go with me?"

"Yes."

I cross Causeway Street. "How soon?"

"Do I have time to pack?"

"No."

"Half hour," she says.

I push the End button and put the phone back in my pocket and look over my shoulder at the Fleet Center and at the squad cars pulling up in front and that is when I see the Jamaicans.

They are on the other side of the street, half a block behind me, watching the cops pile out of their cars. One of the Jamaicans is tall and wide. The other is the one who frisked us at the barbershop. They are moving at the same speed I am. They turn away from the cops and toward me and I snap my head back around, but I am almost certain they saw me see them. I keep walking, sweat dripping down my back, feeling them behind me.

I cross Merrimac Street.

I glance over my shoulder. The Jamaicans are still matching their speed to mine. They are maintaining the same distance.

At Cambridge Street, I reach the corner just as the DON'T WALK sign stops blinking and I slow down and almost stop and then suddenly I dash into the street and hear squealing brakes and slide over the hood of a moving taxi and hear horns screaming behind me and then I am on the other side, running.

Heather's father stands up to meet me. His office is lined with black shelves that hold crystal eggs and lacquered cigar boxes.

"How did you know I'd be here?" he says.

"What do you mean?"

"It's Sunday."

"Oh." I run my tongue along the backs of my teeth. "Heather must have told me."

He looks at me. "Must have," he says.

I take a deep breath. "I need your help." I glance out the window. "By the flower cart."

Heather's father walks to the window and gazes down at the street. "Who are they?" he says.

"I don't know exactly."

"They're pros."

"Yes."

"How'd you make them?"

"I don't know. They just sort of appeared across the street from me."

"I mean, how'd they let you see them?"

"I was looking for them. I knew they were coming."

He shakes his head. "Shouldn't matter."

"But why would they want me to spot them?"

He shrugs. "Maybe they wanted to see whether you'd run. Maybe they figure only a guilty man runs."

We are silent for a while.

Seven stories below us, the big Jamaican crosses the street and walks along the sidewalk and around the far side of the building.

"Why don't they follow me in?" I say.

"They don't know which floor you're on. Also, they'd be worried about the building's security force. And they don't want to trap themselves in case things go south. If they take you in the open, they have escape routes and it's easier for them to avoid the cops. They'll cover the exits and wait to reacquire."

"You learned all this in Vietnam?"

"It's textbook," he says. He lifts his telephone receiver.

"What are you doing?"

"Cops."

I shake my head.

He puts down the receiver. "Sounds like you have something to tell me."

I don't say anything.

He steps away from the window and takes his key ring from his pants pocket and unlocks the top drawer of his desk. He brings out a heavy automatic. He pulls back on the slide and checks the cylinder.

"You keep it *loaded*?" I say.

"Doesn't do much good when it's not." He puts the gun in the waistband of his pants. "You carrying?"

I show him the pistol inside my jacket.

"You any good with that?"

I shrug.

"Who put these guys on you?"

I shrug again.

"This have anything to do with that fairy you hang around with?"

"You mean Kelly?"

"How many fairies you know?"

"But Kelly's just cool."

He snorts. "For a catamite."

"No," I say. "It's his *job*. Kelly sells cool. I sell cheekbones."

He looks at me. "I don't know what the fuck you're talking about. I don't much care. All I want to know is why there are two hard guys waiting for you outside my building."

"It's kind of a long story."

"Give me the broad strokes."

"They think Kelly took out a friend of theirs."

"Did he?"

I stare at him.

Heather's father nods. "I guess that's not too surprising."

"Will you help me?"

He frowns. "You ever do any wet work?"

I take a breath. "Not really."

"Stay close to me. When it happens, hold low and put your man down. Nothing fancy. Keep shooting until he drops."

I am having trouble breathing. "Are we going now?"

He shakes his head. "We'll wait until the game breaks. The more confusion, the better."

When it's time, Heather's father says, "Get yourself frosty. They won't go easy."

"You can tell that by watching them stand on a street corner?"

"That's right," he says. He taps his middle finger against the handle of the gun in his waistband. "Let's go have a little roughhouse."

In the lobby we fall in step with a group of gray-suited corporate lawyers and pass with them through the enormous revolving door. Outside, the street is seething. The sidewalk in front of us is a sea of bobbing heads. We move with the crowd.

I am peering over the people around me, watching the Jamaican leaning against his flower cart on the opposite sidewalk. He is staring into the crowd, trying to keep sight of the door. Heather's father is directly in front of me, crouched slightly, also watching the Jamaican.

Heather's father glances at me over his shoulder. He says, "Cross at the corner. We'll take him as soon as we hit the other side."

I nod. Everything seems far away. I no longer feel shoulders jostling against mine. I no longer feel feet scraping the backs of my heels.

I imagine what would happen if a V-shaped flight of F-4s passed over us and dropped flaming orange sheets of napalm. I see the commuters around me turn black in the heat. I see their melting faces. I imagine an earthquake in which the skyscrapers above us disintegrate into a concrete avalanche. I imagine a world without skyscrapers where we would huddle close together and wait for lions or saber-toothed cats to charge us from the underbrush. We would scatter, lungs burning, tingling-hot all over from the adrenaline burst, and the lions would go after the youngest or the sickest or the weakest and they would bring him down with airborne strikes that break his legs and they would rip him apart.

I imagine meteor showers.

We are almost to the corner when I see Kelly. He is in a second-story window across the street. I do not see his rifle. He nods to me.

I lean toward Heather's father. "We may have a problem," I say.

"You mean your boy in the window?" he says. He does not turn around.

"You saw him."

"When we got out here."

"Why didn't you say anything?"

"I didn't know it was an issue."

"He may not be a friendly," I say.

"Is he a hostile?"

"Possibly."

He turns his head now. "Is there something you're not telling me?"

We have reached the corner.

I say, "I believe there's been a series of misunderstandings and misinterpretations."

"Leading to what?"

"Kelly is probably going to try to kill you."

He stares at me. "Why would he do that?"

I don't say anything.

Heather's father says, "Because you told him to?"

The light changes and we begin moving across the street.

"I've recently come to reexamine some things," I say.

When Kelly appears next to me, Heather's father is still on his knees. The smaller Jamaican is lying next to the flower cart. There is a hole in the center of his face. His cheeks are caved in toward it. The big Jamaican is on the ground next to us. On the ground next to him are the white and gray and blue-veined coils of his guts. He has been cut nearly in half by the exit wound from Kelly's hollowpoint. His face is smooth and unmarked. His eyes are wide open.

Kelly says, "Let's get what we came for."

"I don't think this is what Heather wants."

"Sure it is. You said so."

"I know that. I think I made it up."

"That's crazy."

"Yes," I say.

He shrugs. "I suppose it doesn't much matter. It was never really about her."

"What was it about?"

"Getting back to nature."

Heather's father says, "You don't have to do this."

Kelly draws his pistol. "Don't flatter yourself. It was never really about you either."

I say, "You've already made your progress. You don't need this."

"We need to finish what we started."

I shake my head. "You're being too literal."

"It's what separates us from the animals."

"I thought what separated us from the animals was that we know we're going to die."

"What separates us from the animals," he says, "is our ability to ask what separates us from the animals." He aims his pistol. Heather's father closes his eyes. "The danger," Kelly says, "is to become all talk and no action."

I close my eyes before I fire—holding low, squeezing-not-pulling—so I do not see Kelly's face when the bullet hits him. I imagine him looking at me with enormous, shocked eyes and reaching out his hand and taking a shaky step toward me and I fire again and again with my eyes closed until I hear his body fall.

He is still alive. He sounds like he is trying to clear his

throat. I imagine the way he looks on the ground, flopping like a landed fish, drowning in the air.

I turn away before I open my eyes.

Heather's father is leaning against me. We are shuffling along Purchase Street, trying to seem casual. I have draped my jacket over him to hide his shoulder. Taking the jacket off revealed my gun harness, so I unstrapped it and threw it in a garbage can on Federal Street. I have the pistol in my pants pocket.

There are sirens everywhere now. The cruisers are stuck in the traffic from the Central Artery construction site. The sidewalk is full of people who do not know what has happened. We are lost in the crowd again.

Heather's father drags himself along, stepping as lightly as he can so as not to jostle his shoulder. We do not speak.

Heather is sitting in her Mercedes with the line of taxis in front of South Station.

She says, "Get in."

I open the back door and help her father inside and slide in next to him. Heather pulls away from the curb.

Her father says, "Where are we going?"

"What is he doing here?" Heather says. "What's wrong with him?"

"It's sort of a long story," I tell her. "We can't go home."

"No," her father agrees.

"We need to get out of the city for a while."

"What if they shut it down?"

"The whole city?"

"They could."

"But they don't even know what to look for. They don't know what we're driving."

"Chancy," he says.

· · ·

Heather's father closes his eyes and leans against the back of the seat. We creep onto the bridge beside the Children's Museum and sit in the steaming line of stopped cars.

Heather's father is taking deep breaths.

Heather turns her head toward me. "Do it," she says.

"Do what?" I say.

"Kill him."

I feel the inside of the car begin to spin. I open my mouth but no sound comes out.

"What's wrong?" Heather says.

"I thought I imagined it."

"Imagined what?"

"That you asked for this."

"Why would you think that? This is what you wanted."

"Me?"

"You said you wanted to take care of me."

"I do."

"Then he's served his purpose."

"So he has to die?"

"You want me, you want money. He has both. I want a man who doesn't *ask* for everything. I want a man who *takes*."

"Are you sure you want this?"

"Really, I want it for you. I want you to feel like you can be the man in my life."

I rub my neck.

"I'm establishing my independence," she says.

Heather's father says, "You must know she's crazy." His eyes are still closed.

"Shut up," Heather says. She turns back to me. "Kill him."

"I don't know," I say.

Heather's father says, "This can't be the first time you've seen it. She used to sprinkle detergent in the birdfeeder."

"Do it," Heather tells me, "so we can start our new life."

Her father says, "She was thirteen the first time she tried to kill me."

"Why don't you stake out some territory for yourself?" Heather asks me. "Be a man. Get in the *game*, for Chrissake. You can't let people walk all over you. Let's break free. Let's set out on our own."

"Let's," I say.

"Do it, then."

"Why can't we just leave?"

She says, "We have to cut all our ties."

Her father says, "In an hour she'll love me again. She'll blame you for killing me. Every day you'll be wondering who she's going to ask to do *you*. Indecision, kid. It's what separates man from the animals."

"Regret," I say.

"That too."

I take a deep breath and unlock my door.

"Where will you go?" Heather says. "I thought you were on the run."

"I'll have to think of something."

"You're nothing," she sneers. "You always need someone else to do your work. Maybe I'll get Kelly to do it. I'm sure *he* has the balls. Maybe I'll even throw a little pussy his way."

"Good luck with that," I say. "Today we've been selecting against silk-suit thrill killers."

As I am opening the door, I hear Heather say, "I don't need you anymore."

"I love you," her father says. "I want to help you." His voice cracks.

I close the door and leave them there.

Walking back along the bridge, I imagine the beginning of the universe.

THE ART
OF THE
POSSIBLE

You date pretty, brown-haired, apple-cheeked girls who will seem like virgins even after they have children. You stay away from drugs. You drink just enough not to stand out. You use football to get yourself to school, but not to pay for it (your school doesn't give athletic scholarships)—for that you take out loans and get work-study jobs hauling trash and sweeping floors. Your hair is cut short, but not *too* short. You work for various campus political organizations—all of which are liberal, but not *too* liberal.

You are handsome, but not *too* handsome. You are tall, but not *too* tall.

After college, from which you graduate one year early, you go straight to law school and then to the state attorney's office and you establish residency in a district with a congressman who you have heard is about to make a run for the Senate and when he does you run for his seat. And you win it. Election day is two weeks after your twenty-eighth birthday.

You're going to make a name for yourself championing the common man. You're going to get on the Judiciary Committee during your second term. You are not going to cave to big business. You are going to be a senator. You will keep all of

your promises; you will never sacrifice your ideals for political gain. You will be president by the time you're forty.

You are going to do some good.

Y ou are pretty sure it's Wednesday, but it might be
Monday, and you're dressed in a navy overcoat
and black oxfords and you are striding, strong-jawed, project-
ing quiet confidence, along the edge of a vacant lot in the
center of your district where a construction crew is breaking
ground for a low-rise affordable-housing complex. You are
walking with the contractor, both of you wearing bright orange hard hats, leading a phalanx of reporters. Really, the
phalanx is one longhaired photographer and a beat reporter
from the city paper with coffee stains on his shirt.

You are wondering when your father will call.

Later, you will be interviewed at a local television station
with a blue bedsheet hanging behind you for background.
You will talk about the new housing complex and the economic boon that it will be for your district. You will talk
about your commitment to your constituents.

You will be forthright.

The reporter waddles up from behind you and says, "How
much longer are we staying?"

On your other side, the contractor is still talking about his
building plans. He does not seem to notice the interruption.

You give the reporter the medium smile with just a hint of
teeth and incline your head toward him for increased intimacy and say, "Until you have what you need."

He snorts. "You think I need to walk around a goddamn
parking lot to write this shit? I could have written it sitting
on the toilet."

Your smile widens just a bit and you chuckle and give the
reporter a look that tells him that you acknowledge the
ridiculousness of the situation and that you regret any incon-
venience it has caused him—you feel his *pain*—but that

simultaneously you feel the grave burden of your responsibility to the people you represent. You are a servant of the people. You are the voice of the people.

You could tell him about Betty Friedkin, who is seventy-eight years old (a proud American senior, you would call her) and living on her Social Security and who has trusted you to stand up for her against those Washington fat cats; you could tell him about Jamir Winslow, twenty-nine-year-old African American father of four (*proud* African American father), who is worried about his recent trouble with the state police and wants you to get behind the new federal civil rights bill, which contains strong language against racial profiling, that the fat cats are trying to block; you could tell him about Angela Martinez (proud Latin American—no, you think, that's not quite right, but you don't like the sound of "Hispanic American" and you don't think you've ever heard "Latin American American," although it would seem to make sense—mother of an indeterminate number of children), who wants you to clean up the water and the air and the streets and television—also, you think she wants you to stand up to the fat cats in Washington, but you can't be sure because you've never actually met her. You haven't actually met *any* of these people, but you have been *fully* briefed. You've got your hand on the pulse. You are willing to go the extra mile.

You give one hundred and ten percent.

Wes has been talking to the longhaired photographer, but when he saw the reporter come up alongside you he crept forward so that now he is hovering just over your left shoulder. He says to the reporter, "All I'm thinking about is the single-malt I left in the car. I'm hoping we can kill it on the ride back."

The reporter smiles at him and fades back to walk beside the photographer.

You lean close to Wes and say, "Why aren't you wearing a hard hat?"

"They're just for the pictures," he whispers. He looks at the sky. You follow his eyes. He says, "They haven't started building. There's nothing to fall on you."

Wes is not a bodyguard, but he has a big semiautomatic pistol slung under his left arm. You are not sure that he would be able to use it if the moment arose. Still, you are comforted knowing it's there. Although you very rarely think about the possibility of assassination.

Theo, your security man, trails the group, not smiling. He looks like he could be distantly related to you.

You pass a drugstore on the way to the car. You shake hands with a few people who are wandering in or out. You clap some shoulders. A gray-haired man in a plaid shirt tells you that he met your father once.

"They don't make them like that anymore," the man says. "He'd always shoot you straight."

"Yes," you say.

The car is a black Lincoln Navigator. You have had a row of seats added where the trunk used to be. You have had the original backseat turned around so that the two rows face each other. You sit next to the reporter while the photographer sits across from you snapping pictures. Theo drives. Wes sits beside him, half turned, leaning on the back of his seat, listening to everything you say.

Today is Wednesday (you saw the front page of a newspaper on the rack outside the drugstore before you got into the car). In two weeks, you will be thirty years old. You have not slept in six days.

After the television interview, you lock yourself in a canary-yellow stall in the station's men's room and chew a small handful of pearl-colored Benzedrine tablets. You sit on the closed lid of the toilet and press your palms against your forehead. Your throat is raw.

You hear footsteps in the hallway. You hear the sigh of the air spring on top of the bathroom door and then the footsteps are inside the room. They scrape along the tiles. A shadow appears outside the door of your stall.

Wes's voice says, "You all right?"

You are silent.

Wes says, "Maybe you ought to lie down for a while."

You look up at the closed door. You listen to Wes breathing.

He says, "I have something for you."

The outlines of the door are very clear.

You say, "Any good?"

"Do I ever let you down?"

You smile slightly. "Where is she?"

"In the hallway."

You groan. "I don't know if I can stand up."

"Don't worry," Wes says. "I'll bring her."

The shadow disappears and you hear the footsteps again and the sigh of the door and then the footsteps are in the hallway, getting softer. The footsteps stop and after a few seconds they are replaced by the harsh clacking of high heels. You reach out and unlock the stall door and listen to the high heels clattering into the room.

The girl who pushes open the door of your stall is dirty-blond and smooth-faced. She has wide hips and a narrow waist. She is wearing a gray skirt.

She says, "You were great."

You blink at her. "I haven't touched you."

"The interview."

"You saw it?"

"You were on after my weather report."

You frown. "I thought I knew the . . . ah . . . the meteorologist here."

She nods. "Veronica. She's in Peoria now. And I'm a weather girl."

"What?"

"I'm not a meteorologist."

"Right. Sorry about that."

"It doesn't matter." She smiles. "You know, since I got here I've wanted to meet you."

"I'm a rookie congressman. How do you even know who I am?"

"I like politics. Also, I've always been interested in your father."

"Oh."

She steps into the stall and closes the door behind her.

"What's your name?" you say. Your voice is hoarse.

"Annie."

She reaches behind her and slides the bolt.

You say, "It's good to meet you, Annie." You have to stop yourself from moving to shake her hand.

She says, "Just relax."

She kneels in front of you and smooths her skirt over her thighs and you lean your head back against the wall over the toilet. She is unzipping your fly and you think about speaking on the Senate floor and the way you'll thunder and the way you'll look on television (although it'll mostly be C-Span). You try to imagine what it is you'll be thundering about, but Annie has pulled your pants down low on your hips. She is unbuttoning the fly of your boxer shorts and now you can see yourself in the Rose Garden and you can see yourself in the White House press room, looking stern (the commentators will say that you have gravitas), and you can see yourself during the State of the Union getting a standing ovation from the *entire* audience (*both sides* of the aisle, *across* party lines—you are a *uniter*). You can see a black-and-white photograph of yourself as you stare out the window of the Oval Office, dressed in your shirtsleeves, contemplative, concerned, stoic. Annie has opened the fly of your boxer shorts and reached in and pulled you out and you watch her head begin to bob up and down. And then you don't think about anything at all.

You are at a horseshoe-shaped booth at the back of the diner and Wes is funneling people toward you a few at a time. You are using the medium smile with open mouth. You had your teeth whitened at the beginning of the campaign season.

Every time you shake, you grip the top of the other person's forearm with your left hand. You are giving casual intimacy. You are jovial. You have seven jokes that you are telling in sequence. Three of them are self-deprecating. (These show that your power has not gone to your head.) Four of them are about the president. (These show that you cannot be intimidated.) You have two dirty jokes that you do not tell as part of the sequence. You tell these only to old white men. You lean close to them and whisper. Sometimes, after the punch line, you slap the men lightly on the chest with the back of your hand.

You say, "I'm running for reelection as your representative in Congress. I want to go on fighting for you against the special interests and the Washington fat cats. I sure would appreciate your support."

You like this last sentence. It sounds like something your father would say.

The Benzedrine is washing over you in waves. Your eyes are wide open. You imagine that you can hear lobster-shaped microbes crawling through the fluid in your brain.

You watch the pink glow of the sunset through the long windows at the front of the room.

Wes comes over to the booth and says, "That's enough."

"Are we leaving?"

He nods. "We're taking the act out into the street. We'll catch some of the rush-hour crowd."

Wes nods to Theo, who has been standing in the corner watching your table. Theo pulls himself off the wall and leads you out. You wave at everyone who looks at you as you walk to the door. You shake hands with the people who are close enough.

Wes whispers, "Harrison."

You say loudly to the man behind the counter, "Mr. Harrison, I wish you'd give me the recipe for that apple pie. The wife keeps asking for it."

Harrison, who has a pasty-white bald head dotted with liver spots, smiles and shakes his head. "Trade secret."

You look at the people around you and say, "Looks like I'm sleeping on the couch tonight."

There is laughter. At the door, you turn back toward the room and give thumbs-up with your right hand held high above your head (thumbs-up with your hand held low is a cliché). You keep your arm slightly bent to make the gesture less formal.

On the street, you use the high-intensity smile. You do a lot of waving. People stream past you. Wes talks to the people who are waiting to talk to you. Wes is also using the high-intensity smile.

A woman with deep wrinkles creasing her cheeks, hair bleached blond, says that she never heard your father tell a lie.

"He was genuine," she says.

"Yes," you say.

"He could charm the panties off a nun." She laughs. It sounds like choking. "He was honest, though. An honest man."

She moves past you down the street.

During a lull, when the three of you are alone, Theo says, "Green jacket."

"What about him?" Wes says.

"He hasn't moved since we came out here. He keeps trying not to let me catch him looking at us."

"What do you think?"

"Don't know yet."

You glance at the man they're talking about. He is dressed in a fatigue jacket. He is probably in his mid-forties (proud forty-year-old American veteran). He is leaning against the side of a Laundromat on the opposite sidewalk. While you are watching, a girl in a tight gray skirt suit passes the Laundromat. Her hair is brown and flows around her face. You watch her as she moves down the street.

"You see that?" Theo says.

"The girl?" Wes says.

"He didn't look at her."

"Maybe he's a fag."

"Homosexual," you say automatically.

Theo nods, not looking away from the man in the green jacket. "Maybe."

"Homosexual American," you mutter. "*Proud* homosexual American veteran."

Theo says, "Start going for the car. Don't rush."

Wes puts a hand on your back to guide you. Theo keeps his body between you and the man across the street. You are still waving. Your smile does not falter.

Green Jacket is moving. He is walking parallel to you on the opposite sidewalk.

Wes says, "Can we make the car?"

"Maybe," Theo says.

When Green Jacket begins to cross the street, you are not more than fifty feet from the Navigator.

Theo says, "Go."

Wes takes hold of the back of your suit and starts running, pushing you in front of him. You look over your shoulder and watch Theo move to intercept Green Jacket. They come together in the center of the street. Theo grabs the man's wrist and spins him around. Theo kicks out Green Jacket's legs and knocks him facedown onto the pavement and falls on top of him. People on the sidewalk have stopped to observe the action. Some of them watch Wes hustle you past them.

As Wes opens the sliding door of the Navigator and shoves you in, you give the bent-arm thumbs-up. The sky is dark.

Through the tinted back window, you watch Theo stand and pick Green Jacket up from the asphalt. Green Jacket looks angry. He is yelling. Theo says something to him. He stops yelling and turns to walk away. The onlookers begin moving again.

"Shit," Wes says.

"You'd rather it was a hit?"

He shrugs. "It would have gotten us some press."

Theo opens the driver's door and slips in behind the wheel. He starts the engine and pulls away from the curb. He says, "Guy was planning to spit on you."

Wes says, "You frisk him?"

Theo glances at him. "Of course." He turns back to the road. "He was clean."

"He gonna sue us?" Wes says.

"Doubtful."

"Why doubtful?"

Theo shrugs. "He doesn't even know who we are."

"What the fuck are you *talking* about? You just said he was ready to spit on us."

"On *him*," Theo says, jerking his head back at you. "But he doesn't know who he is. Just figures he's *somebody*."

"Jesus Christ."

"Guy's a fuckin' loony tune, you ask me. Plus he was shit-faced. At *least*. Probably won't even remember it in the morning."

"Homeless?"

"We didn't get that far, but it wouldn't surprise me."

Wes shakes his head. "Sooner or later, every wack job wants to be Oswald."

You say, "Doesn't he know about my antipoverty program?"

"He didn't seem too enfranchised."

You shrug. "At least we won't be losing his vote."

Wes says, "We need to get you some sleep."

You imagine tiny decomposers devouring the old skin cells on Wes's face. If you watch him long enough without looking away, you can see him gradually dying.

Your wife is sitting on the sofa in the living room when you get home. She is reading a newspaper. She does not look up at you. You cross the room and lean down and kiss the cold skin of her cheek.

She says, "Your father's coming over."

"Jesus," you say. "Tonight?"

She nods. "He called an hour ago."

"Why didn't you call the cell phone?"

"I didn't want to interrupt. Besides, I was getting the house picked up."

"Where's Ashley?"

"In her room. Maria's getting her ready." She looks up at you now. "How was it?" She has her hair tucked behind her ears. She is wearing a green skirt and a white V-neck sweater. She looks like she has no pores in her face. She photographs extremely well.

You take a deep breath. Then you give her the medium smile with the left corner of your mouth curled up, which she finds charming. She smiles back at you. You bend down and kiss her on the mouth. You give her the open-lipped kiss with no tongue.

She says, "You look tired. I thought you only had to go this hard the first time. Doesn't the incumbent get to rest?"

You say, "The more I win by this time, the more attractive it makes me as a Senate candidate two years from now. That's what we're campaigning for."

"Is it really going to happen?"

"Yes. Are you ready for it?"

"I was born for it."

"That's true."

She folds the newspaper and lays it down next to her and stands up. "I'm going to put on some perfume." She walks out of the room. Her walk is graceful and elegant and sexy enough to be feminine but gives no hint of her ever taking her clothes off or of there being anything between her legs or of the sounds she makes when you run your tongue around her nipples.

The Benzedrine is wearing off. The speed crash is making your body feel unbearably heavy. You walk as though you're underwater.

You call the cell phone from the phone in the hallway. Wes picks up on the second ring.

"My father's on his way over here," you say.

"He going to endorse us?"

"I don't know. I didn't talk to him."

Wes pauses. "Is something wrong?"

You hold the receiver in your right hand and use the index and middle fingers of your left hand to pinch the bridge of your nose. "I'm just a little worn out."

He says, "I'll be back there in two minutes."

"No," you say. "It's better if it's just the two of us."

Your father says, "You look like shit."

"Thanks, Pop."

"Are you sleeping?"

You shrug.

You are standing in the oak-doored vestibule of your house. Your father is on the stone porch at the top of the stone steps. His bodyguards are standing at the bottom of the steps next to a black Mercedes sedan.

Your father is thick-lipped and taller than you. His shoulders are very wide. He is wearing a tan raincoat and a brown fedora that covers his bald spot.

You say, "Aren't you going to come in?"

He slides past you into the house. In the entrance hall, your wife is standing with your daughter, Ashley, both of them facing the door and giving the high-medium smile with teeth.

You lock the door. You close your eyes and wait for the dizziness to pass.

When you come into the entrance hall, your father is leaning down toward Ashley.

"Put your hand out," he is saying.

She does.

He reaches into his coat and brings out his key ring and hands it to her. "There you go," he says.

Ashley giggles. She is wearing a flowered dress and white stockings and black shoes with gold buckles. She has blond hair and brown eyes.

He frowns. "Isn't that what you wanted?"

Ashley shakes her head.

He takes the keys back from her. He straightens up and makes a big show of patting his various pockets. "I don't know what else I can give you." He reaches into his coat again. "The only other things I have are these." He brings out a handful of caramels wrapped in gold paper.

Ashley claps.

"You want *these*?"

She nods.

"How old are you now?" your father asks her.

"Almost five."

"How close?"

She stares at her hands for a few seconds, her mouth moving. Then she turns and whispers loudly to your wife, "Mommy, how long until I'm five?"

"Two months," your wife says.

Ashley turns back to your father. "Two months."

He scowls. "Well, I guess we'll give it to you. Put your hand out."

He crouches down again and counts five caramels into her hand and puts the rest into his pocket.

"What do you say?" your wife says.

"Thank you, Grampa," Ashley says. "I love you." She kisses him on the cheek. He hugs her.

He stands up and hugs your wife. He kisses her on the cheek.

"I'm glad to see you," she says. She looks down at Ashley. "Time to say good night."

Ashley shakes her head. The high-medium smile has disappeared.

Your wife says, "Don't make your grandfather think you don't have any manners."

Ashley shakes her head again.

You say, "Getting enough sleep is important, especially for little girls. I knew a girl in high school named Emily Thomas who never slept more than four hours a night. She had to drop out. Now she's got three kids and no husband. She's a drain on our country's overextended welfare system. With these new fat-cat welfare-reform bills she may lose her only source of income."

They are all staring at you.

You say, "We don't need any more Emily Thomases."

Your father turns back to Ashley and says, "I thought you were almost five. Five-year-olds don't throw tantrums when it's time for bed."

She nods.

"Maria," your wife calls over her shoulder.

Maria appears wearing blue jeans and a gray sweater.

Your wife says, "Bedtime."

Your father says, "Good to see you again, Maria."

Maria says, "It's good to see you again, Governor."

"I'm not the governor anymore."

She frowns. "I thought you kept the title for life."

"You do, but it's a little embarrassing. It's like a woman keeping her husband's name after they're divorced."

Maria smiles. She takes hold of Ashley's hand and they walk to the stairs.

Your wife says, "I'm going to bed also."

She kisses your father again.

"They're dropping like flies," he says.

When the two of you are alone, you say, "Should we sit down?"

He shakes his head. "I'm not staying."

You give him the medium smile. "All business."

"Shouldn't I be?"

You shrug. "I am."

He nods. "Why didn't you ask for my endorsement last time?"

"I wanted to break in on my own."

"And now that you're in, all the pride is gone?"

Your eyelids are sagging. "It seems more expedient this way."

He says, "I liked that you wanted to do it by yourself. I respected your not wanting me to campaign for you. I respected your not wanting me to pay for your school."

"I don't care about respect anymore."

"What's happening to you?"

You look into his eyes. You are earnest and determined. Your head feels packed in cotton. You say, "My dreams are coming true."

Your father looks at you for a long moment. "I'm sorry," he says.

When he's gone, you sit on the bright white tile floor of your bathroom feeling your stomach churn. You listen to the buzzing of the fluorescent light over the sink. You wonder whether you should have spent some time in the army.

You kneel in front of the toilet and feel the nausea all over you, but you do not vomit. You grip the black porcelain sides of the bowl and stare at your reflection in the water. Your face is blurred by tiny ripples. You have dark purple fatigue bruises under your eyes. Your skin is pale. Still, you recognize the face. This surprises you somehow.

Behind you, in the hallway outside the bathroom, the wooden floor is creaking. The creaking comes closer and closer and then stops and you hear the muted slaps of bare feet on the bathroom tile. Then the footsteps stop and there is only the hum of the lightbulb.

Your wife says, "Aren't you coming to bed?"

You can imagine her face—mouth closed, eyebrows drawn together with concern, eyes wide with urgency and love. In the outside corner of one of her eyes, there might even be the beginnings of a tear.

You do not turn around. "Soon," you say.

"Please come with me."

You can imagine her eyes closing with sadness.

"Soon," you say again.

"At least look at me," she says. She is using the loving tone with a hint of pleading.

You close the lid of the toilet in front of you. You take a deep breath and push yourself up with your arms and turn around and sit on the closed lid.

Your wife is dressed in her white nightgown. The curves of her body make gray shadows in the fabric. Her face is almost as you pictured it, although she is using sadder eyes than you imagined. As soon as you are looking at her, she allows one of the tears to trickle out and along her cheekbone and past the corner of her mouth.

"I love you," she says. She sighs. Her cheeks draw up toward her forehead and she makes more tears that collect at the bottoms of her eyes, ready to spill.

You frown. You say, "Careful not to give too much too soon. Always try for the slow build. Also, it's better to err on the side of understatement."

She sniffs. "What?"

"Real emotion makes people nervous. It's important to reflect quiet calm. Ideally, you should be sitting down behind a big desk. It makes you look powerful but stable. It's vital to stay placid. Passion is too Mussolini."

She is silent.

"We've talked about this," you say.

"I know," she says. She pushes out a few more tears that leave wet streaks on her face.

"If you weren't ready for this, you should have said something earlier."

She is really pouring on the tears now. "But I thought things would still be the same between *us.*"

You spread your arms wide and give her the welcoming smile. "They are," you say.

BLUE
YONDER

The girl sat at one of the outdoor tables with a much younger girl who looked like her in miniature. They both had blond hair and enormous round eyes. The little girl wore a flowered sundress and sat as tall as she could, straining upward, her chin barely clearing the tabletop. The older girl wore a white blouse and high-heeled sandals and a black skirt that hung below her knees. She sat leaning forward, with her elbows on the table and one soft, smooth, tanned calf draped over the other. Her hair was gathered in back and held together with a silver clip. Her sunglasses had tortoise-shell frames and she wore them pushed back high on her forehead.

When the waiter brought my coffee, I motioned him close to me and said, "Do you know that girl?"

The waiter, whose name was Ricky and who spoke English with extreme care, said, "No, mister."

"She's never been here before?"

"No, mister," Ricky said. "I have not seen her."

I nodded. "Tell me your real name, Ricky."

"You don't want to know."

"Tell me anyway."

He told me.

"You're right," I said.

He smiled. "Will you eat?"

I shook my head and he took away my menu.

I did not want to be caught watching the girls, so I only glanced at them occasionally and the rest of the time I watched the people moving into the Public Garden. The sky was steel blue and cloudless. The street was all couples and families, and businessmen who walked side by side very fast. There was a group of boys trying to climb the statue of Washington. Washington sat rigid in his saddle while the boys grabbed at his boots and at the horse's neck.

The older girl was speaking on a cell phone now and I stared at her for a while and then I forced myself to turn back to the park and I noticed Lucien walking on the other side of the street. He was whistling in that nervous way he had and, although I couldn't hear it, I thought that the tune was probably from *Threepenny Opera* because that was almost always what he whistled. When he saw me, he stopped whistling and dashed across the lanes of traffic, between the speeding cars.

"Mr. Tolstoy, I presume," he said when he reached me, his chest heaving.

"Mr. De Quincey," I said.

He frowned. "No, no. All wrong. I haven't had any opium since I was seventeen and even then I could take it or leave it. Also, he was never a painter."

"Sorry," I said. "Short notice."

He flopped into the chair across from me.

"Mr. Basquiat would be better. Or perhaps Mr. Cézanne."

"They certainly would be."

Ricky appeared beside us. "It has been a long time, Mr. Lucien," he said.

Lucien smiled and spoke to him in French.

"Only English, please," Ricky said.

"You'll get rusty," Lucien warned him.

"No one speaks French back home," Ricky said. "Only the government."

Lucien shrugged. "I'll have an espresso then, Ricky—or is that too much Italian for you?"

"Don't be angry, Mr. Lucien. I'm only trying to improve myself."

"I know. I'm sorry, Ricky, I shouldn't be that way. Bring me an espresso, please."

Ricky walked back inside. Lucien said, "Are you working?"

"Some," I told him.

"I have been finding excuses to stay away from the studio. I despise it."

"The studio or finding the excuses?"

"Both."

Far down the street, a construction crew was repaving part of the sidewalk. The men in the crew wore orange vests. Their trucks poured gray exhaust. We could hear the faint, high-pitched beeps that the cement mixer made as it was backed into position, its cylinder turning lazily.

"In with the new," Lucien said.

Ricky brought Lucien's espresso and disappeared again.

"When did you leave the hospital?"

He smiled. "You've been thinking about how to ask me."

"Yes."

"You shouldn't worry so much. It ages you."

"You were released?"

"It's voluntary, anyway," he said.

"I thought it was only voluntary checking in."

"If your money's the right color, anything you do is voluntary."

"That's bullshit," I said.

He waved his hand dismissively. "Whatever it is, there's no point talking about it."

I looked at him for a while, not saying anything, and then he reached into his shirt and brought out a long, cream-colored cigarette.

I shook my head. "Can't do that here."

"I forgot," he said, and put the cigarette back inside his shirt. He sighed. "This really is a terrible city."

"Why are you here?" I asked him.

"Are we philosophers now?" he said.

I stared at him.

He shook his head. "So serious," he said. "You mean, why am I here and not in New York?"

"I mean, if you're leaving the hospital why come back *here*?"

"Too much New York. Even a month is too much. Also, there are no artists here."

"There are some."

"Some," he agreed. "But you can avoid them." He sipped at his espresso. "Why are *you* here?"

"Where would I go?" I took a deep breath. "So why no artists?"

He shrugged. "It seems lately as though the world is full of talentless men who suffer all the responsibility of possessing a really major talent."

"Why do you care about the deluded?"

"Because there is no difference between the way they think about what they do and the way I think about what I do."

"So?"

"So what is there to separate me from them?"

"The work."

He smiled without meaning it. "But I am judging my work and they are judging theirs and we are coming to the same conclusions and what if I am one of the deluded and everyone is laughing behind my back."

"No one's laughing."

"I used to think that if you knew when you woke up every morning that you were supposed to do a certain thing and you thought that you could be great at it then you *could* be great at it. But it isn't true."

"No," I agreed.

"Well, I don't want to wake up one day when I'm fifty and realize that I'm only a decent painter."

"There are worse things to be than a decent painter."

"Not if you are a decent painter who thought he was going to be a great painter." He looked at the sky. "I won't be a failure."

He lowered his eyes. "I had to agree to work with a doctor here," he said. "I mean, for them to let me leave I had to let them palm me off on somebody."

"You don't have to talk about it."

He put up his hand to stop me. "I gave you as my emergency contact. I hope that's all right. You're the only person I know who's still here."

"You know plenty of people."

"I am *acquainted* with plenty of people. I barely *know* anyone."

"Of course it's all right," I said.

"Jack," he said, "tell me I'm going to be a great painter."

"You will."

He grinned. "I wonder whether you would lie to me if we were talking about writing."

I drank some of my coffee, which was cool now, and looked at Washington. Lucien sipped at his espresso again and put it down and looked around and that was when he noticed the girls for the first time. He looked back at me.

"You see this?" he said.

"Since before you got here."

"What have you been doing about it?"

I shrugged. "I get too nervous talking to women I don't know. Especially when they look like that."

"My God," he said. "How old are you now?"

"Twenty-four."

He sighed. "You're squandering your youth."

"I don't think you have the right to talk about my youth. You're not even six months older than me."

He smiled. "But I am an old man."

"Well, why don't you gather yourself then—while you still may—and go over?"

"No," he said. "Why don't *we* go over?"

The girls were more beautiful the closer we got. When we reached their table, they looked up at us with their immense eyes and for a moment I could see nothing but the eyes of the older one and the way a few loose strands of her hair hung forward into her face. My heart was beating fast, as I had known it would, and I was afraid to speak because I wasn't sure whether I could catch my breath.

Then Lucien said, to the little girl, "Excuse me, madam, but you appear to have something in your ear."

The girls stared at him.

"Allow me," he said and reached behind the little one's head and when he pulled his hand back he was holding a quarter.

"I believe this is yours," he said to her.

She held out her palm and he dropped the coin into it.

"Very nice," the older girl said.

Lucien shook his head. "That's nothing. Now, if you want to see *real* talent—" He reached behind the little girl's head again and again brought out a quarter, but this time he put it in his mouth and bit down on it and then he was holding half a quarter with jagged teeth marks along its edge. The girls looked on, openmouthed. Lucien blew hard on the torn quarter in his hand and then suddenly it was whole again. The little girl gasped. The older girl applauded.

"Will you sit down?" she said.

I pulled over two chairs from the neighboring table and we sat. We introduced ourselves.

Kate, the older girl, said, "Where did you learn that?"

Lucien shrugged. "Around."

The little girl, whose name was Nina, looked at Lucien and said, "Where are you from?"

He smiled. "Where do you think I'm from?"

She frowned. "England?"

"Close," he said. "I'm from Denmark. Do you know where that is?"

She shook her head.

"Why aren't you tall and blond and pale?" Kate asked him.

"Good genes."

"You don't have much of an accent."

"I have enough," he said.

"So, how do you know each other?"

"We went to school together."

"Where?"

He told her.

"So," she said, "are you bankers or lawyers or trying to rule the world?"

"Trying to *make* the world."

"Lucien's a painter," I said.

"Is he good?" she asked me.

"He is good," I said.

"Jack is a writer," Lucien told her, "and even if you never see him again, you'll tell your grandchildren about the day you met him."

She looked at me.

Ricky came over and we ordered another round. The girls were both drinking orange juice.

"So," Lucien said, "are you two sisters?"

"I'm her aunt," Kate said.

Lucien watched the cars as they passed and said, "Don't they sound like the ocean?"

"What do you mean?" Kate asked him.

"The tires," he said.

"I thought painters were supposed to *see* differently," I said, "not *hear* differently."

"It just occurred to me," he said.

"I think I see what you mean," Kate told him.

The crew was finished with the sidewalk and had moved into the street. The cement mixer had been pulled away and replaced by a dump truck that was pouring hot tar. The men were spreading the tar before the paving truck came through with its enormous roller.

Nina tugged at my shirt. "Are you strong?" she asked me.

"Why?" I said.

"You look strong."

"So do you."

She nodded vigorously. "I am. I can even beat most of the boys in my grade at arm wrestling."

"Well, then, I know who to call when somebody's giving me a hard time."

She giggled.

"So what have you been doing this afternoon?" I asked her.

"We were shopping with my mother but she was taking too long."

"Is she meeting you here?" Lucien asked.

"No," Kate said. "We're spending the afternoon together."

"We should all go somewhere."

She smiled. "Where should we go?"

"I don't know," he said. "Where do people go?"

"We could ride the swan boats," I said.

"Wonderful," Lucien said. "*That's* what people do. I just don't have a sense of them lately. I'm only doing abstracts and landscapes now; no more portraits."

Nina turned to her aunt and said, "Can we?"

"I suppose so," Kate said.

We signaled to Ricky for the check.

"If I *were* painting portraits," Lucien said to the girls, "I would use both of you as subjects." They smiled. "And Jack, too," he said, turning to me. "Of course, Jack. It should be against the law for someone to be so talented *and* look like that. God ought to choose one gift or the other."

"It doesn't bother *me*," Kate said.

Lucien smiled. His eyes were bright. "You know," he said, "maybe it would be better if just the three of you went. There are some things I really should get done."

He stood.

"Are you sure?" I said.

"Sure, sure." He ran two fingers around the tiny bald spot on the back of his head. "You know, when my hair starts really thinning I'm going to shave it all off. I hope I won't look like a cancer patient." He clapped a hand on my shoulder. "Value your youth, young Tolstoy."

He kissed each of the girls on the hand and saluted us and then walked down the street in the same direction he had been heading when he had first seen me. We were quiet as we watched him get smaller and smaller and pass the construction site where the new-poured tar was flat and steaming. He turned the corner and passed out of sight and that was the last time I saw him until the night I was called to identify him. And when the sheet was pulled back I could hardly recognize him because of what the pistol had done when he fired it inside his mouth.

We stayed at the table for a while before we went to the swan boats. We laughed about things I can't remember. Kate kept touching my forearm. We listened to cars that sounded like the ocean.

THE DEATH OF COOL

Any of the people you pass on the street could pretend to trip and stumble into you and sorry sorry my mistake pour a glass full of cyanide onto your bare forearm. They could push you into traffic. They could swerve their cars into you. They could pull out a nine-millimeter Browning automatic or a snub-nosed thirty-eight or a twelve-gauge Remington shotgun with the buttstock filed down and the barrel chopped to let it fit inside a holster and do you wild wild West. They could shoulder you inside the sliding door of a waiting van and take you blindfolded to an abandoned warehouse and lock you in a coffin full of rats.

From the roof of any skyscraper, someone could be sprinkling pennies that the acceleration during the drop will turn into bullets raining on the sidewalk. Someone could smash a jar of hantavirus on the tracks at one of the downtown subway stops and let the trains carry the death from station to station. Any of the people stepping onto the bus you're riding could have bricks of plastic explosive taped to their chest. They could have covered the explosive with nails and bolts for shrapnel.

You are at their mercy. You are alive because they want

you alive or because they do not care whether you live or because they do not notice you.

You walk with your eyes down. You try to stay under the radar.

You depend on the kindness of strangers.

I lock my door. I take a breath. I speed-walk along the hallway of my building and almost make the stairs before I have to turn around. Back outside my apartment, I check the door and then sprint away from it toward the stairway and this time I get as far as the second-floor landing. I go back and check the door again. I rattle the knob so that I hear the bolt clicking against the inside of the locking mechanism. I take another breath.

I say to the empty hallway, "It's locked."

I go through versions of this routine every morning. You can never be too careful.

I hit the street and start walking.

Any time you slide into the backseat of a taxi, the driver could seal the doors and windows with a button on the dash and trap you inside a Plexiglas cage. After that, you're his. He could pump in chlorine gas through vents in the floor. He could take you to a car compactor. He could point you at the harbor and use a rock to hold down the accelerator. He could let in thousands of inch-long driver ants that would take less than fifteen minutes to strip all your flesh and turn you into a pile of dry white bones.

Public transportation is even worse.

Three days ago, the man waiting next to me on the subway platform got pushed in front of the train. He ended up facing me. The side of the train had pinned him against the side of the platform. Most of his upper body was sticking out of the gap.

The train doors were still closed. Passengers were crammed against all the windows, trying to see what had happened. I thought how strange it was, given the nature of my work and how many dead bodies I'd seen, that I'd never actually watched anyone die.

Then the man blinked.

My mouth opened. No sound came out.

The man said, "It doesn't hurt."

I knelt down beside him.

"I know I'm dying," he said.

A wide-eyed transit cop appeared above us.

The man said, "There's so much to do."

The transit cop said, "Do you have any family we can call?"

The man was silent.

My eyes burned. I said, "You don't have anything to worry about. Obviously, they'll receive the accidental death and dismemberment bonus."

The transit cop said, "If you tell us how to reach them, we can bring them here to say good-bye."

My vision blurred. I said, "If they can show you were on your way to work, they may have a claim on the benefit for death due to homicide while the policyholder is actively engaged in his or her employment. Generally, it's intended for soldiers and policemen, but there's a case pending in Nevada that's trying to get the morning commute included under the legal definition of the workday. They'll want to watch for that decision."

The man was looking around frantically. Now all he kept saying was, "Did anyone see who pushed me?"

I said, "Of course, if they could get this classified as business travel they'd make out like bandits. I admit that's kind of a long shot."

Another cop appeared. He was taller than the transit cop. He had thick pink forearms.

The big cop said, "I have a couple witnesses who say they got a pretty good look at the guy."

The man's eyes widened. "What was he like? Was he tall?

Was he thin? What was he wearing? Did he have a mustache?" He lowered his voice. "Was he black?"

The cop sighed. "Seems like he was just some homeless guy. Some nobody."

"But he can't be," the man said. "He *can't* be."

The EMTs arrived. One of them gave the man a sedative and the cop motioned me away.

"Did you see anything?" he asked.

"I just felt him get shoved past me and then someone started screaming."

"Doesn't matter. I'm sure you wouldn't have recognized the guy." He shook his head. "Must be weird knowing you got killed by someone nobody knows."

"There's no chance he'll make it?"

He shook his head again. "He's all smashed up and twisted around under there. The train's holding his guts in. As soon as we pull it away, his organs will all whoosh out. I've seen it before. It happens sometimes with the push victims. They're trying to stop their momentum so they fall closer to the platform. Every so often they get stuck. The suicides usually jump out pretty far and the impact breaks them like an egg."

I grind my teeth against my tongue. "So if we just left the train there and closed the station we could keep him alive indefinitely. But we're going to let him die so as not to delay rush hour."

The cop stared at me. "He can't live like that for more than a few hours. And it's important to end it before the shock wears off."

My hands were shaking. I couldn't stop them. "So he's finished."

The cop nodded. "Whenever I ride the train, I make sure to stand against the wall while it pulls in. I don't let anybody get behind me." He frowned. "Of course, that doesn't protect you from a bomber or some loony who wants to stick an ice pick in your throat. But I guess you can't worry about *everything*."

. . .

My office is on the fifty-fifth floor and for the last few days, since that morning in the subway, I have been taking the stairs. There's no limit to what they could do to your elevator.

I step out of the stairwell, and after nine hundred seventy-two eight-inch risers I'm barely even sweating. Your best weapon is your physical condition. An army is only as good as its feet. Even before a few days ago, I would never have let myself go.

The receptionist smiles as I pass her. She has curly brown hair and enormous breasts that don't sag. A few years ago, when I was still in college, I would have taken her home and dripped maple syrup all over her and stroked her belly button with a feather. Now, before I did that I would have to perform a full background check—call the IRS, lift her fingerprints from the phone receiver and run them through the FBI database. If the only things you know about somebody are what they've told you, then you don't know anything.

My boss is half-sitting on my desk, sipping his coffee. I never drink coffee. An army marches on its stomach.

My phone is ringing. My boss picks it up. "Claims," he says.

He listens. Then he says, "You want Sales. It's three-five-eight-oh . . . Same exchange . . . That's right."

He puts the phone down and looks at me. "Did you walk up again?"

I don't say anything.

He sighs. "Didn't we have this conversation yesterday?"

"It's not like the stairs are so much better. Someone could always just block the fire doors and drop in a handful of nerve-gas pellets."

"I'm not sure I understand."

"Someone could place charges that would destroy the support structure and send you plummeting all the way down through parking levels and sub-basements until you melt against the damp cement floor at the bottom."

"But what are the *chances* of that?"

"Not too high," I say. "But they exist. Last year, triggered stairway collapses were responsible for fifty percent of homicides by indoor dropping."

"Those are just numbers."

"Life is numbers."

He nods. "But in order to get *through* life, you need to accept small possibilities of catastrophe. That's risk management."

"What about risk elimination?"

"There's no such thing." He frowns. "I suppose you could shut yourself in your apartment and have someone slide your food under the door."

"I've thought of that," I tell him. "You'd still have to worry about poison in the food and about rocket attacks or aerial bombardment. Besides, what's the point of living unless you can find a way to be in the world? I'm not going to let them close me out of my life."

"Who?" he says.

"But I'm also not a sap. I'm not going to ride their goddamn *elevator*." I move closer to him. "You know that old myth about jumping just before the thing hits? It's bullshit."

He stares at me.

"For one thing, how would you know the right moment to jump? Even if there were windows, the timing would be almost impossible. Also, in a frictionless system the elevator would be falling at exactly the same rate you are. You wouldn't be able to generate any force against the floor. And even if you managed to jump, you'd probably just smack against the ceiling and then ping-pong around while the whole thing collapses from the impact and crushes you. It wouldn't do you much good."

My boss stands up off of my desk. He shakes his head. "Have it your way," he says.

• • •

rina Christina Molesky, widow of recently deceased policyholder Alexander I. Molesky, sole beneficiary of a term-life package with an after-tax value approaching three and a half million dollars, does not offer me anything to eat. She doesn't have the Honduran housekeeper, who keeps flitting around us while we sit at the glass-topped kitchen table, brew me a cup of tea. She doesn't tell her to bring out a pitcher of ice water.

Instead she says, "I already told everything to police."

"I understand that," I say.

"Now I have to tell everything again."

"Your husband had an abnormal amount of insurance for a man of his age and medical history. That, coupled with the nature of his death, raises a red flag."

"I do not see red flag."

"A suspicion."

"What suspicion?"

Alexander Molesky, thirty-eight-year-old male nonsmoker with a benign preexisting respiratory condition caused by prolonged childhood exposure to coal dust while working in mines in the Ukraine, father of two, had been president and cofounder of the Mad Russians Car Repair and Limousine Service as well as co-owner of an electronics store, a road-paving company and two junk and demolition yards until Saturday night, when he was found facedown in a gravel parking lot with a plastic bag over his head and both his thumbs missing. The total of his annual life insurance premiums had been twenty-seven thousand dollars.

I'm keeping close track of the maid with my peripheral vision because as soon as I look away she might dash forward and hit me with a syringe full of Dilaudid. They would let me flail around for a while until I passed out. Then they would drag me over to the oven. They would remove the racks. They would wrestle me inside and lock the door and set the dial to Self-Clean.

I say, "It's a long-standing principle of common law that

no one will be permitted to take advantage of his or her own iniquity."

"I am not seeing you."

"It's my job to make sure no one benefits from doing wrong."

She is biting her lip. "Why you're telling me this?"

I take a breath. "Any potential beneficiary who intentionally causes the death of the decedent will be denied the insurance to which he or she might otherwise be entitled."

"You think I murder my husband?"

I shrug. "Twelve percent of male homicide victims in the United States last year were murdered by or at the behest of their wives or domestic partners."

She stares at me.

I say, "For women that number is more like seventy-eight percent."

Her eyes leak tiny tears.

"This isn't personal," I tell her. "Look at the numbers."

"Numbers say I kill my husband?"

"Not necessarily. But you *could* have."

It's not the dying that bothers me. Everybody does that and, mostly, it's not as bad as you think. Some people just drop dead. (This is usually attributed to SCF, sudden cardiac failure, which accounted for 48.7 percent of last year's heart-disease deaths.) But when you're murdered, another person has become your God. They have forced you to bow down to them. And you'll never get even.

Maybe your waitress has ground up glass into your orange juice. Maybe your roommate will toss a plugged-in toaster into the bath with you. Maybe your wife has pumped up the water pressure in your house so when you turn the knob the showerhead howitzers through your skull. She'll fuck your best friend on the floor of your living room, rolling around on piles of money from your annuity payments. She'll spread rumors about you and talk about how she loved you in spite of your shortcomings.

She'll laugh.

I meet Sadie in the lobby of the Four Seasons and, as far as I can tell, I wasn't followed. During the walk over, I doubled back on my route twice. I boarded a city bus and, just as the doors were about to close, I jumped back down to the sidewalk. I went inside a Japanese restaurant and then darted through the swinging door into the kitchen and past white-jacketed sushi chefs who didn't even have time to turn around before I was through the emergency exit and out into an alley.

Sadie is wearing a short gray skirt. She has her sunglasses pushed up on top of her head. She is talking into a cell phone. When I reach her, she gives me a silent kiss and keeps talking into the phone. She smells like honey.

The bellhops stare at Sadie as they move around us. Hotel guests in chinos and short-sleeved polo shirts sneak peeks at her when their wives aren't watching. When we move into the bar, young lawyers with loosened ties glance over and then laugh together.

Any of them who wants her badly enough could follow me into the men's room and slide a three-inch blade into the space between the top of my spine and the bottom of my skull. If he used the right implement, the wound would hardly bleed. He could arrange me on one of the toilets with my feet on the floor and my pants around my ankles. Then he could lock the stall door and slither out through the gap at the bottom. No one would find me for hours.

We sit at a table near the door.

I say, "Somewhere in this room there's probably a guy who can outfight me. He could make me beg for my life."

Sadie looks up at me. "Let me call you back," she says into the phone.

I sweep my eyes around the room. "I'm tired of letting the law protect me. I'm tired of hiding behind the skirts of some cop. I'm tired of trusting in the other guy's morality." I shake my head. "There's no guarantee in that, anyway."

She gives me big eyes. "Baby," she says, "I don't know what you're talking about."

"I'm talking about self-reliance. I'm talking about the State of Nature. I'm talking about, if some guy can own me like that, how can you want me more than him?"

"I'm nervous about what this job is doing to you."

"You're supposed to love me, forsaking all others."

She takes a deep breath. "I think maybe it's time for a change."

"Either you're lying to me, or you're going against the order of things."

"Why don't you think about going to work for your father?"

"We talked about that," I say.

"You know you'll end up there sooner or later."

I am silent.

"Or, forget about your father," she says. "I'm sure one of your college friends would be happy to get you in at Goldman or Bear Stearns or Morgan."

"This isn't about where I *work*."

She takes a breath. "Is this because you're nervous about moving in with me?"

"I just want to know I can protect you."

She smiles. "That's sweet."

"Also, what if you're not who you say you are?"

"What?"

"I mean, obviously I've met your parents and I've seen where you allegedly grew up, but what if it's all a show? What if you're all just acting? What if everybody's in on it but me?"

Sadie's eyes are wet. She says, "There's something wrong with you."

"I used to have a dream where I was walking on a street somewhere and suddenly everyone turned toward me and started stalking me like zombies. The entire world was zombies, except for me. They were pouring out from everywhere to join the chase. I ducked down alleys. I raced through backyards and even through houses. At night, I broke into this skyscraper and hid under a desk on one of the high floors while helicopters shined spotlights in the windows."

"I think you need to talk to somebody."

I nod. "I think you might be right."

A waiter materializes to take our drink orders.

Monroe Grady says, "I hope you're not here about the Molesky thing. It's a gangland killing. A fucking infant could read this one."

I shake my head.

"What, then?" he says.

I don't say anything.

He sighs. "How long have we known each other?"

"A while," I tell him. "Four years?"

"And haven't I always shot you straight?"

"I think so."

"And don't you trust me?"

"That's an awfully complicated question."

He chews his bottom lip.

After a long time, I say, "I'm interested in learning how to defend myself."

"Those self-defense classes are mostly for girls."

"I'm looking for something . . . a little more serious."

He steeples his hands in front of him and taps his index fingers together. "How serious?"

"All the way."

We are at Monroe's desk in the middle of the homicide

unit, surrounded by cops who might all turn on me at once and throw me inside one of the soundproofed interrogation rooms. They could line the doors and windows with water-tight tape and then flood the place. They could watch through the two-way mirror as the water rises and I start to panic. They could turn on the hidden microphones and listen to me drowning.

Monroe says, "Are you sure this isn't about the Molesky thing?"

"What do you mean?"

"I mean, are you here because you're worried about getting mixed up with those people?"

"Everybody's mixed up with everybody."

"But these Russian guys are dangerous."

"Everyone's dangerous. Besides, they're Ukrainian."

He rolls his eyes. "Whatever. It's all ex-KGB hardcases. They're worse than the Colombians."

I shrug.

"That doesn't worry you?"

"No more than anything else."

"Then I don't understand what you're asking me."

"I guess I'm looking for general rules."

"Safety rules?" he says. "Well, for one thing, you're always safer in a public place."

"But not *completely* safe."

He spreads his hands. "I don't know if completely safe is possible. You piss off the wrong guy and he decides to grease you no matter what the consequences to himself, there's not a lot to do."

"But you can make it hard on him."

"Sometimes the most you can do is give yourself a chance." He takes a breath. "But that's the rare case. Mostly, with a few simple precautions you give yourself the upper hand." He leans toward me. "First," he says, "be certain you're seeing all the angles. Once you know where the danger might

come from, you can take steps to protect yourself. Always
have an emergency plan."

I nod. "Well," I say, "I suppose the key is not to let them
get control of you in the first place. Once they have you
locked in the room and they start pumping the water, it's
already too late."

He leans back away from me. "The water?"

I nod again. "Obviously it would be tough to smuggle anything through the metal detectors. It would be better to lift a
service revolver from inside somebody's desk."

"Wait," he says. "I'm not following."

"You'd need to be set to go as soon as the situation starts
to deteriorate. You'd have to get through the room as quickly
as possible. Once you stopped moving, they would call the
SWAT team and then you'd be forced to take hostages. After
that, it's only a matter of time."

He is staring at me. "I think you may have misunderstood."

"You'd talk to the negotiator for a while and you'd make
demands and he would stall and they would talk you out or
wait you out or they'd decide you weren't going to crack and
they'd roll flash-bang grenades in through the air vents and
they'd make a three-point entry with assault-team members
dressed in black jumpsuits. When they have resources like
that," I say, "you can't afford to let them get coordinated."

Monroe is shaking his head. "You came here for my
advice. My advice is just make sure you're aware of your surroundings. Be ready for anything."

"Don't be a victim," I murmur.

I used to sleep with an aluminum baseball bat beside my bed. Saturday afternoon, I replace it with
a Smith & Wesson riot shotgun. I set the police lock on the
front door. The police lock is an iron bar that sticks into a
hole in the floor. To get past it, they'd need to take the door

apart. They could use a sledgehammer. They could use a blowtorch. Either of those takes time. If they used a shaped charge to blow the door off its hinges, the lock might still hold.

Each of my windows is alarmed. I have installed motion detectors on the fire escape.

I will hear them coming.

In a perfect world, I would install security cameras in the hallways and the stairwell and in the street facing in every direction. I would have an antiaircraft battery on the roof. Every night, in a perfect world, I would booby-trap the living room windows with white phosphorous grenades. I couldn't do this to the windows in my bedroom because I would be too close to the blast area and a detonation would incinerate me.

Late Saturday afternoon, someone pushes my buzzer. I stare at the intercom for a long time before I press the Talk button and whisper, "Who is it?"

I press the Listen button.

Sadie's voice says, "It's me."

I buzz her in and wait with my eye against the peephole. I watch her appear at the top of the stairs and come toward me. I look for any sign of movement behind her. She reaches my door and knocks. I keep watching the stairway. She knocks again.

"Let me in," she says.

I undo the police lock and open the door and pull her inside and slam the door closed and reset the police lock and jam my eye back against the peephole. The hallway is still empty. I turn around. Today Sadie smells like gardenias.

"We need to talk," she says.

I say, "Every time I have to talk into the intercom, it gives away my position."

"I think we should see about getting you some help."

"How would you know you could trust them?"

"I've gotten some recommendations."

"I looked into it myself. I'm afraid it's hopeless."

Her face relaxes. "That's great that you've been looking. I thought you were going to say there wasn't a problem."

"Of *course*, I understand there's a problem." I shake my head. "Most of the available guys are Africans or South Americans who just drift from revolution to revolution and pretty much sell themselves to the highest bidder or attach themselves to the side that happens to be winning at any given moment. They have substandard training and suspect loyalty."

Past my window over Sadie's shoulder, the sun is setting. The sky burns pink and orange. Beside her, the television flashes and hums.

I say, "The English guys are mostly ex-SAS, so they obviously have the training, but they're prohibitively expensive. Also, they might have their own agendas. Same goes for the Americans. The fact is, it's a disreputable business that sometimes attracts disreputable people. You could get some crazed Nazi who's waiting for you to fall asleep so he can go to work on you with a chain saw. It's not worth the risk. There's too many freaks out there."

Sadie is silent.

Beside her, the anchorman shuffles his papers. He looks up from his desk. Normally, he says, a particle accelerator is built in a straight line.

Sadie steps toward me and touches my cheek. She is crying.

Speeding up the particle to any substantial velocity requires a great distance.

She pulls herself close to me and gazes up with wet eyes. "I love you," she says.

Because the largest particle accelerators are not even two miles long, their maximum velocity is low.

She says, "I want you to know that I'm not going to abandon you."

A cyclotron or synchrotron solves the distance problem by

moving the particle around in a circle over and over. This may one day allow a particle to achieve velocities approaching the speed of light.

She strokes my face. "I wish you could tell me that you'll snap out of it soon and everything will be all right."

But some theorists predict that accelerating a particle to such an extent will produce enough energy to create a small black hole.

Sadie says, "I'm so worried."

The anchorman pauses. He sets his jaw and looks stoic. The prospect of such an outcome, he says, would give the experiment a tiny but real possibility of destroying the Earth.

Monday morning, I bring a gun to the office because I'm ready. I'm ready if one of my former coworkers bursts in with an automatic rifle and starts executing secretaries. I'm ready if one of the custodians comes after me with the ax from the wall-mounted fire safety kit. I'm ready if the lobby explodes and flames shoot through the elevator shafts and the stairwells fill with black smoke. In that case I would go out the window.

Velcroed to the underside of my desk is a LALO, fast-open, base-jumping parachute rig. In thirty seconds, I can be strapped in and running full-out toward the floor-to-ceiling glass of the north wall. While I run, I will put a few slugs through the center pane to weaken it and then I will cover my face with my forearms and smash through into the sky.

My boss is sitting in my chair when I come back from the men's room. As I approach, I start fiddling with the zipper on my pants. It doesn't fool him. He says, "How many times have you washed your hands today?"

"I'm not sure."

"Try to understand my position."

I nod.

"I need you to be able to take care of yourself. I need to know that I can rely on you."

I nod again.

He leans back in my chair. "Do you remember what I said to you when I offered you this job?"

"You said you were worried I would be bored."

"Is that what's happening?"

"No."

"Do you feel you're having some sort of breakdown?"

"I'm questioning my assumptions."

If he makes a move, I can use my first shot to shatter his kneecap. Even the worst tough guy can't take that smiling. Probably my boss would drop his coffee and crumple to the floor. I would stand and walk around my desk and put the next shot straight into the top of his head.

"How's the Molesky thing?"

"Not bad. I'm meeting with his partners this afternoon."

"You think that's necessary?"

"They called me. They want to meet in some park down by the waterfront."

"And you think that's safe?"

"I'll be careful."

He nods. "I suppose you're right. It's just, they seem so unsavory. Why have contact with them if you don't have to?"

"I won't live in fear," I tell him.

One of them has a pasty-white chemotherapy complexion and steel-wool chest hair. The other is young and dark. They wear thick gold chains and silk shirts with the necks wide open.

They are sitting together on a green bench with cement feet. They are surrounded by trees. Looming behind them over the trees is the Mad Russians Car Repair and Limousine Service garage. It is the only building I can see.

The paler one stands to meet me. He slaps his hand against one of the trees. "To protect from parabolic microphone," he says. He puts out his hand. "I am Victor." We shake. "This is Michael." Victor leans toward me. "Michael, he don't speak English so good like me." Victor sucks on his teeth. "They frisk you already, yes?"

"Yes."

"I know they did. Otherwise you would have not get through. We own this park. They use metal detector, too?"

"Yes."

"Maybe you think we too careful?"

"No."

"Well," he says, "everybody is careful about something. Some man want to know all the time where is their woman. Some people afraid to drive car. I have a friend he don't like to fly because he don't understand how plane stay up. He is all the time waiting to fall, waiting to fall." He shrugs. "Me, I like fly."

"Me, too."

"Please sit down," he says.

I sit.

"Look down at your chest."

On my chest is a small dot of red light, the size of a pencil eraser.

"You know what this is?" he says.

"Yes," I tell him.

"You not scared?"

"Not really."

"How come not scared? Because you know I am businessman so probably I don't kill you?"

I shake my head.

He smiles. "Because maybe you think you are like Superman?" He beats a fist against his chest. "You think bullet no hurt if it hit you?"

"No," I say. "It would hurt."

"So why you not scared?"

"Because there could always be a rifle pointed at me. Why should it be scarier just because I can see it?"

He says something in Russian. Michael says something back.

Victor turns back to me. "We think you are maybe very brave man."

I shrug.

He says, "I hope you not offended by rifle. Is necessary these days. These days, you frisk somebody, he still have bomb in his shoe and he blow himself up with you. Is crazy."

"Maybe he has packets of Sarin gas in his tooth fillings."

Victor holds up his hand. "So please you don't make sudden move because rifle always there. Because I don't know if you crazy."

"I'm not crazy," I say.

He takes a breath. "Is difficult way to live. People think is difficult in Russia, but in Russia you don't have to be scared of badman because you know why? Because is businessman. He want something. You give him, then probably you okay. But you find man who say I kill you because I enjoy or because God tell me, then you have crazy man and you can't say what he do and what he don't do."

At night it is completely dark in this spot. You can see stars that you never see from anywhere else in the city. They look like glowing powder. I know this because I was gazing at the sky last night while I duct-taped handguns to the underside of each of these benches. I had to put one on each because I didn't know where I'd be sitting.

Victor says, "And these crazy man is everywhere now. Okay, maybe not so much here. A few, but maybe not so much. Yes. Okay. But we has business all over the world. We go Africa. We go Uzbekistan. Sometimes Pakistan."

Packed into the dirt around the cement feet of each bench is enough C-4 to take the thing out of the ground and send pieces of its occupants flying all over. I have radio detonators hidden in the heels of my boots.

"Okay," Victor says, "so maybe we decide don't go, is too dangerous. You need protect yourself. But also you need take advantage of opportunity. Maybe everybody else scared to go so you go and you beat competitors and nothing bad happen. So maybe is good thing world is dangerous place because is easy to get success if you know how to be brave."

Somewhere on the ground behind me, covered with leaves, I have a 7.62 mm Dragunov SVD rifle with a forty-magnification starlight night scope. The rifle is fully assembled and wrapped in an oilcloth.

Victor is looking at me. "You are afraid of these man I mention?"

I shrug.

"You should be," he says. "If you Russian, if you American, they want kill you. I go Afghanistan when I am young man and I see these people crazy. And now they kill you when you go in restaurant or when you fly on plane or when you at work. But sometimes, you so worried about people like this you can't see how dangerous is the people right in front of you."

If it starts to break down, I will roll over the back of my bench and crouch behind its cement foundation. I will have to move very quickly and roll at an angle so as to ruin the sniper's aim. In the same motion, I will cover my ears and touch off the C-4 under Victor and Michael's bench. The cement will shield me from the concussion. The smoke from the explosion will blind the sniper. I will grab the pistol from under my bench to use against the bodyguards who will converge on me. I will pull the rifle out of the leaves and sling it across my chest in case, at some point, I have to take out the sniper.

I will have to remember to keep moving. If I hole up, they might send in dogs to find me.

"Is this why you asked me here?" I say.

"You know why I ask you here. I ask you here to talk about Sasha's murder."

"What about it?"

Victor smiles. "You meet Irina? She is very beautiful, no?"

"She's all right."

"And you meet also her maid? So, on night that Sasha disappear, this maid see him leave house with a man she know is old friend of Mrs. Molesky. She say she seen this man many times. He come to house, sometimes to see Sasha and they drink tea together and they make chess and they friends. So, okay. But also, she say, this man come sometimes when Sasha away. He come to see Mrs. Molesky, but she don't know what they do together. Maybe they also drink tea. Okay, so, but this maid she don't like go to police because maybe they make trouble for her because maybe she is not really citizen. So, I wasn't always citizen, but I take test and I say she could do same thing and then she don't have to be scared. But for now, I tell her, we wait to tell police and first I go find this man and I ask him if maybe he know something about what happen to Sasha."

He clears his throat. "So, we find him and we ask and he say he don't know nothing. And I say but you was with him on the night he get killed and maybe you see something and then he don't want to say. So we ask him again and he still don't want to say."

He says something in Russian. Michael smiles.

"So, we ask again and this time we really ask and this time he tell us. He say, he love Irina and she decide she want him to kill Sasha and pretend is some kind of gangster who kill him. Some kind of Marlon Brando. Okay, so he find this other man to help him and they take Sasha and they kill him and then they cut off thumbs and they put him in parking lot and they wait for police to find and say, Marlon Brando do this."

He spreads his hands. "So, we go and find other man and we tell him say if it's true and he don't want to say either. But then we ask him until he do say and it's true."

When he finishes, we are silent for a while.

"Why did you want to tell me this?"

He nods. "Here we come to this part: I want to know who get this money if Irina do not."

"Probably it would be split evenly among the children."

He nods.

"Of course, before I make that determination, I'll have to talk to Mrs. Molesky again."

He smiles. "Maybe she no be there when you go."

I don't say anything.

He says, "I like you. You are brave man. You are young. I hope you don't have to tell police what I just say about Mrs. Molesky."

"I like you, too. I'm glad you didn't push things too far."

He frowns. "I think maybe I don't follow you. I just want to make sure everything okay about Irina."

I sigh. "Are you the beneficiary of her life insurance?"

He narrows his eyes. "I don't think so."

I nod. "Then it's really not my business."

There is a tiny but real possibility that tomorrow will be the beginning of the revolution. If the system collapses, you will be ready to fill the void and prevent the slide into anarchy. You will assign jobs and ration food and gasoline and establish a command-and-control structure. You will provide for basic needs. You will build the whole world from the ground up. You will be king.

Of course, you hope none of this will be necessary.

Of course you hope that.

HIGHWAY

Eddie would not stop staring at the radio. He said that the V of the metal antennae reminded him of a girl with her legs spread. The radio sat on a narrow shelf above the grill. The man working the grill was so big that he was blocking Eddie's view. Eddie leaned forward in his chair and stretched his neck, trying to get a better angle. Carl reached across the table and snapped his fingers next to Eddie's face.

Eddie drew himself upright, startled. "Hey," he said. "What'd you do that for?"

"You're embarrassing me," Carl said.

"I was just having fun."

"You were acting like a goddamn retard."

Eddie's eyes narrowed. "I ain't no retard."

"Well, that's what everybody in here thinks now, watching you carry on like that."

"They don't think that," Eddie said.

"Have it your way. I thought you wanted to be normal."

"I do."

"Well, I'm just trying to help you."

"I know. I just forgot."

Carl shook his head. "Sometimes I don't know why I bother. Maybe I should leave it alone."

"No, please."

"Some people just don't want to change. I don't have to stay where I'm not appreciated."

"Please," Eddie said, reaching out to touch Carl's forearm. "Please, I'll be better."

Eddie and Carl sat by the door at a blue Formica table. Beside them was the high window that ran the length of the front wall of the diner. On the other side of the window was the parking lot and the white sun and the black line of the highway that disappeared, flat and uncurving, into the distance in both directions.

The waitresses wore blue dresses and white aprons. The three of them sat together at the far end of the room. They were the only other people in the diner. One of the waitresses was thin and old and hard. One of them was fat and old and hard. The third had smooth skin and dark blond hair that fell to her shoulders. When Carl put down his menu, the third waitress slid out of her chair. She swayed her hips slightly as she walked.

She stood beside the table and smiled at Carl. "What can I get you?" she asked him.

"What's good here?" Carl asked.

She shrugged. "It's all good."

He grunted. "That's quite a boy you have behind the counter."

"Luther?" the waitress said. "He's just like a big teddy bear."

"That so?" Carl said.

"He's the best cook we've had since I got here."

"When was that?"

"Two years ago."

He nodded. "And before that you were captain of the second-best cheer squad in the state."

"Third-best." She stared at him. "How'd you know that?"

Carl said, "We'll both have orange juice and coffee with cream—sugar in one—and I'll have the Denver omelet and he'll have the scrambled eggs and sausage and a side of French toast."

The waitress said, "How'd you know about the cheerleading?"

"His eye-cue is one sixty-three," Eddie told her. "That means he's a genius."

She smiled at Eddie. "Where'd they test you?" she asked Carl. "Army?"

"Something like that," he said.

"Where were you stationed?"

Carl frowned. "All over."

"My brother's at Fort Leavenworth. You ever get up there?"

"Time to time."

"What were you doing you had to move around so much?"

"I'm not really supposed to talk about it," he told her.

"Mysterious," she said.

He stared at her.

"My name is Celia."

"That's beautiful."

"Thank you." She stared at him again. "Don't you have a name?"

Eddie glanced at him.

"My name is George," Carl said.

"And your friend?"

"Steve," he said before Eddie could answer.

"Nice to meet you both," she said.

When the waitress was gone, Eddie said, "I don't even *like* the name Steve."

Carl said, "I almost called you Lenny."

"I don't understand. Why's that funny?"

"Never mind."

Eddie scowled. "Hey, I didn't know you was in the army."

Carl ignored him. He was remembering the way it felt to run over the groundhogs or rabbits or even the occasional coyotes that tried to dash across the road in front of his car. He would swerve toward them, leading them slightly, hoping to get them just at the bottom of the spine. If he hit them right, he would crush their back legs and then he could watch in the rearview mirror as they poured blood, scrambling to stand. Sometimes, if the road was empty, he would pull to the side and sit on the hood and listen to the sounds the animal made as it tried to drag itself away. Sometimes he would stand over it on the hot black asphalt and spit in its fear-widened eyes or grind his heel on its mangled legs. But none of that was as good as the feeling just before the hit when he saw the thing disappear under the bumper and waited for the thump of the tire going over and maybe the ringing of the head against the underside of the car.

He watched Celia as she moved behind the counter and gave their orders to the enormous cook.

"You think she liked you?" Eddie said.

"Sure."

"You going to try her?"

"I don't know."

Celia brought the orange juice and coffee. Carl watched the muscles in her legs. When she was next to him again, he examined her soft, hairless arms.

"Who gets the sugar?" she asked.

Carl pointed at Eddie. Celia set down their drinks.

"You must like it here," Carl said to her.

"Why do you say that?"

"Just a sense I get."

She nodded. "I love that everybody who comes in here is going somewhere."

"Makes you feel full of possibilities."

"It makes me feel like there are all these worlds around me that I'm not a part of."

"Makes you feel bigger and smaller at the same time."

She looked at him and did not say anything.

"Why don't *you* ever go?" Carl asked her.

"Where would I go?"

"Anywhere."

"You can't just go *any*where."

"We are," Carl said.

"You don't know where you're going?"

He shook his head. "We're just going."

Eddie was shifting restlessly in his chair.

Carl said, "You got a jukebox in here?"

Celia shook her head. "Just Luther's radio."

Eddie frowned. "It ain't even turned *on*."

Celia said, "I'll see if he can find some music for you."

She walked away from them and spoke to the cook. He nodded at her and turned on the radio. It was tuned to a blues station.

"That all right?" the cook said.

"It's all right," Eddie told him.

Eddie closed his eyes. His shoulders slumped forward slightly and he did not look quite so big.

The song ended and the station went to a newsbreak. When the lead story began, Eddie's eyes popped open and he said, "Turn that up."

Carl looked at him quickly. Luther glanced over his shoulder at them and turned up the volume on the radio. The announcer said what he had been saying all morning.

One of the old waitresses said, "I read where the cops think it might be the same fellas who set that girl on fire in Pennsylvania."

The other said, "I heard they raped the girls after they was dead."

"I heard they made the boy watch them do it."

"I heard he was still alive when they cut his thing off."

"Hell in a handbasket," the first one said.

Luther said, "Order up, Celia."

Celia brought their food on three plates. She had Eddie's

French toast balanced in the crook of her left arm. When she had put down the plates, she said, "I always told my mother I wanted it to make the news when I died."

Eddie looked up at her.

Carl said, "By the time that happens it won't do you much good."

"But it's how you know you were important," she said.

"But you don't want it like that," he said. He nodded at the radio.

"No," she said, "not like that."

She pulled a ketchup bottle from inside her apron and set it on the table. "I just want to be remembered."

"Those folks will be remembered." He nodded at the radio again. "Their names are on the front page of half the papers in the country."

She shuddered. "I don't think it's worth it."

Carl thought he saw Luther glance at him again. The newsbreak ended. Eddie poured a lake of ketchup in the center of his eggs and laid down neat lines of maple syrup on his French toast and began to eat.

When Celia was sitting at her table again, Carl stood and walked to the counter. Eddie was so concentrated on his food that he did not look up. Carl climbed onto one of the red swivel-top stools. Luther was spooning lard onto the grill from a white bucket.

Carl looked both ways to make sure there was no one near him. "You ever do any Lewisburg time?" he said quietly.

Luther did not turn around. "What makes you think I done time?" His voice was very soft.

Carl snorted.

Luther spread the lard with his spatula. He nodded. "No," he said. "Never Lewisburg."

"These people know?"

Luther glanced at the waitresses. "These people don't know nothing," he said.

"Luther your real name?"

Luther did not say anything.

"You know why I want to talk to you?" Carl asked him.

"I suppose I do."

"Eddie give it away with the radio?"

Luther shrugged. "A lot of things give it away."

"Yeah," Carl said. "Anyway, it appears we have a problem."

"Maybe."

"You know how to play Helen Keller?"

Luther nodded.

"So maybe we finish here and get back on the road and keep driving and you keep flipping your pancakes and the people here keep knowing nothing about nothing."

"I can live with that," Luther said. "But you have to leave the girl."

"What do you care about her?"

Luther shook his head. "She don't deserve that."

Carl glanced at Celia, who was pretending not to look at him. "What if I say no?" he said.

Luther turned around, the spatula still in his hand. He looked even bigger from the front. "Then you're right. We do have a problem."

"You think you can put us both down?"

"I think we can find out."

Carl stood up and walked back to the table. Eddie was still working through his eggs. Carl sat down across from him and poured ketchup beside his omelet. They ate in silence for a while.

When the state police car rolled off the highway and into the parking lot, Carl reached across the table and touched Eddie's hand. Eddie looked up and saw the car. He continued to eat, but more slowly.

Carl leaned back and unzipped his jacket and let his right hand fall into his lap.

The cops wore campaign hats with wide brims and powder-blue shirts with short sleeves. The first one in was short and thick with blond hair cut very close on the sides of his head. His partner was almost as tall as Eddie. The partner had brown hair and dimples.

The cops walked to the counter and did not sit. The short one said, "How you doing, Big Luther?"

Luther said, "Yourself?"

"Can't complain," the cop said. "I'll have an egg sandwich."

The tall cop said, "Make it two."

Luther went back to the grill.

The short cop swaggered toward the waitresses. The tall one leaned against the counter and looked at Carl and Eddie. Carl was picking at his omelet with his left hand so he could keep the right one in his lap.

"How you boys doing?" the cop said.

Carl smiled at him.

The cop said, "You from around here?"

Carl shook his head. "San Diego."

The cop frowned. "You don't look too San Diego."

Carl said, "What do you want me to do?"

The short cop was looking at them now.

"Where you fellas going?" the tall cop said.

Eddie put down his fork.

Carl said, "There some kind of problem?"

The tall cop said, "You been watching the news?"

"We've been on the road."

"From San Diego."

"That's right."

"That your Ford in the parking lot?"

"Yeah."

"How come you don't got California plates?"

"My sister's car."

The tall cop smiled. "You got all the right answers, don't you?"

Carl said, "We do something wrong?"

"I don't know," the tall cop said. "Did you?"

Eddie's hand was under the table.

Carl could feel the muscles tightening in his stomach.

Luther said, "Two egg sandwiches." He was holding a brown paper bag dotted with dark blotches of grease.

The tall cop paid him and took the bag without looking away from Carl and Eddie.

Luther said, "These boys been in here last night, too. I think they stayed at the Super 8. No way they could be the ones done them folks up north. They wouldn't have time for the drive."

"That's true," the cop said. He stood up from the counter. "You got a kind of a smart mouth," he said to Carl.

The short cop fell in behind him, looking mean.

Carl watched them through the window as they got back into the cruiser.

"Will they run the license?" Eddie asked him.

"They might. If they do, they'll probably wait until they're out of sight."

"Should we go?"

Carl waved to Celia. She came over.

"Are you done?" she asked.

He nodded. She took the check pad from the pocket of her apron and tore off the top slip. She put it on the table and kept her hand on top of it. She was smiling. She said, "I didn't know you were in here last night."

Carl was looking at Luther, but he was bent over the grill again with his back turned. Carl took a long breath and shifted his look to Celia. "I think you might make the news tonight."

Her smile wavered. "Why do you think that?"

"Because you've been talking to me."

The smile returned. "A girl talking to you isn't news."

Carl said, "Sometimes you make the news for being dead; sometimes you make the news for being alive."

She waited but he did not say anything more and she turned and took the dishes behind the counter.

In the parking lot Carl knelt in front of the Ford, holding his screwdriver. Eddie stood behind him, blocking the view from inside the diner. Carl removed the license plate and replaced it with one from the set he had stolen at the last rest stop. Then he and Eddie walked around to the back of the car and did the same with the rear license.

Carl pulled out of the parking lot and onto the on-ramp and merged with the traffic, which was heavier now than it had been when they pulled off. There were cars all around them. In the Ford, with the new plates, they looked just like everybody else.

THE ROPES

For the first day or so, even when I had visitors the doctors kept my room in velvet darkness and sometimes I couldn't tell whether I was awake. When I was sure I was awake, I wouldn't remember ever having slept. There were no clocks in my room. I had tried once to check the time on the digital watch one of the nurses had left on my bedside table, but the green light from the watch's face burned like a welding torch in the center of my brain.

It hurt to talk. Most of the time it hurt to open my eyes. I lay on my back and watched the glowing shapes that floated through my vision.

I couldn't remember the fight. The last thing I remembered was walking along the concrete aisle with the crowd screaming all around me. Spotlights made the ring rise up in front of me like a blue island in a sea of black. I wasn't sure how much to trust my memory, because the scene would always end just before I started up the stairs to the apron and it would always be followed by the same dream. In the dream, I was lashed to cliffs that overlooked the ocean. The dream was just as vivid as the memory. I could feel the waves crashing below me while gulls pecked at my heart.

I remembered bits and pieces of the day that led up to the fight. It had started out well for me. In the early morning, I had made love to a pretty green-eyed girl whose grandfather's great-grandfather had, indirectly, given orders to mine. Hers was Ulysses Grant. Mine, Thomas J. Folsom, had been with the Irish Brigade at Fredericksburg. It would have been more fiendish—or at least more interesting—if her grandfather's great-grandfather had (indirectly) killed mine. But Thomas Folsom was not even scratched at Fredericksburg. The Irish Brigade, however, took almost fifty percent casualties in a charge on the stone wall at Marye's Heights. The Union Army came at the wall in waves all afternoon. Before each charge the men would draw up wills and leave them with Headquarters Company. By the end of the day, they had lost more than seven thousand men in front of that wall. They never took it. I took Christina Grant-Stevenson at her parents' house in her childhood bedroom under a thumbnail moon.

After three days I could keep my eyes open most of the time and one of the nurses cracked the blinds in front of my window to let in a gray trickle of sunlight. The headache was constant. My eyes leaked. Everything I could see was blurred and doubled and squashed together. I had jumbled pictures of my mother sitting beside my bed and sometimes of my father sitting with her, but those scenes could have taken place fifteen minutes ago or fifteen years ago and I wouldn't have known the difference.

• • •

Toward the end of the week, the headache would go away for long stretches and I would feel almost clear again. I could eat a little. I could lift myself out of bed. I could walk some, but my balance still hadn't come back and when I went anywhere I had to hold myself up with my hands against the wall.

I was sitting up in bed when Connelly came in. He wore a white track suit with green trim. He was holding a tweed watch cap in his hands and mashing it nervously. My mother closed the book she was reading and stood. She looked too long at Pete Connelly. Then she turned to me.

"I'm going to the cafeteria to find your stepfather," she said.

Connelly nodded to her as she passed him. She didn't acknowledge it.

He chewed his lip.

"You want to sit?" I said.

He sat in the chair my mother had left.

"Congratulations," I said. "I hear you took the whole thing."

He shrugged.

"You trying for the Olympics next?"

He shook his head. "Turning pro." He squinted at me. "Your face don't look too bad."

"I guess not," I said.

"They have to pack your nose?"

"No."

"That's good. You ever have that?"

I shook my head.

"I've had my nose broke three times," Connelly said, "and it never hurts getting broke like it does when they pack it. They cram the gauze in so tight it makes your eyes swell up like a frog's. You feel like your head's gonna pop."

"Glad I missed it."

He nodded and then swiveled his head to look around the room. "You're a college boy, right?"

"That's right."

"Don't see too many college boys in Open class. Not at the finals, anyway."

"I won the Novice two years ago."

He stopped examining the room and looked back at me. "Novice ain't Open," he said. "Ain't even hardly the same sport." He took a breath. "You good in college?"

"Yeah."

"That ain't the same sport, either."

"No," I agreed.

"How many years you have left?"

"I graduated a month ago."

"Congratulations," he said.

"Thank you."

"You fight light-heavy there, too?"

"The last three years. As a freshman I fought middle."

"That musta been tough for you to make. You ain't built like a middle." He took a breath. "But you ain't really tall enough for light-heavy, either. You got kind of a tweener build. What's your walk-around?"

"One-eighty, one-eighty-one."

He gave a little whistle. "Goddamn. I'm walking around at one-eighty-eight before breakfast and buck-ass naked. Guy I beat in the local finals in Houston said he dropped down from one-ninety-four. I can't believe you made it past regionals."

"Thanks."

"I didn't mean it like that."

"Never mind," I said. "I know how you meant it."

We were silent for a while.

Then Connelly said, "When they carried you out, I thought you was dead for sure. You wasn't moving or anything. They put one of those orange boards under your head. Your arms was all floppy."

"I'm not dead," I said. I didn't know what else to say.

Connelly said, "If you really had been dead, I don't know if I woulda been able to fight anymore. I was in a neutral corner when they started working on you, so I was by myself, and I felt alone like I never felt before. I felt like the worst person in the world."

"It wasn't your fault."

He narrowed his eyes. "They told me you didn't remember what happened."

"My mother told me about it. Someone has a video."

"You gonna watch it?"

"I don't know."

He nodded. "Anyway, it don't matter if it was my fault. It still woulda been me that killed you." He took a breath. "For a couple hours, I tried to blame you. I said you was just a fool college boy and you had no business here if you wasn't prepared and you couldn't protect yourself. But the truth is if you're here you had to earn your way here and anybody can get hit wrong and so maybe it's nobody's fault. But it's hard to make yourself believe that "

"No one would have blamed you if I'd died."

"Your mother blames me anyway."

"She's my mother."

Connelly looked through the open blinds at the parking lot below my window. "What do the doctors say?"

"They don't understand this stuff too well. They say once the swelling goes down in my brain, I'll probably get everything back all the way. Motor skills, memory, stuff like that. But now that I've had one like this, I'm much more likely to have another. Or even one of the kind that you never come all the way back from. So I have to take it easy for a while and after that I can live a normal life. But no more boxing."

He looked away from the window and stared at me. "I'm sorry," he said.

"I was pretty much done anyway. I would've liked to take

a shot at the Olympics, but that was probably just college-boy fantasy." I took a breath. "I couldn't beat those guys," I said.

He didn't say anything.

My mother sat next to my bed, reading one of her mysteries. I watched her with my eyes slitted, keeping my breathing slow and regular, careful not to move. After a while, without looking up, she said, "Some girl named Christina came to see you a few times while you were coming out of it. Do you remember?"

"No."

"She seems sweet."

"They all seem that way. It doesn't mean much."

"You don't really believe that. You're just saying it because you like the way it sounds."

"How does it sound?" I said.

"Like your father."

She still wasn't looking at me. She kept turning the pages of her book.

"Have you heard from him?" I said finally.

Now she looked at me. "He called when he read about it in the paper."

"What did he say?"

"He asked how you were."

"What did you tell him?"

"I told him how you were."

"Did you tell Hal he called?" Hal was my stepfather.

She smiled. "Don't change the subject."

"You still want to talk about Christina? I went to school with her. She's from around here."

"You know her well?"

"Not really."

My mother sighed. "That's not an awfully safe way to behave these days."

"I'm careful."

"Apparently not."

"I meant . . . during."

She made a face. "I knew what you meant. Are you going to call her to tell her you're all right?"

"Can we not talk about this?" I said.

"Fine."

She went back to her book. I closed my eyes. We didn't say anything else until my stepfather came into the room much later.

"Hal," I said.

"Alex," he said.

He moved to shake my hand and then reconsidered and stood uncertainly next to my bed. My mother stood and kissed him on the cheek.

"I spoke to the doctor," he said. "They're a little concerned about you flying. Something about the pressure change."

"So, where does that leave us?" I said.

"Well, I was thinking maybe we should just drive."

"To New York? That's two thousand miles."

"I know that." He glanced at my mother. "We could make an adventure out of it. We'd stay in some fun hotel each night. It shouldn't take us more than four days."

"I'm fine to fly."

"Alex," my mother said, "if it's not safe it's not safe."

"What's the danger? A little headache? I can make my own decisions. I'm twenty-one years old."

"Not quite."

I sent them back to their hotel. Then I packed my suitcase and stood it against the wall. A young dark-haired nurse brought my dinner. When she was gone, I called Christina at her parents' house to tell her I was leaving. She didn't seem surprised.

· · ·

After a week in New York, I still wasn't sleeping. My appetite came and went. Car-horn blasts made my heart flip-flop and set off fireworks in my head.

Some nights I would leave Hal's apartment after dinner and walk to Madison Avenue and watch all the people hurrying out together or, if it was late, watch the couples hurrying home together. I would walk into the park, which would be almost deserted, and then walk across to the West Side, praying for someone to jump out in front of me and put up his fists and dare me forward. There would be no neutral corners. There would be no mandatory eight counts. I would put this man on the ground and then stomp him until my bootprints showed on his chest. Thick blood would ooze from his ears. If I were still angry enough, I might lift him up by his hair and smack his face again and again into the pavement until his skull opened and poured gray-yellow brains.

One night, on Amsterdam in the high seventies, I watched a homeless man steal a pair of shoes from an outdoor display. I could have taken two steps to my left and gotten in front of him, but he was mean drunk or mean crazy, or both, and as he passed I could smell his antiseptic, old-sweat, hospital smell, which made me very sad. I didn't move. He jogged away with the shoes clutched against his stomach like a baby.

Walker, my stepbrother, came over from his mother's place in the West Village to take me to a movie.

We sat on the aisle. I used a sip of Walker's soda to wash down one of the codeine-laced Tylenols the doctor had prescribed because the tiniest sounds were like hammers beating against my eardrums. My senses had become so acute that I imagined my blood had been replaced with liquid amphetamines. I was very aware of the warm bodies around me and the way the whole theater smelled like hot butter. I could feel armies of microbes covering all of us and scuttling in huge columns along the cement floor. Walker, who was tall and handsome like his father, slouched in his seat and told me about the end of his sophomore year and how drunk he had gotten. He told me about the summer internship he had just begun at his father's law firm.

He said, "After I graduate, I'll probably put in a couple years as a trader. Your quality of life is really a lot better there than it is as an analyst. The danger is that you get tracked differently and you might not be able to move up as high. But after those two years I'll go to law school. Definitely on the West Coast. Probably Stanford. Again, it's a quality-of-life decision. After that I'll make a determination about which firm to work for, based on opportunity for advancement as well as quality-of-life considerations. Also, I've already started paying into a retirement fund. If you start paying when you're eighteen, by the time you're sixty-five it's like winning the lottery."

"What about the writing?"

He nodded. "I almost forgot. Being a trader will also leave me some time to write on the side. I mean, you only really need to be in the office while the market's open. You also have to entertain clients in the evenings, but I'm sure I'll still find some time. Anyway, I'll give myself those two years to make it with the writing and if that doesn't pan out I'll still have done some serious résumé building." He shook a few M&Ms into his hand and tossed them into his open mouth. "I'm pretty sure it'll work out. I mean, sometimes I take passages from *Gatsby* and make little corrections that any editor in the world would tell you are improvements. I'm not saying it's not a great book, I'm just saying there are some things I do differently that are just objectively better. I've been wanting to talk to you about that." He sipped his soda. "What about you? Do you know what you're gonna do now?"

"No," I said.

During the movie, whenever I felt the nausea coming I just closed my eyes and pressed my palms against my ears and mostly I was all right. Afterward, Walker took me to a party at his girlfriend's parents' duplex on Park Avenue.

Bass from the stereo shook the floor. The air tasted like beer and sweat. I sat in an armchair and talked to a girl who had just finished her junior year at Dartmouth. We had to shout to hear each other over the music.

She was saying, "I just don't know if people realize how fucking good *The Waste Land* is. I mean, they say they know, but it's just so fucking good."

"Yes," I yelled at her, "it's very good."

"It's like Picasso. Or *Middlemarch*. Everybody always tells you how good they are. But they're really, *really* good. It's amazing."

"Are you studying English?"

She nodded. "I think maybe I'd like to be a writer. I keep meaning to be disciplined about it."

"That sounds like a good idea."

"I'm going to Tahiti this summer. I'm going to see some of the places Gauguin painted. I spent last semester in France. I visited his house. He's another one. Do you realize how good he was? How fucking *good*?"

"I think so," I told her.

When I came home, my mother was reading in the living room. I sat down next to her and turned on the television. The television was showing baseball highlights.

"Did you have fun?" my mother asked.

I shrugged.

"It was nice of Walker to want to take you out. It was his idea, you know?"

I took a breath. "I've been thinking I might go visit Dad for a while."

She was silent for a long time. Then she said, "Fine."

"Do you want to talk about it?"

"I told you it's fine. I think it's a good idea."

"I'm happy to talk about it if you want to."

"I'm trying to read," she said.

The bus went along Central Park West past buildings that looked like stretched-out Renaissance palaces—the Dakota, the San Remo, the Beresford—until the park ended and then across and uptown through East Harlem and then onto the raised highway into the Bronx. We passed over dull garages and bodegas with bright signs and the bombed-out skeletons of old warehouses. We passed boarded-up apartment houses and enormous political campaign banners and billboards that carried advertisements for the state lottery and for an amusement park and for a newsmagazine show.

The man next to me had his clothes packed into gray garbage bags that he had stuffed into the roof racks. Two rows in front of us, a baby was crying. When we got out onto the highway, the driver started the movie, which played on tiny screens mounted on the ceiling. I pressed my face against the air-conditioned glass of the window and tried to sleep.

During the layover in Boston, I went into the station men's room and splashed water in my eyes and rubbed at the sleep creases in my face.

In Boston, the baby and the man with the garbage bags got off and were replaced by young couples with straight teeth and matching luggage sets. We drove out of Boston and into the country for a while and then across the bridge to the Cape. We drove through narrow streets between clapboard houses and down to the dock, where the bus sighed to a stop.

The ferry was already docked when I stepped down off the bus. I went inside the Steamship Authority building and bought my ticket. I walked through the back door and up the ramp to the gangplank, which creaked in the wind, and across onto the ferry.

I sat outside on one of the white benches near the bow and waited for the cars to load. Some of the cars were delivery trucks. Some were old and dented. But mostly they were Mercedes and BMWs with new finishes that gleamed in the sun. When the cars were loaded, their passengers pulled themselves up the metal stairs to the deck. Most of them were families dressed in white polo shirts and no socks. As we pulled away, I looked over my shoulder and watched the low wooden houses of Woods Hole shrink into the shoreline and then watched the shoreline shrink into the ocean. Then I turned around and watched the water rushing past.

Gulls flew with the ferry. Sometimes one would land on one of the masts. He would sit for a while and then fly away and start circling again and another gull would take his place.

Two of the truck drivers stepped out of the snack bar in the middle of the upper deck and stood together by the railing. They spoke to each other quietly and laughed and spit into the water.

My father was waiting in the parking lot at Vineyard Haven. He was standing beside his truck, talking to the men who would direct the unloading of the cars. They were all smiling. Behind them the sun was setting. When he saw me, my father stopped smiling and nodded. He said something to the men. They glanced in my direction.

My father came toward me. He was wearing old blue jeans and a short-sleeved khaki dress shirt. He hugged me and I stood holding my bags, not sure whether to put them down.

He stepped back. "You feel all right?" he said.

"Sure."

"How was the trip?"

"Long."

He nodded. He took the bags out of my hands and walked back toward the car.

The night my father had his retina detached by Earnie Shavers in front of a full house at Madison Square Garden, he weighed one hundred ninety-seven pounds. Now he was at least twenty pounds over that. But he carried it well.

"He caught me with a lucky right hand at the end of the fourth," my father would say when he told the story. "The doctor stopped it between rounds. Shavers had dynamite in both hands. I once heard an old fighter say every time Joe Louis hit him with a jab it felt like he was smashing a light-bulb against his face. Well, Shavers didn't have Louis's jab, but when he landed that steam-shovel right it felt like all the lights in Yankee Stadium just got cracked against my skull. It was like a fire alarm going off inside my head. He had the best straight right I ever saw. Foreman had thunder in his right, but he didn't really throw it straight. Besides, I was never in with Foreman. I would put Shavers's right up there with Dempsey's or Louis's or Marciano's. Of course, I was never in with them, either. Anyway, Shavers had big-league power. But he had kind of a soft chin. If he hadn't caught me with that lucky right, who knows?" My father would pause here and look around at his audience long enough for them to take in his ruined nose and the drooping muscles around his left eye. "If the fight had gone on, maybe I would've been able to hurt him." He would smile. "If I'd done that, he would've killed me."

He slid my bags behind the backseat and hopped up into the truck. I climbed into the passenger seat. My father started the engine. As we pulled out of the parking lot, he gave the men on the dock a little mock salute.

"How long you planning to stay?" my father said.

"I'm not really sure." I looked at him. "That okay?"

"Of course it's okay," he said.

We were driving along the two-way road that curved

through the middle of the island. The houses were all set back in the trees. They were invisible from the road.

"How you fixed for money?" my father said. "You want me to get you on with Dave Mayhew? Or Billy Sanders's crew?"

"Maybe. See if Billy can use another roofer."

My father frowned. "You sure? I could ask Billy to let you drive one of the trucks and do some light carpentry or something."

"I'll make a lot more roofing. Plus I'll get a tan."

"We can talk about it later. Maybe you'll take it easy for a couple weeks just to humor the old man."

"I've *been* taking it easy."

He made the turn onto North Road. "How's your mother?"

"She's fine."

"She say anything when you told her you were leaving?"

"Not really."

He chuckled. "I'll bet she can't understand why you'd ever want to come back here. She couldn't stand it. When we moved out here, she thought I was a big shot just 'cause I'd seen some money. She thought we were gonna get invited to cocktail parties. Thought she was gonna be chairwoman of the Chilmark sewing circle. But you can't buy your way into that."

"I guess not."

He nodded. "It ain't like as soon as you put a little cash together you get invited down the Cape with Ethel Kennedy. It don't work that way."

"No," I agreed.

"It don't really bother me, you understand. I mean, at the beginning I felt bad for your mother." He grunted. "But she wised up quick, boy. You better believe she wised up."

"Maybe we shouldn't talk about her."

He shrugged. "Whatever you want."

"You tell anybody I was coming in?"

"I told Charlie McClure. He'll tell Tommy."

"Tommy still living at home?"

He nodded. "So's Luke Hanlan. Tommy and Luke're working for Billy these days."

We turned off the main road onto one of the dirt roads into the woods. The truck bounced over the ruts, just clearing the trees on both sides. We took a few turns and then suddenly the trees opened up into a clearing and there was my father's house. We parked on the gravel in front. Behind the house was a huge yard with a swimming pool and a hot tub. Past that, the trees closed in again like a wall.

"The truck looks funny parked in front of this place," I said.

My father smiled. "I know," he said. "It looks like the caretaker's truck."

In his sweltering office outside Oak Bluffs, Billy Sanders said, "I'd pay you just like I pay all the other carpenters. Obviously it's not like the roofers, but your old man says you might still be having some problems with your balance and I can't be responsible for that. Also, there's a few things we have to get straight. For one, you wear long pants and steel-toes on my jobs. I know some of the other guys are lax about that but that's not my problem. Also, I ever catch you stoned, you're gone right there. That kind of shit puts everyone at risk. If I have to, I'll start piss-testing everybody twice a month."

"I can live with that," I told him.

"I'll bet you can."

He started me at a tiny reshingling job in Oak Bluffs. In the course of that first morning, I discovered that the shock that traveled up my arm every time I swung my hammer made me feel like my eyes were bleeding. The second time I puked, Billy sent me home.

The rest of the day I lay on my father's couch, popping codeines and watching television. I imagined what it might be like to unscrew my head and crack open my skull and use steel wool to scrape the bruises off of my steaming brains.

The next day Billy sent me to Boston with Tommy McClure to pick up a load of Italian marble. On the ferry on the way back to the island, we ran into a pair of Sun Transport drivers. They sat with us at one of the indoor tables.

"How come Sanders didn't get us to move that stuff around for you?" one of them said. "He doesn't like his jobs done right?"

"He didn't want it to end up on the floor of some bathhouse," Tommy said.

"There you go," the other one said.

"There I do go," Tommy said.

"Who's your friend?" the first driver said. "I ain't seen him around."

"He's Galahad Kincaid, the famous race-car driver. He's here on his honeymoon."

"I'm the man who shot Liberty Valance," I said.

The first driver sighed. "You gonna tell us who he is?"

"Sure," Tommy said. "He's Alexander Folsom, the famous prizefighter."

The driver rolled his eyes.

"No, really. He's the kid who almost got killed at the Golden Gloves. It was on the news. You musta seen it."

The first driver stared at me. "That really you?"

I shrugged.

He said, "Didn't your father go the distance with Jerry Cooney?"

"Quarry," I said.

"What?"

"It was Jerry Quarry."

He nodded. Then he glanced at his friend. "Must be tough," he said, "being Ron Jeremy when your old man's Johnny Wad."

I shrugged again. "I don't really think about it much. Besides," I said, "your wife doesn't seem to feel the difference."

All four of us laughed at that. The first driver pounded me on the shoulder. The other passengers didn't look at us.

When the announcement came over the loudspeaker, we walked down inside the cargo bay and sat in the truck while the ferry was brought into its slip. The cars were unloaded one row at a time. When it was our turn, I drove across the ramp and out of the parking lot and through the intersection at Five Corners.

When we got to Edgartown, Tommy said, "Slow, now. I sometimes miss the driveway."

I slowed the truck. We passed a deer-crossing sign.

"On the left," Tommy said.

I eased the truck onto the dirt path through the woods and drove straight until the trees opened onto an overgrown field. The road curved around to an iron gate in the middle of a tall hedge. I stopped in front of the gate and Tommy jumped down and unlatched the gate and swung it open. I drove through. He closed the gate and jumped back up beside me. We were on a cement driveway in the middle of an enormous lawn. The lawn slanted up gradually to the edge of a cliff and behind that was the ocean. Just in front of the edge of the cliff was the biggest house I had ever seen. A few hundred feet away from the house was another house maybe half its size. Scaffolding covered the smaller house like vines.

Tommy said, "You're not gonna believe this place, kid."

The big house was five stories tall and had a huge deck in back facing the ocean. From the front of the house, you could see an immense piece of the island. You could see other houses built into the cliffs and long empty private beaches and huge fields filled with grazing cows. But you couldn't see any of the cars passing on the road below. The view of the road was blocked by the hedge and the trees.

Billy waved us over and we began unloading the boxes of eighteen-by-eighteen-inch filled-travertine tiles and straining to lay them softly on the dolly. When the dolly was full, we rolled it up the ramp and into the foyer of the smaller house. The walls of the foyer had already been painted linen white. We rolled the dolly across the plywood subfloor of the foyer and into the living room and stacked the boxes against the wall.

As we were loading another set of boxes onto the dolly, a new-looking Lexus SUV came through the iron gate and along the driveway and pulled up in front of the big house, spraying gravel. I used my forearm to wipe the dust and sweat out of my eyes.

Tommy glanced at me and didn't say anything.

The girl who got out of the SUV had dark brown hair that fell to her shoulders. She wore sunglasses and gray knit shorts and a yellow tank top. Her legs were tan all the way down past her ankles.

The hammering on the roof stopped. Billy Sanders was standing near the entrance to the smaller house, by the base of the scaffold. He pretended not to notice any of it. The girl walked up the stone steps and into the house. The hammering started again.

"Jesus Christ," Tommy murmured. "Jesus, my good Christ."

I shrugged. "Plenty around like her."

He snorted. "Not around me."

"She's too short for you. Also, girls like that don't age well. They shrivel up like raisins. They end up having to buy new faces every few years."

"Just once I want to know what it's like to be with a girl like that."

"It's like being with any girl."

He shook his head. "I'll bet her pussy tastes like peaches and cream."

"Vinegar," I said.

"You're a cynic," Tommy told me.

Billy Sanders shuffled over to us. "How's your head?" he asked me.

"Fine as long as I stay out of the sun."

"What do you think happened yesterday?"

"I'm not sure. Good days and bad days."

He nodded. "Any time you need a break, just say so." He scratched his chin. "No need to be a hero."

There were never fights on the island. It did not have the seamy side of Gloucester or Provincetown, where every so often two fishermen would carve each other into jigsaw puzzles outside some waterfront bar. In those places, especially during the off-season, there would be times when one of the fishing boats would chug back into the harbor one man short. The crew would tell stories of freak squalls and rogue waves taller than the mast. As far as they could figure, the lost man must have been washed overboard in the dark. It was impossible to investigate cases like that. As long as the crew kept telling the same story, the event joined the legend of the place and the name of the vanished man joined a list on a monument in the town square built to honor locals lost at sea. Most of the time, of course, the story was true. But once in a while the thing would smell wrong and everyone would know it and nothing would ever be done about it but the feeling of it would hang over everything like a fog. In a place like that, you could feel the violence in your sweat.

The island was not that way. There was alcoholism in the local population and there were lean winters as in any summer town, but the place was not threatening. This was a source of disappointment for me during the days I spent imagining how I would meet the girl from the big house in Edgartown. I wanted to pull her out from the middle of a brawl between Portuguese fishermen. I wanted to save her from a mob of drunken sailors. I wanted to discover her being harassed by a giant longshoreman and step between them and push her behind me.

The longshoreman would grin like a crocodile. He would swing at me with a fist the size of a cinder block. I would step to the side and let him stumble past me and hit him on the ear with the heel of my hand, which was what my father had taught me to do if I ever had to fight without gloves. He would come at me again and I would step inside his next punch and bring my elbow straight down on the bridge of his nose. Blood would pour like a dam had broken. Then his knife would be out. I would keep my eyes locked on the knife hand. When he slashed, I would suck myself up away from the blade. We would circle for a while. He would be tired by now because he was so big. Eventually, he would move too slowly with the knife and I would grab his wrist and pull myself toward him and thumb him hard in the Adam's apple. That would be the end of it. The knife would clatter to the pavement and he would sink to his knees. I would take the girl's hand and walk down the street with her, leaving the enormous longshoreman on the ground behind us, holding his neck with both hands, trying to grunt the pain away.

It didn't happen like that. What happened was that I ran into Thatcher Harrison at the supermarket in Vineyard Haven.

I was with my father. He was leaning forward on the handlebars of his shopping cart, pushing it absently in front of him. We were in the freezer section.

My father was saying, "Get a couple of the family-size lasagnas. We're almost out. Also, get the big pack of chicken cutlets and that ice cream you like."

Thatcher came around the corner at the far end of the

aisle. He didn't notice me. He was talking to a young girl who kept trying to climb into his cart. When he came close, I said his name and he jerked his head toward me. Then he smiled. "Alex," he said.

We shook hands. I introduced him to my father. He introduced the girl, who turned out to be his sister.

"How long are you here?" he asked me.

"Not sure."

"Don't you have to get back to start your job?"

"No job," I said.

He gave me the phone number at his parents' house on the island. I gave him my father's number. We said good-bye and they moved past us down the aisle.

"He lived on the floor below me," I told my father.

"Looks like a frat boy," he said.

"Not his fault."

"Also, what kind of name is Thatcher?"

"He's all right," I said.

My father shrugged. "Have it your way."

That night, while my father and I were eating canned beef stew and instant biscuits, sitting on the couch in the living room so that we could watch the baseball game, Thatcher called to invite me to a party.

Two-tenths of a mile after the sign for East Chop, I passed the stone wall and the cluster of mailboxes that Thatcher had used as landmarks in his directions. At the light blue mailbox, I turned onto the dirt road into the woods. The road curved around to the right and then I could hear the music. When the trees opened, I saw the ocean and the glow from the fire. The flat stretch of sand in front of the dunes was filled with cars. I parked my father's truck off the road next to a green Land Rover. I walked between the parked cars toward the fire.

Open coolers full of ice and beer rested on the sand at the

foot of the dunes. The big stereo sat next to them on a lawn chair. In front of the stereo, down toward the water, was the bonfire. People were strewn all over, dancing or lying on blankets in the sand or drinking and talking in tight circles.

I walked down one of the dunes and took a beer from the cooler. The flickering of the fire made my stomach churn. My vision blurred. I felt as though I was on the pitching deck of a ship. I sat down in the sand and held the cold, sweating beer can against my forehead.

Thatcher sat down next to me. He was wearing jeans and a blue dress shirt with the sleeves rolled up. He had a navy sweater tied around his shoulders. "I was hoping you'd come," he said.

"This your party?"

"Not really. Some friends of mine own this beach."

"How nice for them."

"Isn't it?" He smiled. "You want to come let me introduce you around?"

"Give me a second."

"You still recovering from that thing?"

"I hope so. I'm still feeling it, anyway."

"Must be rough."

I shrugged. "I'm used to it now. It's part of my day-to-day. If it went away, I think I might actually miss it."

He looked at me. "You really believe that?"

"I don't know. Maybe I just said it."

We sat and drank together. The light from the fire played tricks with my vision and when I first saw her I thought it was my imagination. It would have been easy, through the heat shimmer, to have seen her face on another girl. I stared for a while. The face didn't change.

"Who's that?" I said.

Thatcher squinted into the firelight. "Which one?"

"In the white sweater. Talking now. Just touched the elbow of the girl next to her."

"Jamie Mitchell."

"What's funny?"

He shook his head. "Nothing."

"That bad?"

"You up to another beating?"

"For her?"

He shrugged. "I'll take you over."

We stood. I brushed the sand off my jeans.

Jamie Mitchell was standing with several other people. They were close enough to the fire that I could feel the heat on my skin as we walked toward her. When we arrived, the group stopped talking and looked at us.

"This is Alex," Thatcher said. "We went to college together."

The people in the circle introduced themselves. A kid with curly hair and a shell necklace said, "Where are you staying on the island?"

"My father has a house near Menemsha," I told him.

"What does he do?"

"As little as possible."

I looked around the circle and paused too long when I came to Jamie. I lowered my eyes. My heart was beating so hard I thought it might choke me.

"I love your sweater," she said.

I was wearing an old gray cable-knit sweater of my father's. "I think it's called a fisherman's sweater," I said.

She nodded. "I've never seen one like it."

The curly-haired kid said, "It's like the kind Picasso used to wear."

"Those were striped," someone said.

"I mean the *style*," the kid said.

"Also, Picasso's were more jerseys than sweaters. I think they were Cuban or something."

"I don't know about Cuban," someone else said and then the conversation was away from me.

Jamie moved over so that she was standing next to me. "I know you," she said.

"That's not impossible."

"You're working on my fiancé's house."

"Your fiancé," I said.

"Well, it's not really *his*. It's his family's."

I didn't say anything.

"You look like an athlete," she said.

"So do lots of people," I said.

"He's a boxer," Thatcher said.

"Not anymore," I said.

Thatcher turned to me. "You didn't tell me that."

I shrugged.

"What happened?" Jamie asked me.

"I got hurt."

"Were you a good boxer?"

"Yes."

"Could you have been a professional?" she said.

"Anyone can be a professional. All you have to do is pass the physical."

"Could you have been a champion?"

"No."

"Could you have come close?"

"No."

"I thought you were good."

"I am."

"I don't think I could ever hit anybody," she said.

"Almost everybody thinks that before they do it." I took a breath. "When I was five years old, my father brought me home a tiny pair of gloves. He showed me how to put them on and lace them up and make sure they were tight enough. Then he got down on his knees in front of me and told me to hit him."

Jamie's eyes were wide. "Did you?"

"Not at first. I just stared at him. Then he said, 'Hit me. You won't kill me.' "

"So you hit him."

I nodded. "All you need to learn is that you can hit him

and he can hit you and that it might hurt but you're not going to kill each other."

"Except sometimes," she said.

I nodded again. "Except sometimes."

The next day was Sunday and the hours stretched out like a desert. I went down into my father's basement and lifted his weights for a while. When I was done, I went running. I ran through the headache. The sun was heavy on my shoulders. My breath came in gasps and moans. Cramps seared my chest. When I got back, I walked back and forth along the porch with my hands on my hips. My throat felt raw. I coughed a few times and spit into the bushes.

I sat on the couch and thought about how I didn't have anything. The thought didn't give me any of the delicious self-pity thrill I was expecting. My father wandered downstairs from his bedroom. He flopped down across from me in his armchair.

"Why wasn't I a better fighter?" I said after a while.

He stared at me. "I didn't think you cared too much about that."

"Sometimes I wanted it so badly I thought I'd go crazy."

"Maybe you just want it now that you can't do it anymore."

"Why didn't you ever come watch me?"

He shrugged. "Who needs to watch two middle-class college boys fight? Fighting's what you do when you can't think what else to do. Middle-class boys always have something else. They don't need it enough to be good at it."

"What about Ali?"

"Ali's *black* middle class."

"That makes no difference to me."

"I'll bet it makes a difference to him."

I chewed my lip. "Anyway," I said, "why didn't you come watch me just because I was your son?"

He shifted his weight, which made the chair creak. "I don't need to watch my son try to be a thug."

"Then why did you teach me at all?"

"I also didn't want you to be one of those lily rich boys who doesn't know how to take care of himself. But there's a long way between that and being able to handle the real bangers."

"The guys I saw at the Gloves weren't bunnies."

He nodded. "Look what they did to you," he said.

I didn't call Thatcher Harrison for her phone number or to ask him to arrange another meeting. I didn't go to work every day at the house in Edgartown praying for her to show up. I was happy not to be seeing her again. I was happy during the bright mornings and the hot, lazy afternoons and I was very happy at night when I would lie in bed and dream I had been washed overboard and dragged away by the tide.

Thursday evening, my father and I met Billy Sanders and Dave Mayhew at the bar in Oak Bluffs. We sat at a table by the window. We all ordered beer.

The waitress squinted at my driver's license when I gave it to her. "Happy birthday," she said. She gave the license back to me.

"I remember my twenty-one," Dave Mayhew said when the waitress had gone.

"I don't," Billy Sanders said.

"I was with two girls at once," Dave said. "It was the only time."

"How much that cost you?" Billy said.

"Didn't cost me nothing."

"Like hell. You're not Sinatra."

Dave smiled. "My old man paid."

"Nice of him," my father said.

"I thought so."

"That the plan for tonight?" Billy said. "I could give him tomorrow off if he's having trouble walking."

"Having trouble walking anyway," I said.

"That's true. Good thing your father's got friends in high places."

"Like who?" Dave said.

Billy ignored him. "Otherwise you'd be out of luck. We don't really need a gimp on the job. Especially not one who can only work every other day." Billy had been drinking before he came to meet us. I hadn't noticed it until now.

"Go a little easy," my father told him.

"It's his birthday. Didn't you always take some on your birthday?"

"Sometimes. But that doesn't mean he has to."

This time when I saw her I was sure I was imagining it. We were on our third round of beers. I was looking across the street through the fading light and really it could have been almost anybody with the right body. She was with another girl. They were waiting in line outside the old wooden building that held the carousel. I watched them until they were out of sight inside the building.

When I turned back to the table, Dave Mayhew was smiling. So was my father.

Billy said, "That wouldn't be the girl who's marrying Greg Cunningham, would it?"

"How do you know I wasn't looking at the other one?"

He stared at me. "It *was* her, wasn't it?"

"It might have been," I admitted.

He shook his head.

"Your problem," I said, "is you've got no imagination."

He frowned.

My father said, "I spent my twenty-first birthday in jail."

We looked at him. He wasn't smiling anymore.

Dave said, "You never told me that."

My father shrugged. "It's not much of a story."

"Was it about a girl?"

"Why would you ask that?"

"I don't know. It seems as likely as anything else."

My father nodded. "But it wasn't jailbait and it wasn't any kind of restraining-order business."

"No," Dave said, "it wouldn't be that."

"As far as the cops were concerned, it wasn't about her at all. For them it was about her husband and whether he was gonna die."

"He come close?"

"Pretty close. He stayed in the coma almost three days."

"Rich man?"

"Rich man's son."

"He hit you first?"

"He didn't hit me at all. But he *swung* first."

"I suppose you told them that."

"Sure. But I had turned pro by then. My lawyer said it was the same as if he'd thrown a punch at me and I had pulled out a gun and shot him."

"What'd they want you to do?"

"Not use my hands, I guess. Maybe if I'd have just kicked him I would have been all right."

"You would have had to take off your shoes," Billy said. "Otherwise, the legal issue is still the same."

"I'm not sure he would have been willing to wait for that. He seemed quite anxious to get at me. Anyway, it wasn't really my hands that did the damage. It was the curb that got him on the way down. The cops didn't think too much of that distinction."

"Hard to blame the curb," Dave said. "It was just standing there."

"So was I," my father said. He sighed. "To be honest, I probably should have thought about the curb, but I hadn't fought outside a ring since I was fifteen. I forgot that on the street when they go down they don't just hit the canvas."

"Canvas can still hurt them if they hit wrong."

"Not like pavement." My father sipped his beer. "I was pretty dumb back then. You know, the thing that bothered me most in the lockup wasn't wondering how long I might be there or how I was gonna feel if he died. What really got under my skin was that the other prisoners didn't know who I was."

"You mean because if they'd known who you were they'd have left you alone?"

"They left me alone anyway. Everybody there was pre-trial. They were all on best behavior. I just wanted them to know who I was. I wanted them to know we might have come from the same kind of place but I was somebody now. I wasn't like them."

Dave frowned. "You were young."

"Yeah."

"If you went to jail now, they'd know you," I said.

My father shook his head. "No, they still wouldn't. But it wouldn't matter to me so much."

"Smart man," Billy said.

My father took a deep breath. Then he smiled. "Handsome, too," he said. "Rare for a white pug these days."

Dave smiled back at him and nodded. "After the fifties, the white guys got pretty unfortunate. Faces like chew toys and clumsy and no class."

"There were still some," I said. I was happy to be talking about something else.

"Some," Dave said. "But mostly they were like that Chuck what'shisname that knocked down Ali."

"Wepner," my father said.

Dave nodded again. "Wepner."

Billy said, "Why haven't I heard of him if he knocked down Ali?"

"Ali didn't stay down," Dave told him.

"Sometimes they won't," my father said. "It can be awfully discouraging."

"Right after the knockdown, Wepner was in the neutral corner and he leaned out and said to his manager, 'Start the car. We're going to the bank. We're millionaires.' "

"Premature," my father said.

Dave grinned. "The manager said, 'You might want to turn around before we start counting our money, 'cause he just got up. And he looks pissed.' "

"He was, too. He knocked Wepner out of the ring."

"Not all the way. But he took him apart. After the ref called it, Wepner almost couldn't make it back to his corner."

"At least he didn't make any excuses."

"Like Liston did. Neither of them could stay in with Ali, though."

My father shrugged. "Neither could most people."

We drank. I watched the carousel building. When Jamie and the girl with her appeared in the doorway, I pushed my chair back and said, "I have to go."

My father looked at me. "Where?"

I stood. "Thanks for the beers. I'll find my own way back."

"What should I tell your mother when she calls to say happy birthday?"

"Tell her I'll call her when I get back if it's not too late."

He waved his hand. "I'll let the machine answer," he said.

I was across the street and standing in front of her before I realized I didn't have anything to say. The other girl was staring at me.

Jamie smiled. "Hello," she said.

I felt her voice in my stomach. "I don't know if you remember me."

"Don't be silly."

I gestured toward the bar. "I was having a drink with my father," I explained. "I saw you out the window."

"Is that him on the left?"

"That's right."

She nodded. She turned to the other girl. "Stephanie Durham. Alex"—she turned back to me—"I forget your last name."

"Folsom."

I shook Stephanie's hand.

"I'm about to take Stephanie home," Jamie said. "You probably need to get back."

"Not really. I was feeling a little strange in there. Like my head was full of paint."

"Alex was injured in the ring," she told Stephanie. "He's a boxer."

"Really?" Stephanie said.

"No," I said, "but I used to be."

"Well," Jamie said, "would you want to take a ride? Stephanie lives in Chilmark."

"Maybe."

"The air might be good for you. If I stop in Menemsha, would you walk out on the jetty with me?"

"I don't see why not. It's down the road from my father's house."

She smiled. "It's my favorite place in the world."

We drove on the road that twisted along the north side of the island. There were forests on both sides and the road had been cut in between. It was easy to imagine the island before the road was here. It was easy to imagine the time when the seas were frozen and the island was lifted by glaciers the size of countries and laid down again and lifted again and laid down until the ice melted. It was easy to imagine the time before that when dinosaurs grazed over the ground where the yacht club now stands and stomped giant footprints into the private beaches.

We dropped Stephanie and got back on the road into Menemsha. We parked at my father's house and walked down toward the water. The sky was dark now. The air was full of mosquitoes.

"Your father was a boxer, too?" Jamie asked.

"You mean, because of his face?"

"Yes."

I nodded. "He was a boxer."

"Was he born here?"

I shook my head. "East Boston."

"When did he come?"

"When he stopped boxing."

"He brought your mother?"

"And me, but I was just a baby."

"And you lived here year-round?"

"Until she left him."

We walked along a fence past a yard with several dogs tied up inside it. The dogs turned their heads with us as we passed them.

Jamie said, "You graduated with Thatcher?"

"That's right."

"Do you know what you're going to do now?"

"I don't like to talk about it."

"What do you mean?"

"I don't like a lot of talk about plans. Most things you either do or you don't do. It doesn't help much either way to talk about it."

"I agree. Let's not talk about it."

"It doesn't leave much to talk about."

We passed Larsen's, the fish market, which was dark inside. The air tasted like salt. This close to the beach, there were no more mosquitoes. We walked through the parking lot beside the dock. We walked onto the sandy part of the parking lot and then up onto the sand and then onto the huge square stones that had been crammed together to make the jetty. We walked all the way out to the rusted light tower. In front of us we could see the blue light of the buoy and hear its bell ringing as the waves jostled it. In the darkness the water was like the top sheet on an enormous bed.

"I used to come here when I was a little girl," Jamie said.

"Pretty far from Edgartown."

"My family's house is out near Gay Head. I go to Edgartown to visit Gregory."

"I haven't seen you there lately."

"He usually only comes up on the weekends. He works during the week."

"Doing what?"

"Banking."

"Where?"

"New York."

"I meant, which bank?"

"Oh. Does it matter?"

I smiled. "Probably not. How did you meet him?"

"Our parents are friends. I've known him forever."

"How long have you been engaged?"

"A year."

I scraped my teeth against my lip. "I've never known anyone my age who was getting married."

"It's not so rare."

"I was shocked when you told me."

"Didn't you see my ring?" she said. "It's as big as the Ritz."

"I don't usually notice things like that."

We were silent for a while.

"We could talk about boxing. I've always wanted to know about it."

I shook my head. "No good."

"You shouldn't look at me that way," she said.

"What way?"

"You know."

"It's too dark for you to see how I'm looking at anything."

"There's a moon," she said.

"So you drove me all the way out here just because you felt sorry about my poor head?"

"Don't be mean. I'd like to be your friend."

"A girl like you is drowning in friends. What's one more or less?"

The air was cold off the ocean. Jamie was hugging herself to stay warm. "I like you," she said. "You're more interesting than most of the people I know."

I wanted to lean over and kiss her and smell her hair and carry her back to the house and lay her down on my bed and feel how warm she was. But I didn't know how to do any of that.

Some time later, I walked her back to her car and watched her drive away.

When the phone rang the next evening, I knew it wouldn't be her. Still, I wasn't surprised when I lifted the receiver and heard her voice.

"Thatcher gave me your number."

"Yes," I said.

"Can I come see you?"

"Of course."

"Right now?"

"If you want."

"You don't want me to?"

I listened to the ticking silence.

"I really do want to be your friend. I think maybe you got the wrong idea last night."

"Did I?" I said.

I strained to hear her breathing.

"I'm used to getting everything I want," she said after a long time. "I've never had to resist my impulses."

I didn't know what to feel. Until then, I had never quite believed any of it was true. "So why not just never see me again? Why make it hard on yourself?"

"Exposure is the only cure, I think. Anyway, it's a good test. Resisting temptation is part of what it means to be an adult."

"I don't know what it means to be an adult."

"Can I come over there?"

"Yes," I said.

I went into the living room to wait. I couldn't sit still. I paced in front of the window. Every time I heard a car engine I held my breath. My father sat in his armchair and shook his head.

When Jamie's SUV pulled into the driveway, my father said, "You're on your own." He dragged himself out of his chair and shuffled up the stairs to his bedroom.

She walked quickly toward the house with the light fading behind her. She was wearing a flowered sundress and white canvas sneakers. I met her at the door.

"Do you want to come in?"

"Come out," she said. "It's so beautiful."

We walked to the far end of my father's lawn without speaking. Next to us, the pool was steaming.

"Do you want to go swimming?" I said.

"It's a little cold for that."

"It's heated."

"Even so."

I imagined for a moment that the sound of the crickets was really the sound of the trees' breathing.

"Doesn't your fiancé usually come in on the weekends?"

"They were having weather problems in New York."

"He flies," I said.

"Of course."

"Of course."

She looked away from me. "I want you to teach me to fight."

"You know, sometimes I feel like that's all anybody ever wants to talk to me about."

"It's interesting," she said. "It's also safe. Anyway, I don't want to talk about it, I want you to teach me."

"Now?"

"Why not?"

I took a breath. "I haven't really been practicing."

"But you didn't forget how." She sighed. "You can't live your whole life treating yourself like you're made of china."

I ran my tongue over my bottom lip. "Make a fist," I said. She smiled.

"Keep your thumb bent and down to the side. If you keep it straight out like that you'll break it." I walked around behind her. "Now, keep your right hand locked against your jaw. Keep the left up too, but out in front of you and turned out a little. Keep your elbows in tight to your body. When you punch, you start and end in this position. Don't pull your hands back or drop them down before you throw and don't leave them stuck out for show after they land. You get back to this position as quick as you can. Make sure you're off balance as little as possible. Make sure your legs never cross. Keep your chin down. Always be ready. When you punch, explode from your legs and through your shoulder and throw your fist straight out like a bullet out of a gun."

She tried that a few times.

"You have to step into your punches," I said.

"That feels unnatural."

"As you get better, the step gets smaller. When you're good, the step is so small you almost can't see it."

"So why learn it this way?"

"At the beginning you have to take a real step to learn how to throw with your weight behind it."

She frowned.

"My father used to say imagine there's a ditch in front of you filled with alligators. Every time you punch, you have to think about stepping over the ditch."

She sighed. "When do I get to fight *you*?"

"I'm not sure you're ready for that."

"I thought you said you'd teach me."

"Not in one night. Where's your patience?"

"I don't have much." She turned toward me. "Come on. Tell me how you'd fight you. If you were me."

I looked at her. Then I said, "You'll want to stay inside to take away my reach advantage."

"What's 'inside'?" she asked.

"Inside just means close to me."

"So I have to stay close to you."

I felt the tingle along my spine. "Right," I said. "But first you have to *get* inside."

"How?"

I shrugged. "There's no one way. Mostly, you have to be willing to pay the price. I'll be trying to keep you off me by jabbing, which holds you at the proper range for my overhand right. Some people say jab a jabber, which means your job would be to counter with your own jab and use that to cover you so you can get close to me. Another way would be to just bull in under my jab. You'd have to eat a few if you did that, but probably you'd have to eat a few no matter what. Anyway, once you're inside you'll have to crowd me so I can't create enough distance between us to use my right hand and so you can keep us fighting inside where the shorter fighter has an advantage because it's easier for him to work to his opponent's body."

"Her," she said.

"What?"

"Easier for *her*."

I smiled. "If you can stay inside against a tall opponent, there's a chance he'll just fold, because the really tall guys usually aren't effective close in."

"You're not all that tall. You're not even six feet."

"Tall enough. Taller than you, anyway. But, unfortunately for you, my left hook is my best punch, which means I'm more dangerous inside than out. The only way to give yourself a chance is to try to beat me to the punch and throw your own left hook inside mine. If yours lands first and hits me as I'm putting my body into mine, then you'll be using my own power against me."

"Kind of like jab a jabber."

"Kind of," I said.

We walked back to the house with our bodies very close to each other but not touching. When we hugged good-bye at the door, she wouldn't let go. I looked at her.

"One of your eyes is smaller than the other," she said.

"I realize that."

"It's not noticeable unless you're really close and really looking."

"Yes."

She was looking up at me with big eyes.

Much later, when my headaches were gone and the summer had ended and Jamie's wedding was coming like a train, my days would blend together. I woke up. I ate. I worked. I lay in bed with Jamie and pulled the covers over us and the hours didn't pass and the world disappeared. I slept. At the end of every day there would be a moment when I thought I couldn't take it.

"You can't marry him," I would say then. "I love you."

"It's not that easy," Jamie would say.

"It should be," I would tell her.

But that night, in my father's living room, I didn't know about any of that. I said, "I'm going to kiss you."

"All right," Jamie said.

"Unless you tell me not to, I'm going to kiss you."

"Yes."

"Do you want me to?"

"Yes. You know I do."

I kissed her with my hands around her waist. She had one hand on the back of my neck. When we took a breath, I leaned back and looked at her face. I moved in again and kissed her again and then we were tearing at each other like animals. I was happy and desperate and delirious and frustrated all at once. Still, some part of me was very calm.

I took her to bed.

"Talk to me," she whispered after a while.

I pressed my lips against her ear, burying my face in her hair. "It's mine," I growled.

She gasped and pulled herself toward me even harder.

"It's mine," I told her.

"It's yours," she said between breaths.

My teeth were clenched. "It's always mine."

She held herself against me so that her back wasn't touching the bed. "Oh, my God," she said.

I licked her ear.

"Oh, my God," she said. "I'm coming."

She moved her hips against me. I felt the wave rising inside me, so I closed my eyes and thought about pain. Jamie's arms tightened around my neck.

"I'm coming," she said.

I felt the wave rising again. I imagined smoldering cities that bled rivers of refugees with burnt-paper skin hanging off them like rags. I pulled my head back out of Jamie's hair and opened my eyes to make sure she was still there. Her eyes were shut. Her lips shook like she was about to cry.

"I'm coming," she said. "I'm still coming."

This is real, I thought. But, really, it didn't matter.

A NOTE ABOUT THE AUTHOR

Benjamin Cavell attended Harvard College, where he was a boxer and an editor for The Harvard Crimson. Rumble, Young Man, Rumble *is his first book.*

A NOTE ON THE TYPE

The text of this book was composed in Trump Mediæval.
Designed by Professor Georg Trump (1896–1985) in the mid-
1950s, Trump Mediæval was cut and cast by the C. E. Weber
Type Foundry of Stuttgart, Germany. The roman letter forms
are based on classical prototypes, but Professor Trump has
imbued them with his own unmistakable style. The italic
letter forms, unlike those of so many other typefaces, are
closely related to their roman counterparts. The result is
a truly contemporary type, notable for both its
legibility and its versatility.

Composed by Creative Graphics, Allentown, Pennsylvania

Printed and bound by R. R. Donnelley & Sons, Harrisonburg, Virginia

Designed by Iris Weinstein